Drugs, Athletes, and Physical Performance

Edited by

John A. Thomas
University of Texas Health Science Center
San Antonio, Texas

Plenum Medical Book Company • New York and London

Library of Congress Cataloging in Publication Data

Drugs, athletes, and physical performance.

Includes bibliographies and index.

1. Doping in sports. 2. Drugs—Physiological effect. 3. Anabolic steroids—Physiological effect. I. Thomas, J. A. (John A.), 1933- . [DNLM: 1. Drugs—pharmacokinetics. 2. Exertion—drug effects. 3. Sports Medicine. QT 260 D7943]

RC1230.D784 1988 615′.7′088796 88-22381

ISBN-13: 978-1-4684-5501-4 e-ISBN-13: 978-1-4684-5499-4

DOI: 10.1007/978-1-4684-5499-4

Softcover reprint of the hardcover 1st edition 1988
233 Spring Street, New York, N.Y. 10013

Plenum Medical Book Company is an imprint of Plenum Publishing Corporation

Contributors

Suzanne Barone, National Institutes of Health (N. I. D. D. K.), Bethesda, Maryland 20892.

Howard D. Colby, Department of Biomedical Sciences, University of Illinois College of Medicine at Rockford, Rockford, Illinois 61107.

Richard Cotter, Clintec Nutrition, Travenol Laboratories, Inc., Deerfield, Illinois 60015.

Charles R. Craig, Department of Pharmacology and Toxicology, West Virginia University Health Sciences Center, Morgantown, West Virginia 26506.

Raymond A. Dombroski, The University of Texas Health Science Center at San Antonio, San Antonio, Texas 78284.

Michael J. Glade, Department of Pharmacology, Northwestern University, Chicago, Illinois 60611.

Donald B. Hoover, Department of Pharmacology, Quillen-Dishner College of Medicine, East Tennessee State University, Johnson City, Tennessee 37601.

David L. Horwitz, Department of Medicine and Department of Dietetics, University of Illinois at Chicago, Chicago, Illinois 60612.

Edward J. Keenan, Departments of Pharmacology, Surgery, and Medicine, School of Medicine, The Oregon Health Sciences University, Portland, Oregon 97201.

Edward T. Knych, Department of Pharmacology, University of Minnesota School of Medicine, Duluth, Minnesota 55812.

Penelope A. Longhurst, Department of Biomedical Sciences, University of Illinois College of Medicine at Rockford, Rockford, Illinois 61107.

Michael P. McLane, Department of Surgery and Department of Physiology, Loyola University Medical Center, Maywood, Illinois 60153.

Nancy A. Nuzzo, College of Pharmacy, University of Illinois at Chicago, Chicago, Illinois 60612.

Marc Salit, Baxter Healthcare Corporation, Round Lake, Illinois 60073.

Carol Grace Smith, The University of Texas Health Science Center at San Antonio, San Antonio, Texas 78284.

Paula H. Stern, Department of Pharmacology, Northwestern University, Chicago, Illinois 60611.

John A. Thomas, Department of Pharmacology, University of Texas Health Science Center, San Antonio, Texas 78284.

Michael J. Thomas, Department of Pharmacology and Toxicology, West Virginia University School of Medicine, Morgantown, West Virginia 26506.

Donald P. Waller, College of Pharmacy, University of Illinois at Chicago, Chicago, Illinois 60612.

Galen R. Wenger, Department of Pharmacology, University of Arkansas for Medical Sciences, Little Rock, Arkansas 72205.

Preface

The use of performance-enhancing substances by athletes is not a contemporary epidemic. In fact, athletes purportedly resorted to such measures over 2000 years ago. Even at the ancient olympic games, athletes employed special diets and concoctions to enhance their performance. In ancient Rome and ancient Egypt, gladiators and athletes ingested various potions in order to improve their physical endurance. In most instances, such early examples of substance abuse by athletes involved relatively innocuous chemicals, and one might presume that any enhanced performance could be attributed largely to a placebo effect. Nowadays, aside from the ethical issues, these performance-enhancing substances are far more potent and hence toxic to the body. The many performance-enhancing chemicals, drugs, and hormones exert a variety of complex pharmacological actions, but all are meant in some fashion to improve physical ability. Their pharmacological effects ranges from improved muscle strength, as in the case of anabolic steroids and growth hormone, to central nervous system stimulation, as in the case of caffeine or amphetamine. Analgesics or other pain-killing drugs may also be used to suppress an existing injury in order that the athlete may compete.

The recent history of international competition is replete with numerous examples of drug use by athletes. Unfortunately, there have also been many examples of deaths due to drug overdose and of the disgrace of being disqualified from Olympic competition. France was perhaps the first nation to introduce antidoping laws, and it was followed thereafter by several other countries. Despite such laws, doping-related incidents continued, due not only to the intense pressures to win, but also to a wider selection of abused substances and the difficulties of detecting them in body fluids.

With advances in technology came the analytical methods necessary to identify various substances that were prone to abuse by athletes. So pandemic has the abuse of drugs become that such detection procedures have now been invoked in other subpopulations, including both athletes and nonathletes. Society has become increasingly aware of the impact of drug use on public safety as well as on public figures such as athletes.

Drugs, Athletes, and Physical Performance provides an understanding of how various drugs and hormones affect the body's physiology. It describes how some of these drugs act upon specific target organs or groups of cells and how they are metabolized by organs of excretion and eliminated in the urine. Some of the substances described are, in fact, endogenous to the body (e.g., growth hormone); some are close chemical analogues of the body's male sex hormones (e.g., anabolic steroids). Other substances described are clearly legitimate classes of drugs that have been designed for a specific therapeutic purpose yet are being misused for the sole purpose of improving physical performance. Certain classes of drugs described in this volume have been defined as so-called recreational drugs (e.g., cocaine), and certainly their abuse is not restricted to athletes. Nutritional supplements (e.g., vitamins and minerals) and adequate fluid balance are discussed in terms of their importance in physical performance. The effects of physical performance and exercise on different physiological systems such as the immune system and the reproductive system are also described. Finally, the effect of exercise on insulin requirements is described in the physically active person with diabetes mellitus. *Drugs, Athletes, and Physical Performance* includes new insights into how drugs, chemicals, and hormones can affect body performance and to what extent such substances can adversely alter biological function(s).

John A. Thomas

San Antonio

Contents

5. *Calcium*

Michael J. Glade and Paula H. Stern

6. *Muscle Relaxants*

Donald B. Hoover

11. Exercise and Immunity

Marc Salit

12. Reproductive Consequences of Athletic Training in Women

Carol Grace Smith and Raymond A. Dombroski

13. Human Growth Hormone

Michael J. Thomas and John A. Thomas

Drugs, Athletes, and Physical Performance

1

Vitamins and Athletes

Suzanne Barone

The maintenance of normal metabolic function in the body is regulated by small amounts of chemically unrelated compounds, called vitamins. These substances act as cofactors in many body processes including carbohydrate, fat, and protein metabolism. Vitamins are also involved in human growth. Several of the vitamins are synthesized in the body in amounts sufficient to maintain normal function. Other vitamins, termed essential, cannot be made by the body and must be acquired from an exogenous source. The amounts of these vitamins needed to meet the known nutritional needs of healthy people have been estimated. These recommended dietary allowances (RDA) can be attained by eating a proper well-balanced diet.[1]

During exercise or athletic training, the energy expenditure and metabolic processes of the body are changed. The study of the nutritional requirements, including the vitamin status, of the athlete is becoming an important area of sports medicine.

This chapter focuses on vitamins and the athlete. A summary of the physiological functions, dietary sources, and deficiency diseases of vitamins is given. The utilization of vitamins during exercise is outlined, followed by a discussion of the effects of nutrition on the enhancement of performance, vitamin supplementation, and the toxicities of hypervitaminosis.

1. PHYSIOLOGICAL FUNCTION

Vitamins are classified as either water-soluble (vitamin B complex and vitamin C) or fat-soluble (vitamins A, D, E, and K) substances. The water-soluble vitamins cannot be stored in the body and are readily excreted by the kidneys. The fat-soluble vitamins can accumulate in the body and are generally stored in the liver and adipose tissues. Our knowledge of the physiological function of vitamins has been gained through the use of individual vitamin deficiency studies. The following section will discuss the known biological activities of vitamins, highlighting their role in the maintenance of metabolic function.

Suzanne Barone • National Institutes of Health (N.I.D.D.K.), Bethesda, Maryland 20892.

1.1. Water-Soluble Vitamins

1.1.1. Vitamin B Complex

Vitamin B complex is the name given to a group of compounds that includes thiamin (B_1), riboflavin (B_2), niacin, pyridoxine (B_6), pantothenic acid, cyanocobalamin (B_{12}), biotin, and folic acid. Most of these substances play a role in intracellular metabolic function. In general, the vitamins of this complex are metabolized to active forms which act as coenzymes in many biological reactions. The specific properties of these compounds are listed below.

1.1.1a. Thiamin (Vitamin B_1). Thiamin is metabolized to an active cofactor that is involved with cellular energy metabolism. The cofactor, thiamin pyrophosphate, plays a role in the multienzyme complex that is responsible for the oxidative decarboxylation of pyruvate to form acetyl-CoA, a substrate which is necessary for the Krebs cycle, and ultimately the generation of ATP.[2] Thiamin, in addition to this enzymatic role in the Krebs cycle, is involved in neurotransmission. It is believed that thiamin plays a role in the transport mechanism for Na^+ and K^+ during nerve conduction.[2]

Thiamin and the other B complex vitamins occur in many foodstuffs. Good sources of thiamin include brewer's and baker's yeast, pork livers, cereal germs, whole grain products, nuts, and legumes.

A deficiency of thiamin in the body results in the disease beriberi. The symptoms of this disease include anorexia, weight loss, heart enlargement, tachycardia, and neurological symptoms such as paresthesia and ataxia. Severe thiamin deficiency is seldom seen except in countries where polished unfortified white rice is the main dietary staple. Thiamin deficiency is also associated with alcoholism.

1.1.1b. Riboflavin (Vitamin B_2). The biochemically active flavoprotein forms of riboflavin act as coenzymes in a number of biological oxidation reactions. The two common flavoproteins are FMN and FAD. These substances are essential in many enzyme reactions including those responsible for the metabolism of carbohydrates, fats, and proteins. These substrates are also involved in the activation of other B complex vitamins to their coenzyme forms.

Riboflavin is found in a variety of dietary food. Milk, meat, and leafy vegetables are good sources of this vitamin.

The symptoms of riboflavin deficiency include a localized dermatitis of the face and scrotum, stomatitis, and geographic tongue. A deficiency in riboflavin will also affect the metabolism of glucose, fatty acids, and amino acids.

1.1.1c. Niacin. Niacin or nicotinic acid is metabolized to the dinucleotide analogues, NAD and NADP. The oxidation and reduction of these substances is important in over 40 biochemical reactions, including those concerned with fat synthesis, glycolysis, and intracellular respiration.

Niacin can be obtained from the diet or it can be synthesized within the body from the amino acid tryptophan. Niacin is present in meat, poultry, whole grains, and peanuts.

The disease associated with a deficiency of niacin is called pellagra. The lesions associated with this disease are dermatitis on exposure to sunlight, stomatitis, and cheilosis. Since niacin is produced in the body from tryptophan, pellagra is thought to be a multiple deficiency of other B complex vitamins and dietary proteins in addition to a lack of niacin.

1.1.1d. Pyridoxine (Vitamin B_6). Vitamin B_6 is the name given to three related compounds, pyridoxine, pyridoxal, and pyridoxamine. The most active coenzyme of vitamin B_6 is pyridoxal-5-phosphate (PLP). The coenzyme PLP plays a role in most of the enzyme reactions involved with amino acid metabolism. Vitamin B_6 is a cofactor in the synthesis of niacin from tryptophan. In addition, PLP plays a role in the synthesis of several hormones and neurotransmitters, including norepinephrine and epinephrine.

Vitamin B_6 is found in meats, whole grains, and nuts. The levels found in most vegetables and fruits are rather low.

A lack of vitamin B_6 will produce changes in skin, blood, and central nervous system function. The symptoms of deficiency include anemia, dermatitis, depression, confusion, and convulsions. Since this vitamin is involved in the synthesis of niacin, pellagra-like symptoms can occur with vitamin B_6 deficiency.

1.1.1e. Pantothenic Acid. Pantothenic acid is metabolized into its active form, coenzyme A. This substance is involved in the enzymatic reactions associated with the synthesis of fatty acids and cholesterol and the metabolism of carbohydrates and fats.

The name pantothemic acid is derived from the Greek word *pantos* meaning everywhere,[2] and as the name implies, this vitamin is found in most animal and plant tissues.

Because of the ubiquitous nature of the vitamin, a deficiency syndrome has not been observed or described except in cases of severe malnutrition.

1.1.1f. Cyanocobalamin (Vitamin B_{12}). The active coenzyme forms of vitamin B_{12} play a role in protein metabolism. Cyanocobalamin is also responsible for the normal function of hematopoietic cells.

Vitamin B_{12} is found in most animal products with very high concentrations in animal organ meats, especially liver, kidney, and heart.

A deficiency of this vitamin results in pernicious anemia, characterized by megaloblastic anemia and neurological changes. The absorption of vitamin B_{12} from the gastrointestinal tract requires the presence of intrinsic factor. This glycoprotein is secreted by the parietal cells of the gastric mucosa and aids in the active transport of vitamin B_{12} across the ileum. A vitamin B_{12} deficiency syndrome most often occurs because of lack of intrinsic factor secretion due to genetics or total gastrectomy.

1.1.1g. Biotin. The biotin-dependent enzymes participate in many biochemical reactions including those involved in gluconeogenesis and fatty acid biosynthesis.

Biotin is synthesized in the human intestine by bacteria, and thus the dietary need for biotin is not so great.

A deficiency of biotin is characterized by scaly dermatitis, nausea, and depression. This deficiency occurs when avidin, a biotin-binding glycoprotein found in raw egg whites, binds to biotin, making it unavailable.

1.1.1h. Folic Acid. The active coenzyme form of folic acid plays a role in protein and nucleic acid metabolism. An interrelationship exists between folic acid and vitamin B_{12}: folic acid is involved in the activity of methionine synthetase, an enzyme requiring vitamin B_{12}. In addition, folic acid plays a role in the production of normal red blood cells.

The major dietary source of folic acid is green leafy vegetables such as spinach and broccoli.

A deficiency of this vitamin results in megaloblastic anemia and lesions in the gastrointestinal tract.

1.1.2. Vitamin C

Another water-soluble vitamin is vitamin C or ascorbic acid. Vitamin C plays a role in many important body processes including the synthesis of collagen, the metabolism of steroids and lipids, and the biosynthesis of catecholamines. The entire biochemical function of this vitamin is not yet understood; however, ascorbic acid is essential as an oxidation–reduction system in the functions listed above.

This vitamin is present in many fruits and vegetables, especially the citrus fruits. Vitamin C is destroyed during cooking and can be oxidized by exposure to air during storage.

A deficiency in vitamin C results in the disease scurvy. Symptoms of this disease include fatigue, bleeding gums, weakening of collagenous structure, and hemorrhages.

1.2. Fat-Soluble Vitamins

1.2.1. Vitamin A

Vitamin A, or retinol, is a fat-soluble vitamin that plays a role in many physiological functions including vision, growth, and tissue differentiation. The alcohol, retinol, when reduced to the aldehyde, 11-*cis*-retinal, combines with opsin to produce rhodopsin, a visual pigment that plays a role in dark adaptation. Vitamin A is also involved in bone growth and development in children. This vitamin is essential for maintaining membrane stability and differentiation of epithelial cells.

Vitamin A is present in many foodstuffs including milk, cheese, butter, eggs, and liver. Carrots, spinach, and other highly pigmented vegetables contain carotene, a precursor to vitamin A. Since vitamin A is a fat-soluble vitamin, over 90% of the body's supply is stored in the liver.

A deficiency of vitamin A results in night blindness, xerophthalmia, fetal malformation, and retardation of growth.

1.2.2. Vitamin D

The term vitamin D describes a group of compounds including cholecalciferol (vitamin D_3) and ergocalciferol (vitamin D_2). Vitamin D_3 is formed when ultraviolet radiation from the sun strikes the skin, converting the sterol provitamin 7-dehydrocholesterol into cholecalciferol. Vitamin D is stored in the liver. This vitamin undergoes metabolic hydroxylation to its active form, which plays a role in calcium homeostasis. Vitamin D, calcitonin, and parathyroid hormone work together to regulate plasma calcium levels. In addition, vitamin D plays a role in phosphorus homeostasis. Both calcium and phosphorus are important for bone mineralization.

Dietary sources of vitamin D are fortified dairy products. Milk is artificially fortified with the vitamin to aid in the intestinal absorption of calcium. The major source of vitamin D is through sunlight irradiation of the skin.

A deficiency in vitamin D results in the disease rickets in children and osteomalacia in adults. Both of these conditions are the result of the demineralization of bone due to inadequate serum calcium and phosphate. Rickets, which occurs in the growing bones of children, results in bowlegs, knock-knees, and deformities of the pelvis and spine. Osteomalacia occurs in adults with mature skeletal development. The symptoms include muscular weakness, bone pain, and bone fractures.

1.2.3. Vitamin E

Vitamin E is a term used to describe tocol and tocotrienol derivatives. Of these, alpha-tocopherol is the most potent. Vitamin E is a fat-soluble vitamin with potent antioxidant properties. All the biochemical consequences of this vitamin E activity have not yet been elucidated. It is known, however, that the vitamin can protect polyunsaturated fatty acids from oxidation. Vitamin E, through its antioxidant properties, may aid in cellular defense against the damage of disease and environmental stress.

The major dietary source of vitamin E is plant and vegetable seed oils.

Low plasma levels of vitamin E in adult humans result in a decrease in red blood cell half-life, and neuromuscular deficits. Low-birth-weight infants have difficulty in absorbing vitamin E. Hemolytic anemia, thrombocytosis, intraventricular hemorrhage, and increased susceptibility to oxygen toxicity[2] may result from a vitamin E deficiency in these babies.

1.2.4. Vitamin K

The term vitamin K describes a group of quinones that possess antihemorrhagic activity. The compound phylloquinone is most associated with the name vitamin K. Vitamin K plays an important role in the blood coagulation system. This vitamin is responsible for the activation of four clotting factors (prothrombin, and factors V11, IX, and X). These vitamin K-dependent factors are essential parts of the body's clotting mechanism.

Phylloquinone is found in various green vegetables such as broccoli and spinach.

Other vitamin K analogues are produced by the bacteria of the gut, and therefore the dietary requirement for vitamin K is low.

A deficiency of vitamin K results in an increased bleeding time. The group most at risk for the deficiency are newborn humans. The intestines of these babies are devoid of bacteria, and therefore vitamin K supplementation may be necessary to avoid hemorrhagic disease.

2. METABOLISM, EXERCISE, AND VITAMINS

The endurance training that is part of an athlete's daily exercise regimen results in many physiological and biochemical change in the body. Cardiovascular, hormonal, and metabolic alterations cause increases in aerobic working capacity.[3] Metabolic changes include increases in the activity of enzymes involved in the metabolism of fats and carbohydrates. The enzymes of the Krebs cycle exhibit an increased activity.[3] The capacity of the skeletal muscle to carry out oxidative metabolism is increased,[3] while decreases in protein synthesis occur during exercise.[4] As was outlined in Section 1 of this chapter, many of the vitamins act as coenzymes in the metabolic processes listed above. A major question exists concerning this relationship between vitamins and metabolism and the role vitamins play in the function of physical performance. The approach taken to study this problem has been to restrict the intake of individual vitamins and study the effects of deficiency on physical work and performance capacity.

The vitamins of the B complex have been studied most extensively due to their roles as cofactors in metabolic reactions and the ease of depletion of these water-soluble substances. Since the B complex vitamins are related and are found together in many foodstuffs, most of the early depletion studies involved the restriction of more than one B complex vitamin. The data from human studies that have been collected since the 1940s have been quite variable. In general, the results of most of the studies involving a depletion of thiamin in addition to a possible deficiency of other B complex vitamins showed a decrease in physical performance capacity during the deficient period.[5] Replacement of the vitamins resulted in an improvement in the physical fitness parameters in some studies.[5] In a more recent study, a restricted intake of the four vitamins thiamin, riboflavin, vitamin B_6, and vitamin C resulted in a decrease in aerobic power and anaerobic threshold.[5] No conclusions could be made about the contributions of the individual vitamins to the decreases.

Depletion studies using the fat-soluble vitamins, such as vitamin A, are much harder to carry out due to the storage of these vitamins in the body. Vitamin A deficiency studies carried out over a six-month period failed to show any changes in physical performance.

Even though changes in metabolic and endurance parameters have been found during vitamin deficiencies, it is difficult to make correlations between these data and those of vitamin utilization of the athlete. Vitamin B_6 utilization has been studied recently in nondeficient inactive and trained men fed the same diet, containing two times the RDA of this vitamin. Monitoring the excretion of vitamin B_6 metabolites failed to provide conclusive evidence for an increased demand for vitamin B_6 in athletes.[6] However, it has been demonstrated that riboflavin requirements were increased in healthy, active women to maintain normal metabolism during exercise.[7]

It is difficult to make a general conclusion about vitamin restriction, vitamin utilization, and performance capacity; however the data suggest that reduced consumption of the water-soluble vitamins, particularly thiamin, decreases endurance capacity.[5]

3. VITAMIN SUPPLEMENTATION AND ENHANCED ATHLETIC PERFORMANCE

In the previous section, the relationship between deficiency and performance capacity was discussed. It is not clear from the results of those studies, however, whether an increase in physical exercise could lead to an increase in vitamin utilization and ultimately to a vitamin deficiency in the athlete. It is also not known whether the metabolic systems of athletes are operating at peak capacity. Vitamin supplementation studies have been done to examine these points. Will athletic performance be enhanced by supplementing vitamins above the RDA? The results of studies supplementing vitamin B complex, vitamin C, and vitamin E will be discussed.

Supplementation studies have been carried out using thiamin, niacin, and cyanocobalamin individually as well as in combination with the other B complex vitamins.[5,8] These studies have examined the effects of different levels of supplementation on different muscular work parameters.[5] The results, for the most part, seem to indicate that vitamin B supplementation has no effect on muscular ability, endurance resistance to fatique, or recovery from the exertion of brief or prolonged exercise.[5]

The results of vitamin C supplementation studies have been very ambiguous. Some studies have reported increased mechanical efficiency and physical working capacity with vitamin C supplementations while others have shown no beneficial effect.[5,8] Other investigation has dealt with vitamin C supplementation and the prevention of injury,[8] due to the role the vitamin plays in wound healing. No conclusive evidence exists that ascorbic supplementation will prevent injuries.[8]

The results of the study of the supplementation of vitamin E, a fat-soluble vitamin, have also been variable and conflicting. Some studies have shown increases in aerobic capacity while others have shown no beneficial consequence of vitamin supplementation.[5,8]

The sketchy results outlined above for all of the vitamin supplementation studies are due to experimental inadequacy. Many of the studies did not use a double-blind experimental design. In addition, many used inadequate controls and lacked proper statistical analysis and interpretation.[5,8] Based on these conflicting data, it is difficult to make a final decision about vitamin supplementation and the athlete. However, the general feeling at this time is that general and specific vitamin supplementation has little or no beneficial effect on athlete performance in the absence of a deficiency.[5,8,9]

4. TOXICITY OF HYPERVITAMINOSIS

As the previous section has described, the use of supplemental or "megavitamin" therapy for the purpose of increasing athletic performance is not justified at this time. In addition, large doses of vitamins can produce toxic effects in the body. Because of their water-soluble nature, vitamin B complex and vitamin C are less toxic in large doses than the fat-soluble vitamins (A, D, E, K). However, adverse effects have been characterized for several of the water-soluble compounds. The major toxicities of hypervitaminosis are listed below.

4.1. Vitamin B Complex

Among the B complex vitamins, toxic effects have been characterized for niacin and pyridoxine. High doses of niacin will result in vasodilatation, sensation of heat, itching, nausea, vomiting, and headaches.[2]

Pyridoxine in large doses has been reported to cause sensory neuropathies with the symptoms of numbness and alterations in the senses of pain, touch, and temperature.

4.2. Vitamin A

Acute hypervitaminosis A results in headache, vomiting, muscular weakness, blurred vision, and bulging fontanelles in neonates. A chronic increase will lead to skin dryness, alapecia, anorexia, bone thickening, leukopenia, and hepatocellular damage.[2]

4.3. Vitamin D

Vitamin D intoxication can be a serious problem. Early symptoms include hypercalcemia, anorexia, and joint pain. Irreversible calcification of vital organs such as heart, lungs, and kidneys can lead to death.

5. CONCLUSION

There is no doubt that vitamins play an essential role in the regulation of metabolic function. However, the relationship between vitamins and the level of physical performance of the athlete is still in question. The uncertainty of the results obtained in studies of the effects of vitamin supplementation and deficiency on athletic performance make it difficult to resolve this question. As of now, a well-balanced diet containing the RDA of the vitamins in addition to sufficient calorie intake will supply the athlete with the proper metabolic fuel.

REFERENCES

1. National Research Council, Food and Nutrition Board: *Dietary Allowances*, ed. 9. Washington, DC, National Academy of Sciences, 1980.

2. Machein LJ (ed): *Handbook of Vitamins*. New York, Marcel Dekker, Inc., 1984.
3. Ruderman NB, Balon T, Zorano A, et al: Acute and chronic metabolism changes following exercise: mechanisms and physiological relevance, in Winick M (ed): *Nutrition and Exercise*. New York, John Wiley and Sons, 1986, p 1.
4. Young V: Protein and amino acid metabolism in relation to physical exercise, in Winick M (ed): *Nutrition and Exercise*. New York, John Wiley and Sons, 1986, p 9.
5. Van Der Beek EJ: Vitamins and endurance training. *Sports Medicine* 2:175–197, 1985.
6. Dreon D, Butterfield G: Vitamin B_6 utilization in active and inactive young men. *Am J Clin Nutr* 43:816–824, 1986.
7. Beiko AZ, Obarzanek E, Kalkware HJ, et al: Effects of exercise on riboflavin requirements of young women. *Am J Clin Nutr* 37:509–517, 1983.
8. Wilmore JH, Freund BJ: Nutritional enhancement of athletic performance, in Winick M (ed): *Nutrition and Exercise*. New York, John Wiley and Sons, 1986, p 67.
9. Vitale JJ: Nutrition in sports medicine. *Clin Orthop* 198:158–168, 1985.

2

Fate of Anabolic Steroids in the Body

Howard D. Colby and Penelope A. Longhurst

1. INTRODUCTION

The use of anabolic steroids in an attempt to enhance athletic performance has become a widespread practice in both amateur and professional sports in recent years. The rationale for such use (or abuse) of these agents is based upon the growth-promoting and musculature-developing, or anabolic, effects of the naturally occurring steroid hormones known as androgens. These are the hormones that play an important part in the sexual development of males, that is, the production of various masculine traits. The physiologically most important of the naturally occurring androgens is the hormone testosterone, which is produced principally by the testes. The anabolic steroids used by athletes are various synthetic derivatives of testosterone, substances with longer durations of action and/or greater potencies than the physiological androgens. Some of these compounds have been synthesized with the goal of enhancing the anabolic effects of testosterone relative to its masculinizing actions. Since these synthetic preparations are not native or endogenous to the body, they are classified as exogenous substances or drugs.

As noted above, the synthetic anabolic steroids are both structurally and functionally related to testosterone. Thus, knowledge of the basic physiology of androgenic hormones provides considerable insight into the actions and mechanisms of action of the synthetic anabolic agents used by athletes. In fact, for some of the drug preparations employed, detailed investigations have not been carried out and it is simply assumed that many of their characteristics are similar to those of endogenous androgens. Accordingly, before discussing some of the synthetic steroids used in athletics, we will provide an overview of the physiology of androgens. This information will serve as important background material and provide the basis for subsequently compar-

Howard D. Colby and Penelope A. Longhurst • Department of Biomedical Sciences, University of Illinois College of Medicine at Rockford, Rockford, Illinois 61107.

ing the characteristics of the anabolic steroid drugs with those of the naturally occurring hormones.

2. PHYSIOLOGY OF ANDROGENIC HORMONES[1]

2.1. Structures and Names

All of the naturally occurring androgens belong to the class of compounds known as steroids. The steroids are a group of hydrophobic substances characterized by the ring structure illustrated in Fig. 1. The individual rings are identified by the letters A to D as indicated in the figure for the compound cholesterol. Each of the carbon atoms in the steroid molecule is identified by a number (Fig. 1). The official chemical nomenclature for all steroids is based partly upon this carbon numbering system, but there are simpler and more widely used names for most of the more common steroids. The latter names will be used throughout this chapter. Nonetheless, some familiarity with the carbon numbering system is desirable since the names of many synthetic steroids are based upon structural features or modifications at specific carbons in the steroid nucleus. For example, the anabolic steroid 19-nortestosterone (nandrolone) differs from the naturally occurring androgen testosterone in that the former lacks the 19-carbon atom. Thus, knowledge of at least some chemical nomenclature will make many of the common steroid names more meaningful.

The naturally occurring androgens contain 19 carbon atoms and do not have a side chain attached to the steroid nucleus. The major androgenic hormones are shown in Fig. 2. Testosterone is the most potent of these androgens, and many investigators believe that androstenedione and dehydroepiandrosterone (DHEA) exert their androgenic or masculinizing effects only after being converted to testosterone. As discussed below, the further metabolism of testosterone to the compound 5α-dihydrotestosterone plays an important role in the actions of this hormone.

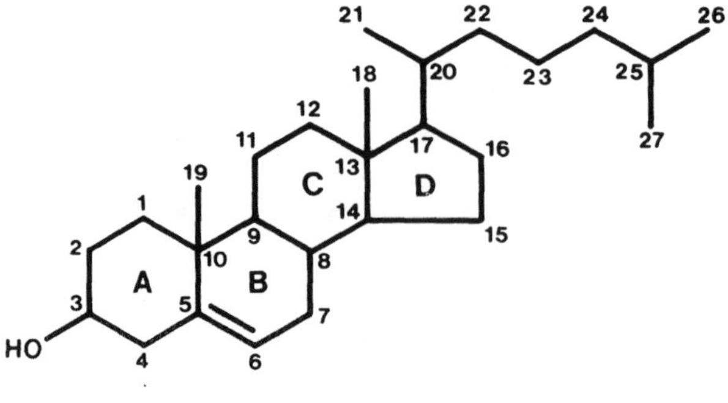

Figure 1. The ring structure and numbering system of the carbon atoms in steroids, illustrated for cholesterol. (From Hedge GA, Colby HD, Goodman RL: *Clinical Endocrine Physiology*, W. B. Saunders Co., Philadelphia, 1987).

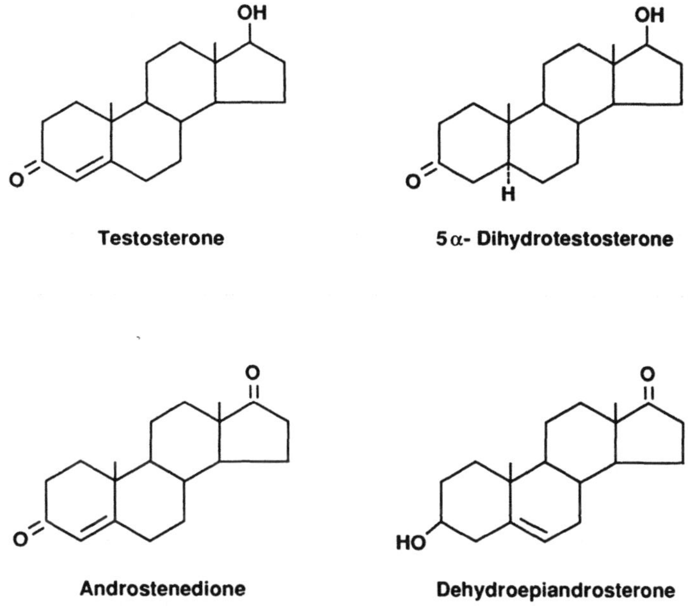

Figure 2. Structure of the androgenic hormones, testosterone, 5α-dihydrotestosterone, androstenedione, and dehydroepiandrosterone.

2.2. Sites and Pathways of Androgen Production

Steroid hormones are synthesized principally in the adrenal cortex, testes, ovaries, and placenta, but the specific secretory products of each of these steroidogenic organs vary considerably. In males, the testes are the dominant site of testosterone production. Androstenedione and DHEA are also synthesized in the testes, but in relatively small amounts, and since these compounds are relatively weak androgens, testicular secretion of testosterone is of far greater physiological significance. In both males and females, the adrenal cortex represents the major source of androstenedione and DHEA. Since very little testosterone is produced in females, adrenal secretion of androstenedione and DHEA provides the major physiological supply of androgenic hormones in women. Small amounts of androgens are secreted by the ovaries, but normally far less than the quantities provided by the adrenal cortex.

The common precursor to all steroid hormones, including androgens, is cholesterol. Thus, adequate amounts of cholesterol are essential for hormone synthesis in androgen-producing cells. All steroid-secreting cells have the capacity to synthesize cholesterol, but many are also able to sequester circulating cholesterol for androgen production. The relative importance of intracellular cholesterol synthesis versus removal of cholesterol from the blood for use as substrate for hormone production varies from tissue to tissue. Regardless of the specific source of cholesterol, most is stored in large quantities in steroidogenic tissues in the form of cholesterol esters. As substrate

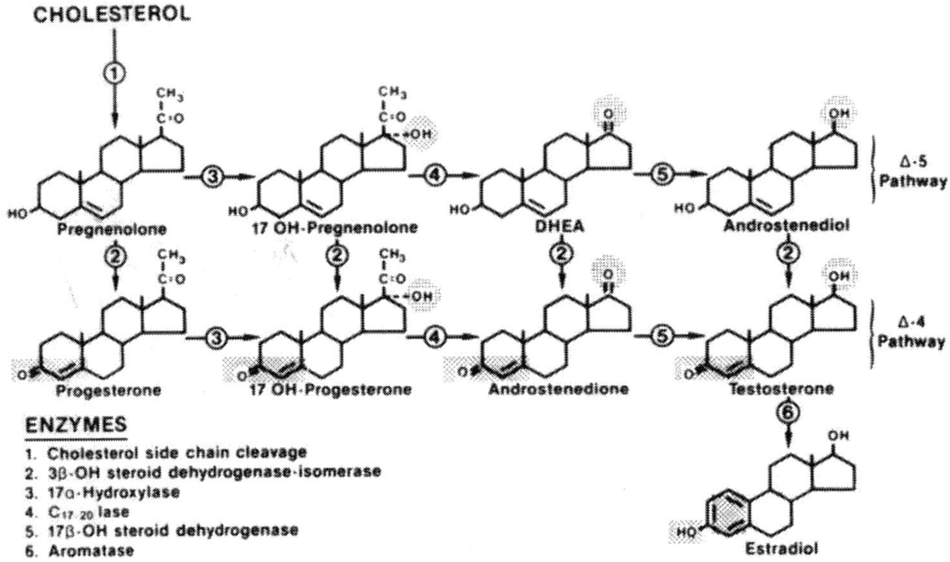

Figure 3. Pathways involved in the synthesis of anabolic–androgenic steroid hormones. (From Hedge GA, Colby HD, Goodman RL: *Clinical Endocrine Physiology,* W. B. Saunders Co., Philadelphia, 1987).

for androgen synthesis is needed, the esters are enzymatically hydrolyzed to generate free cholesterol.

The pathways and the names of the enzymes involved in the conversion of cholesterol to androgens are shown in Fig. 3. The first step in the pathway, the conversion of cholesterol to the intermediate pregnenolone, is common to the production of all steroid hormones. This reaction is the rate-limiting step in androgen synthesis, and, as a result, regulation of androgen production occurs by modulation of this reaction. After the formation of pregnenolone, androgen synthesis may proceed via either of two routes, known as the Δ-4 and Δ-5 pathways. The names of the pathways refer to whether the constituent steroids have a double bond between the C-4 and C-5 (Δ-4) or C-5 and C-6 (Δ-5) positions. The pathway utilized is determined by the relative activities of the various steroidogenic enzymes within the cell. In humans, the Δ-5 pathway appears to dominate for androgen production, but as can be seen in Fig. 3, the enzymatic reactions in the two pathways are very similar. Both androstenedione and DHEA may serve as precursors to testosterone, and, as noted above, such transformations may be necessary for their androgenic activities. Androgens, once produced, may be further metabolized to the feminizing hormones, estrogens (e.g., estradiol); this process is of greatest physiological significance in the ovaries and placenta but may occur to some extent in a variety of tissues including the testes and adrenal cortex.

2.3. Circulation of Androgens in the Blood

A large fraction of all steroid hormones in the blood are reversibly bound to plasma proteins (Fig. 4). It is important to appreciate that it is only the unbound or free

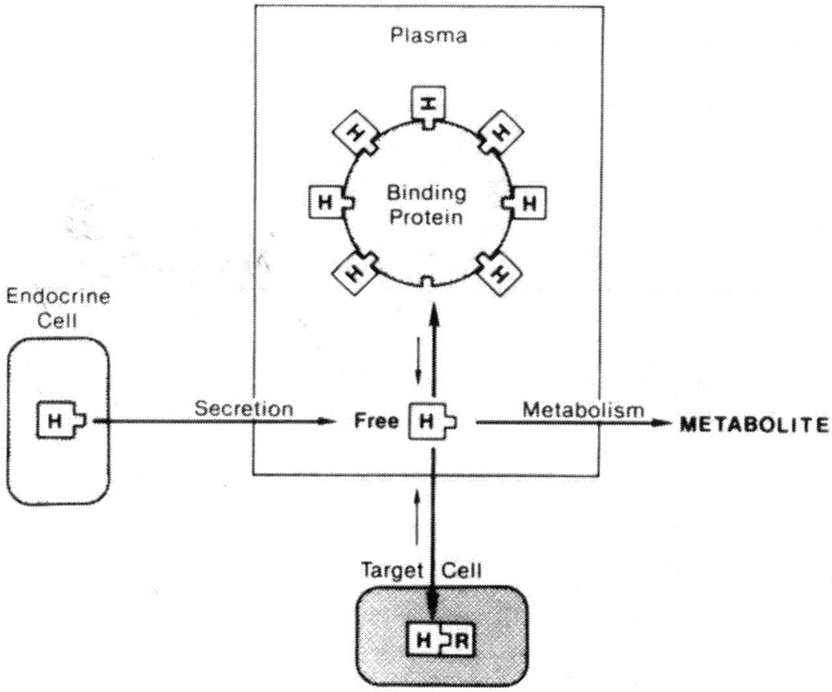

Figure 4. Circulation of androgens in plasma. (From Hedge GA, Colby HD, Goodman RL: *Clinical Endocrine Physiology,* W. B. Saunders Co., Philadelphia, 1987).

fraction of hormone that is biologically active. Thus, most of the circulating androgen pool does not exert any physiological effects. The protein-bound testosterone, for example, comprises approximately 97 to 99% of the total amount in the blood; only the remaining 1 to 3% is able to interact with receptors in target tissues and initiate biological responses (Fig. 4). However, the protein-bound hormone is in reversible equilibrium with the free fraction and provides for a large hormone reserve to replenish the free pool. In addition, protein binding protects the hormone from enzymatic degradation by the liver, thereby extending its duration of action or biological half-life.

Most of the blood testosterone is bound with high affinity to a specific globulin, known as sex hormone-binding globulin (SHBG), which is synthesized in the liver. A significant amount (~40%) is also bound to plasma albumin, but with relatively low affinity. The specific pattern of hormone distribution in the blood varies somewhat from androgen to androgen, but all androgens are extensively protein bound and this binding impacts on their biological activities.

2.4. Regulation of Testosterone Synthesis and Secretion by the Testes

In contrast to protein hormones, there is no known mechanism for the storage of steroid hormones after they are synthesized. Since steroids are highly lipophilic molecules, once produced they simply diffuse across cell membranes into the vasculature.

Thus, synthesis and secretion of steroids tend to be tightly coupled processes, and the secretion of androgens is regulated by modulation of the rate of synthesis.

Testicular androgen synthesis is controlled by a negative feedback control system involving the hypothalamus and anterior pituitary gland (Fig. 5). Gonadotropin-releasing hormone (GnRH) is secreted by hypothalamic neurons into the hypophyseal portal blood vessels, which transport it to the anterior pituitary gland. GnRH then stimulates the secretion of luteinizing hormone (LH) by anterior pituitary cells, and the LH is carried by the blood to the testes. Within the testes, LH acts upon the steroid-producing cells or Leydig cells to increase testosterone synthesis and release into the blood. The increase in testosterone secretion is brought about by LH activation of cholesterol metabolism, the rate-limiting step in steroid biosynthesis. Within the Leydig cells, the actions of LH on steroidogenesis are mediated by the second messenger, cyclic AMP.

The feedback control system for testicular androgen secretion is completed by the inhibitory effects of plasma free testosterone on GnRH and LH release. Thus, as plasma testosterone levels increase, GnRH and LH secretion are inhibited, decreasing testosterone production. On the other hand, if plasma testosterone concentrations decline, GnRH and LH secretion are stimulated, bringing about an increase in testosterone synthesis and release. Thus, this control system is designed to maintain fairly constant blood levels of free or biologically active testosterone. Although various other factors may at times modulate androgen production by the testes, the negative feedback loop described above is the dominant regulatory system. The production of sperm by the testes occurs in different cells (Sertoli cells) and is controlled by different hormones (FSH, inhibin) than those responsible for testosterone synthesis (Fig. 5).

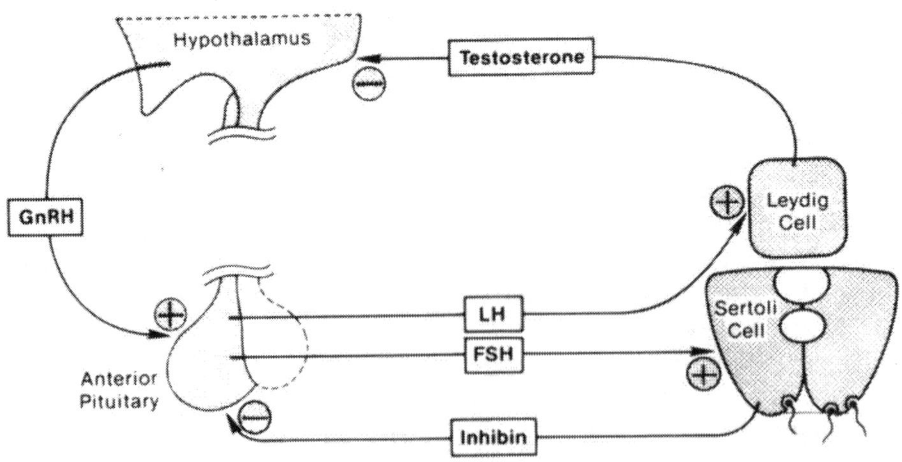

Figure 5. Regulation of testosterone secretion. (From Hedge GA, Colby HD, Goodman RL: *Clinical Endocrine Physiology*, W. B. Saunders Co., Philadelphia, 1987).

2.5. Actions and Mechanism of Action of Testosterone

Testosterone exerts a variety of effects, most of which are related to reproductive function in males (Table 1). Such actions are androgenic in nature. Effects of testosterone on the male reproductive tract include differentiation *in utero,* maturation of the external genitalia at puberty, and maintenance of the internal reproductive tract in adults. Testosterone is also necessary for the development of various male secondary sexual characteristics including the deep-voice characteristic of males, the male pattern of body hair growth (beard, chest hair, etc.), and muscular development. The development of a normal sex drive at puberty requires adequate amounts of testosterone as does sperm production by the Sertoli cells of the testes. As noted above, testosterone is involved in the feedback regulation of GnRH and LH secretion by the hypothalamus and anterior pituitary gland, respectively.

The use of androgenic compounds by athletes is related solely to their effects on protein synthesis. Androgens are anabolic steroids in that they stimulate protein synthesis in a variety of tissues throughout the body. It is this effect of androgens that is responsible for the pubertal muscle development that occurs in males. Testosterone is also important for the pubertal growth spurt in boys but ultimately causes fusion of the epiphyses of long bones, thereby terminating growth. The ideal androgenic steroid for athletic use would be one with high anabolic but low androgenic activity. Although many of the synthetic androgens (anabolic steroids) are purported to have such characteristics, this issue remains a very controversial one with little definitive data available to support or refute these claims. However, all agree that androgenic actions represent potentially serious side effects associated with the use of anabolic steroids, particularly by females or children.

Table 1. Actions of Testosterone[a]

Effects on reproductive tract and external genitalia
Differentiation *in utero*
Maturation at puberty
Maintenance in adult (tract only)
Development of secondary sexual characteristics (at puberty)
Male pattern of hair growth
Deep voice
Increased muscle growth
Other reproductive effects
Development of libido at puberty
Required for spermatogenesis
Inhibition of gonadotropins
Nonreproductive effects
Anabolic actions
Pubertal growth spurt and then closure of epiphyses
Increased secretion of sebaceous glands

[a]From Hedge GA, Colby HD, and Goodman RL: *Clinical Endocrine Physiology*. Philadelphia, W. B. Saunders Co., 1987.

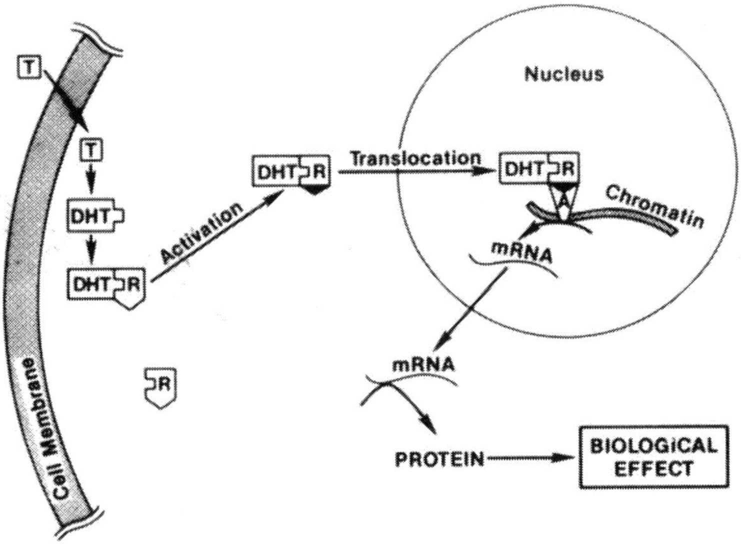

Figure 6. Mechanism of action of testosterone in target tissues. (From Hedge GA, Colby HD, Goodman RL: *Clinical Endocrine Physiology,* W. B. Saunders Co., Philadelphia, 1987).

The mechanism of action of androgens is, in general, similar to that for all steroid hormones and is illustrated for testosterone in Fig. 6. As lipophilic compounds, androgens are able to diffuse freely from the blood into cells and interact with high-affinity and specific receptor sites in the cytosol. The actions of androgens are limited to those cells (target cells) which contain these receptors. In the case of testosterone, conversion to the metabolite 5α-dihydrotestosterone (DHT) by the enzyme 5α-reductase precedes binding to the cytosolic receptor in at least some tissues, most notably the sex accessory organs. The binding brings about activation of the hormone–receptor complex, which increases its affinity for nuclear chromatin. The complex then migrates into the nucleus of the cell and activates various genes, bringing about an increase in protein synthesis. The specific proteins synthesized in response to androgens are characteristic of the particular target cell and are responsible for the biological effects(s) manifested. Most of the available evidence indicates that the same receptor mediates both the androgenic and anabolic effects of androgens; only the target cell differs. Thus, there appears to be little reason to think that the anabolic and androgenic effects may be separable on the basis of androgen receptor differences in different tissues.

2.6. Elimination of Androgens from the Body

Most steroid hormones are structurally modified by a variety of enzymatic processes prior to their elimination from the body. Although such modification may occur in various tissues, the major site of steroid metabolism is the liver. The major pathways for testosterone metabolism in the body are presented in Fig. 7. Metabolism usually results in the formation of products that are less active than the parent compound, but

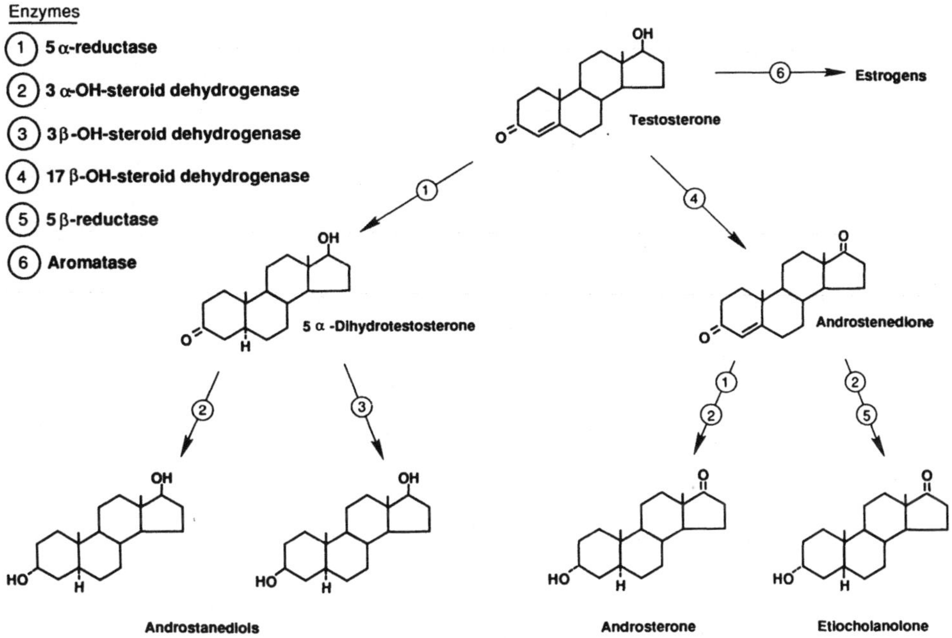

Figure 7. Routes of metabolism of the androgenic/anabolic steroids.

in some instances, the reverse may occur. The latter is illustrated by the conversion of testosterone to DHT, a compound with a very high affinity for the androgen receptor and, thus, a very potent androgen. Metabolism of steroids usually entails a series of reduction reactions followed by conjugation with glucuronide or sulfate moieties. Conjugation increases the water solubility of steroid hormones and facilitates their excretion in urine, the major route of elimination. Thus, the rate of hepatic metabolism is usually closely correlated with the rate of steroid elimination from the body. The major end products of testosterone metabolism are various stereoisomers of androsterone (Fig. 7), which are conjugated and excreted in the urine. The specific profile of metabolites and the rate of elimination from the body vary from androgen to androgen. A number of factors which influence the metabolism of steroids are discussed in the following section on the synthetic anabolic agents.

3. SYNTHETIC ANABOLIC STEROIDS

Synthetic androgen-like steroids have found a variety of applications as either anabolic or androgenic agents. The use of synthetic rather than naturally occurring androgens has been dictated largely by the rapid metabolism of the latter compounds. The rate of hepatic degradation of testosterone, for example, precludes its oral administration and necessitates frequent administration by injection for sustained effects. Many of the synthetic derivatives produced by drug companies circumvent these problems by resisting hepatic inactivation or by being slowly released from injection sites over prolonged periods of time. In addition, some of the synthetic compounds are purported to have greater anabolic but less androgenic activity than testosterone, characteristics which are highly desirable for some applications.

In this section, the various uses of anabolic steroids will be discussed and the general characteristics of the major types of synthetic preparations available described. We will then present some of the specific properties of two commercially available anabolic steroid preparations, representing the two major types of synthetic anabolic agents. Particular emphasis will be placed on comparing the fates of these synthetic steroids in the body with those of the naturally occurring hormone testosterone.

3.1. Uses of Anabolic Steroids[2–5]

The clinical uses of anabolic steroids are listed in Table 2. Many are highly controversial, and in some instances, careful clinical trials have not been carried out to establish definitively the therapeutic efficacy.

Table 2. Uses and Dosages of the Synthetic Anabolic Steroids

Steroid	Route of administration	Usual adult dose	Clinical use(s)
17α-Alkylated			
Ethylestrenol	Oral	2–4 mg/day	Antirheumatic, antiosteoporotic, antianemic
Fluoxymesterone	Oral	M: 5–20 mg/day F: 10–40 mg/day	M: Androgen replacement F: Antineoplastic
Methandrostenolone (methandienone)	Oral	2.5–5 mg/day	Body building
Methyltestosterone	Oral Lingual	10–20 mg/day	M: Androgen replacement F: Antineoplastic
Oxandrolone	Oral	2.5–20 mg/day	Antiosteoporotic
Oxymetholone	Oral	1–5 mg/kg/day	Antianemic
Stanozolol	Oral	2–6 mg/day	Hereditary angioedema
17β-Esters			
Dromostanolone propionate	i.m.[a]	100 mg, 3 times a week	Antineoplastic
Nandrolone decanoate	i.m.	M: 100–200 mg/week F: 50–100 mg/week	Antianemic
Nandrolone propionate	i.m.	25–100 mg/week	Antineoplastic
Testosterone cypionate	i.m.	200 mg every 2 weeks	Growth stimulant
Testosterone enanthate	i.m.	200 mg every 2 weeks	Growth stimulant
Testosterone propionate	i.m.	10–25 mg/day	Growth stimulant

[a]i.m.: intramuscular.

3.1.1. Testosterone Deficiency (Male Hypogonadism)

The principal clinical use of the synthetic anabolic steroids is to treat testosterone deficiency in hypogonadal males. The long-acting testosterone esters, testosterone enanthate or testosterone cypionate, are administered parenterally at one- to three-week intervals to increase plasma testosterone levels. This treatment results in the development or restoration of male secondary sexual characteristics and male sexual behavior, stimulates erythropoietin secretion by the kidney, promotes protein anabolism, and accelerates epiphyseal closure in young males. However, androgen therapy alone does not fully restore spermatogenesis in hypogonadal states.

3.1.2. Catabolic or Protein-Depleting States

Ethylestrenol or oxandrolone is indicated as an adjunct treatment in conditions such as chronic infections, extensive surgery, or severe trauma, all of which represent catabolic states. However, although anabolic steroids can improve nitrogen balance during the first few days following minor surgery, they have not been shown to offer any advantage over parenteral nutrition, and are therefore probably of little therapeutic benefit.

3.1.3. Anemia

Androgens stimulate erythropoiesis by increasing the production of erythropoietin by the kidney and are used in the treatment of anemias which are refractory to other types of therapy. These include acquired and congenital bone marrow failure anemias and renal insufficiency anemias. Approximately one-half of the patients appear to respond to androgen therapy, although some authors suggest that the apparent improvement after androgen therapy is due to spontaneous remission. Therapeutic agents used for this treatment include ethylestrenol, nandrolone decanoate, and oxymetholone.

3.1.4. Carcinoma of the Breast

Large doses of dromostolone propionate, nandrolone decanoate, fluoxymesterone, and testosterone are used to treat inoperable advanced or metastatic breast carcinoma in women. The mechanism by which the androgens bring about remission of breast cancer is unknown. These agents are contraindicated for the treatment of breast carcinoma in males.

3.1.5. Hereditary Angioedema

Hereditary angioedema is an autosomal dominant disorder producing a defect in complement inactivation that results in unopposed activation of the complement cascade and increased blood vessel permeability. The 17α-alkylated steroids stimulate the production of the deficient C1 inhibitor and therefore are of benefit in the prophylaxis and treatment of this potentially fatal disorder.

3.1.6. *Short Stature*

Use of synthetic androgens for the treatment of constitutional delayed growth is controversial. Administration of these drugs prior to epiphyseal closure produces an accelerated growth velocity, probably as a result of stimulation of growth hormone secretion, but may have no effect on the final height. Care must be taken to avoid the use of doses which would produce premature epiphyseal closure and further compromise the final height attained. These agents are not recommended for use in young females because of their virilizing side effects. Oral preparations such as oxandrolone, fluoxymesterone, or methyltestosterone are usually chosen to promote growth.

3.1.7. *Osteoporosis*

Ethylestrenol and oxandrolone are used as adjuncts in the treatment of bone pain and decreased bone strength associated with osteoporosis, although their efficacy in this treatment is questionable.

3.1.8. *Arthritis*

Ethylestrenol is used as an adjunct to improve strength and promote a sense of well-being in patients with arthritis. The efficacy of this treatment is questionable.

3.1.9. *Enhancement of Athletic Performance*[6]

The use of anabolic steroids by athletes to improve athletic performance has become increasingly popular and increasingly controversial. These steroids are used principally by weight lifters, weight throwers, football players, swimmers, and track and field athletes. Many athletes believe that the anabolic steroids improve their performance. However, the results of various tests have consistently failed to show any improvement in aerobic performance, as measured by maximal O_2 uptake, or in running or swimming times. In addition, there are inconsistencies in the literature concerning the effects of anabolic steroids on strength. Increases in strength, as measured by the single-repetition maximal weight technique, have been found in trained weight lifters who continued training during the period of time that the steroids were administered. The use of a high-protein diet concurrent with the steroid administration also seems to promote strength development. However, there has not been any consistent change in strength development observed when other weight lifting techniques have been employed to measure strength. In addition, athletes who had not previously weight trained before administration of the steroids did not show any consistent increase in strength. The anabolic steroids, therefore, appear to produce increases in strength only if they are given to athletes who are already weight training, who continue the training during the period of steroid administration, and who simultaneously receive a high-protein diet. The androgenic steroid most commonly used by athletes is the 17α-alkylated testosterone derivative methandrostenolone. This agent has no clinical uses.

In general, the side effects reported following the use of anabolic steroids in athletes have been benign and reversible. These include changes in libido, aggression, muscle spasm, gynecomastia, and abnormal liver function tests. However, long-term use of the orally active 17α-alkylated testosterone derivatives is associated with various types of more severe liver damage.

3.2. Contraindications for the Use of Synthetic Anabolic Steroids[2]

All steroids with androgenic actions are contraindicated in prostate and breast carcinoma in males because they may stimulate growth of androgen-dependent tumors. Their use is also contraindicated in pregnancy because of potential virilizing effects on the fetus. In addition, these agents should probably not be used in patients with any type of liver disease.

3.3. Adverse Effects of Synthetic Anabolic Steroids[2,4,5]

3.3.1. Virilizing Side Effects

The most common side effect resulting from anabolic steroid therapy is virilization. Although the different anabolic steroid preparations produce virilization to varying degrees, at high doses almost all of them produce some masculinizing effects, including acne, deepening of the voice, hirsutism, male pattern baldness, and clitoral enlargement and menstrual irregularities in females. In elderly males, androgens may produce prostate enlargement resulting in urinary obstruction.

3.3.2. Feminizing Side Effects

As discussed earlier in this chapter, the naturally occurring androgens can be converted to estrogens in a number of tissues. Many of the synthetic androgen analogues can similarly be converted to estrogens and may therefore produce feminizing side effects in some individuals. The most common manifestation of androgen-induced feminization is the gynecomastia that occurs in children or adult males following the use of high dosages of synthetic anabolic steroids as well as in patients with liver disease who receive these agents.

3.3.3. Liver Dysfunction

The 17α-alkylated anabolic steroids can cause life-threatening liver toxicity. The occurrence of peliosis hepatitis and of hepatomas has been reported in patients receiving long-term anabolic steroid therapy. In addition, some patients develop increased sulfobromophthalein (SBP) retention, but this does not appear to be of any clinical significance.

3.4. Structural Features of Synthetic Anabolic Steroids[4,5,7]

One of the major goals of structural modification of the testosterone molecule to produce the synthetic anabolic steroids is to increase resistance to metabolic inactivation by the liver. The short half-lives of the naturally occurring androgens make them difficult to use as therapeutic agents. In addition, some chemical changes such as removal of the 19-methyl group or 5α-reduction of the A-ring of the steroid nucleus increase the anabolic/androgenic potencies of these compounds. The two general types of synthetic anabolic/androgenic steroids that are used clinically are the 17α-alkylated and 17β-ester derivatives of testosterone.

3.4.1. 17α-Alkylated Testosterone Derivatives[2,4,5]

The 17α-alkylated androgens (e.g., ethylestrenol, methandrosterone, methyltestosterone; see Table 2 and Fig. 8) are more effective orally than testosterone as a result of increased resistance to hepatic inactivation. These compounds may also be administered by the buccal–sublingual route. The 17α-alkylated androgens act directly on androgen receptors and do not require removal of the 17α-alkyl group before receptor binding. These compounds are metabolized and excreted with the 17α-alkyl

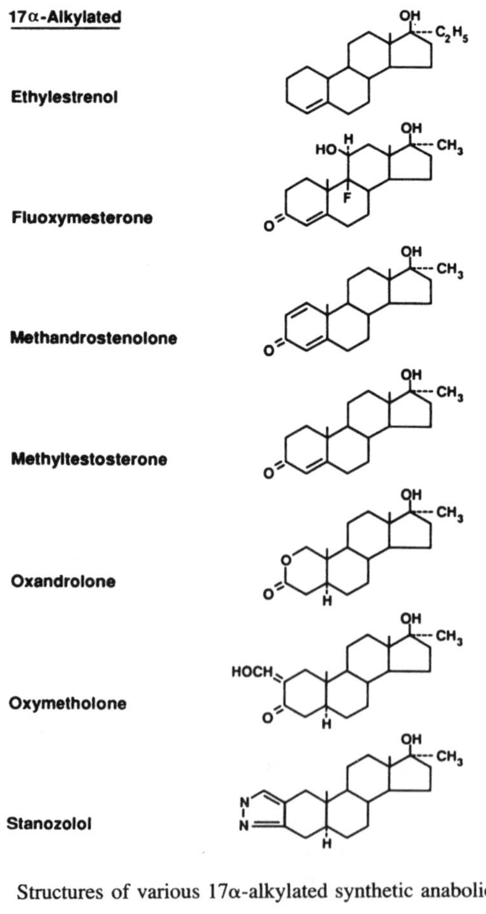

Figure 8. Structures of various 17α-alkylated synthetic anabolic steroids.

groups intact, and therefore, plasma levels of testosterone cannot be used as an index of the efficacy of the therapy. Methyltestosterone and fluoxymesterone exert principally androgenic effects, while for some of the other 17α-alkylated steroids such as oxandrolone, the anabolic effects predominate. The 17α-alkylated steroids are highly hepatotoxic and may produce cholestatic jaundice, peliosis hepatitis, or hepatomas. The reason(s) for the liver toxicity produced by this group of compounds is unknown, but the toxicity appears to be influenced by the patient's previous liver function status.

Methandrostenolone. Methandrostenolone, also known as methandienone, is one of the 17-alkylated synthetic anabolic steroids that can be taken orally because of its resistance to degradation by the liver. The structure of this drug is shown in Fig. 8. Methandrostenolone differs structurally from testosterone in having a methyl group at the 17-carbon position and a double bond between C-1 and C-2. Apparently, both structural modifications confer resistance to hepatic metabolism.

In general, the 17-akyl configuration, which is characteristic of methandrostenolone and structurally related compounds, is retained during the course of drug action and subsequent elimination from the body. Other than differences in hepatic metabolism, most of the basic features of these drugs are very similar to those of the naturally occurring androgens. For example, the circulation of methandrostenolone in the blood appears to be in association with the same plasma proteins to which testosterone is bound. However, the affinity of methandrostenolone for human sex-hormone-binding globulin is considerably lower than that of testosterone. Also, as in the case of testosterone, it is only the free or unbound fraction of methandrostenolone in the blood that has access to receptors in target tissues and is, therefore, biologically active. The lower affinity of methandrostenolone relative to testosterone for plasma binding proteins may facilitate "delivery" of the former to target cells and thereby enhance its biological activity.

The metabolism of methandrostenolone, like that of other steroids, occurs principally in the liver. The two major metabolites identified in the urine of humans treated with methandrostenolone are 6β-hydroxymethandrostenolone and 17-epimethandrostenolone (Fig. 9). Unmetabolized methandrostenolone has not been found in the urine of individuals taking the drug. Both of the major metabolites are excreted as the free or unconjugated compounds. In fact, there have not been any conjugated compounds identified as excretory products of methandrostenolone in humans. It has been hypothesized that both the 17-methyl group and the structure of the A-ring of methandrostenolone contribute to the inhibition of conjugation.[8,9]

The identities of the urinary metabolites of methandrostenolone indicate that the pathways of methandrostenolone metabolism are unusual for anabolic–androgenic steroids. Hydroxylation of the C-6 position is more commonly associated with glucocorticoid metabolism, and epimerization at C-17 rarely occurs. Of perhaps greatest significance is the absence of A-ring reduction of methandrostenolone by the liver. As noted previously, reduction of the C-4—C-5 double bond and of the 3-ketone is the principal route of metabolism of androgenic steroids. Since 17α-methyltestosterone undergoes extensive A-ring reduction prior to excretion, it appears that introduction of the C-1—C-2 double bond into the steroid nucleus suppresses reduction of the A-ring.

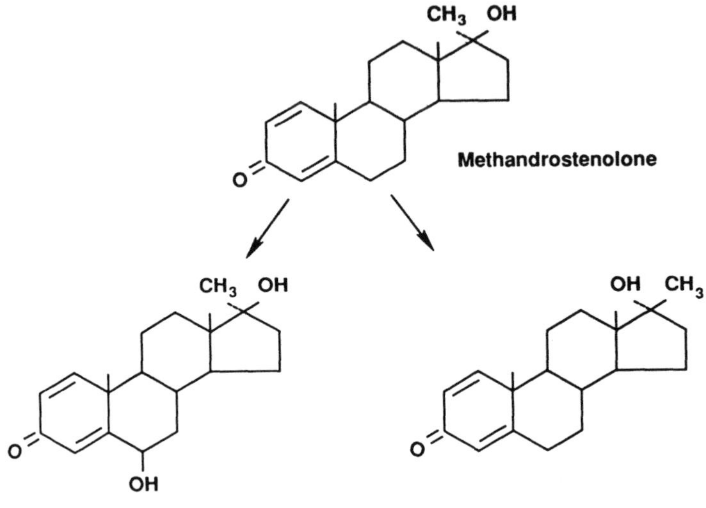

Figure 9. Pathways of hepatic methandrostenolone metabolism.

It is probably this resistance to A-ring metabolism by the liver that makes methandrostenolone an orally effective drug.

The resistance to A-ring reduction may also influence the relative anabolic/ androgenic activities of methandrostenolone. It has been demonstrated that the 5α-reduced derivative of methandrostenolone, like that of testosterone, has a higher affinity for the androgen receptor and is, therefore, a more potent androgen than the parent compound. However, methandrostenolone cannot be converted to the 5α-reduced compound in target tissues because of its resistance to enzymatic A-ring metabolism. Thus, in sex accessory tissues which have high 5α-reductase activity, the potency of testosterone is enhanced by its conversion to 5α-dihydrotestosterone (DHT), but methandrostenolone cannot be similarly "activated." By contrast, in tissues which have very little 5α-reductase activity, such as muscle, there is no such increase in the potency of testosterone relative to that of methandrostenolone.[10] Thus, the relatively greater ratio of anabolic : androgenic activity exhibited by methandrostenolone compared to testosterone may again reflect differences in metabolism in "anabolic" versus "androgenic" target tissues.

3.4.2. *17β-Esterified Testosterone Derivatives*

The 17β-esterified synthetic androgens (e.g., nandrolone decanoate, nandrolone propionate, dromostanolone propionate; see Table 2 and Fig. 10) are highly lipid-soluble compounds which are administered by injection in a lipophilic vehicle. Consequently, they are slowly absorbed from their intramuscular sites of administration, resulting in a prolonged duration of action and permitting several days or more to elapse between drug administrations. In general, the duration of action of the 17β-ester

17β-Esters

Dromostanolone propionate

Nandrolone decanoate

Nandrolone phenpropionate

Testosterone cypionate

Testosterone enanthate

Testosterone propionate

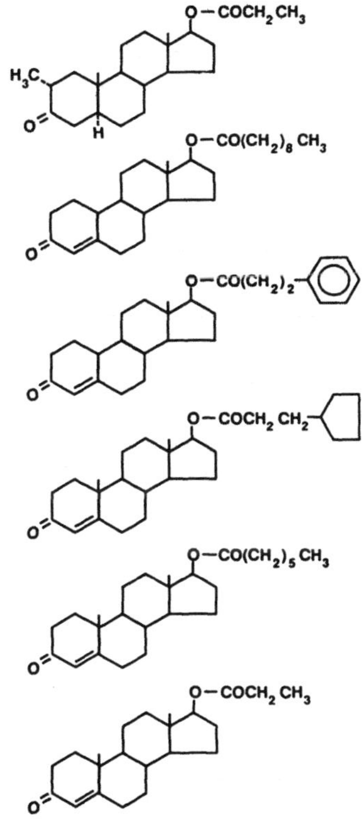

Figure 10. Structures of various 17β-esterified synthetic anabolic steroids.

derivatives increases with the length of the carbon side chain. The 17β-ester androgens must be hydrolyzed to the unesterified forms in order to bind to androgen receptors within target cells and produce their characteristic effects. The hydrolysis may take place in the plasma or in the liver. The products of hydrolysis of the 17β-ester testosterone derivatives can be measured in the plasma to determine the efficiency of absorption and the efficacy of the therapy. In contrast to the 17α-alkylated androgens, the 17β-esters are relatively nontoxic, although acne and gynecomastia have been reported following administration of these compounds.

Nandrolone Decanoate. Nandrolone decanoate is one of the synthetic steroid preparations commonly used when a sustained anabolic effect is desired. Structurally (Fig. 10), this compound is the decanoate derivative of 19-nortestosterone. In animal experiments, it has been found that when injected intramuscularly, nandrolone decanoate is slowly absorbed unchanged from the injection site into the general circulation. In rats, the time required for the amount of steroid at the injection depot to decline to 50% of the initial amount is approximately 130 h for nandrolone decanoate compared to 0.6 h for nandrolone (19-nortestosterone). A comparison of various 19-nortestosterone ester preparations indicated that the half-life for loss from the injection site increased with increasing chain length of the ester. Once in the plasma, the ester is rapidly hydrolyzed by esterases, resulting in the release of the free steroid (nandrolone), which is the biologically active form. Thus, it is the rate of release of the preparation from the injection site that is the rate-limiting step in the delivery of the active anabolic steroid into the circulation.

Results similar to those described above have also been obtained in humans.[11] When healthy volunteers were injected intramuscularly with nandrolone decanoate, a mean half-life of 6 days was found for the release of the ester from the injection site into the general circulation. The ester was not hydrolyzed while in the muscular depot, but once released into the blood, hydrolysis occurred with a half-life of 1 h or less. The combined processes of hydrolysis of the ester and distribution and elimination of the free steroid had a mean half-life of slightly more than 4 h, and the serum clearance of nandrolone was approximately 1.55 liters per hour per kg body weight. These characteristics of nandrolone decanoate disposition are similar in normal males and females when differences in body weight are taken into account.

Once free nandrolone is generated in the blood, its subsequent fate is very similar to that of testosterone. The nandrolone circulates in blood as both protein-bound and free steroid; it is the latter which is biologically active. However, the affinity of nandrolone for human sex-hormone-binding globulin is considerably lower than that of testosterone. Metabolism of circulating nandrolone occurs primarily in the liver, and the enzymatic modifications that occur are similar to those for testosterone. Thus, many of the metabolites of nandrolone are the 19-nor analogues of testosterone metabolites. The major pathways involved in the metabolism of nandrolone by the liver are illustrated in Fig. 11. The major metabolite identified in the urine of men receiving nandrolone decanoate is 19-norandrosterone. Other quantitatively significant metabolites include 19-noretiocholanolone and 19-norepiandrosterone (Fig. 11). As with most steroids, conjugation usually occurs prior to excretion of the metabolites in the urine.[12,13]

All of the available evidence indicates that the actions of the synthetic anabolic drugs, like those of testosterone, are initiated by steroid interactions with the cytosolic androgen receptor in target tissues (Fig. 6) resulting ultimately in an activation of cellular protein synthesis. In addition, the androgen receptors in the sex accessory tissues appear to be identical to those in muscle and various other organs. Thus, the "androgenic" as well as the "anabolic" effects of the synthetic and naturally occurring androgens are mediated by a common receptor which is found at all target sites. Apparent differences in the ratios of anabolic to androgenic potencies of the synthetic anabolic steroids and testosterone, therefore, cannot be attributed to differences in receptor types.

The intracellular metabolism of androgenic steroids in target cells may be an important factor in determining the relative anabolic/androgenic activities of various compounds. It has been demonstrated that steroid 5α-reductase activity is very high in sex accessory tissues but very low in muscle.[14] Thus, anabolic–androgenic steroids such as testosterone and nandrolone are rapidly converted to their 5α-reduced metabolites in the sex accessory organs but remain largely unaltered in muscle cells. These

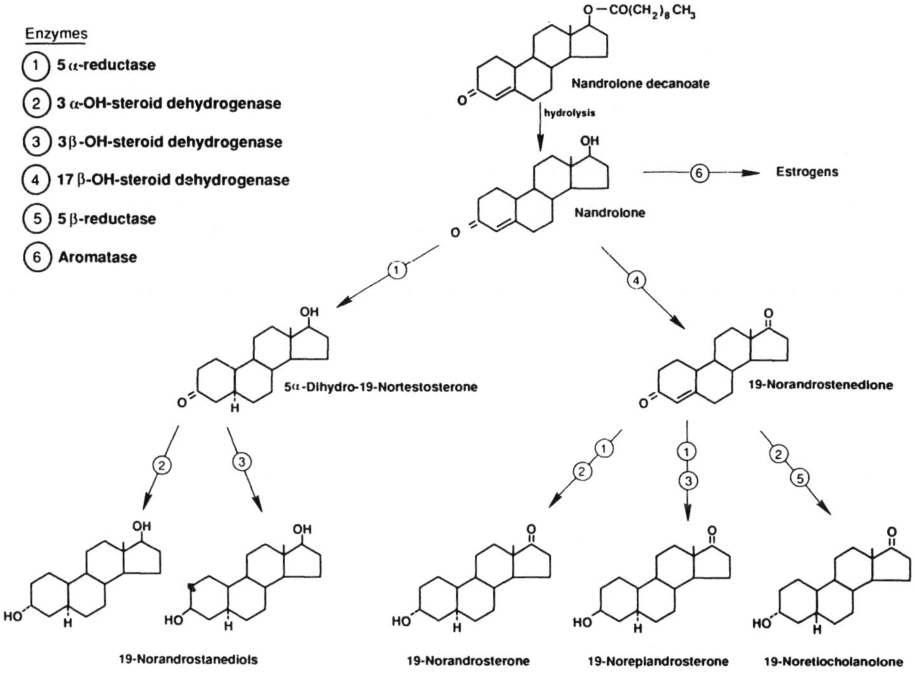

Figure 11. Pathways of nandrolone decanoate metabolism in the body.

differences in metabolism can have an impact on steroid interactions with the androgen receptor and consequently on androgen action. For example, 5α-reduction of testosterone results in the formation of DHT, a compound with a greater affinity for the androgen receptor than testosterone. In contrast, the 5α-reduced metabolite of nandrolone, 5α-dihydronandrolone, has a lower affinity than nandrolone for the androgen receptor. Thus, in tissues with high 5α-reductase activity, the potency of testosterone would be enhanced but that of nandrolone decreased, whereas in tissues with low enzyme activity, the opposite would pertain. According to this hypothesis, the relative potency of nandrolone compared to testosterone would be greater in muscle than in sex accessory tissues. Tissue differences in metabolism and differences in the affinities of the metabolites for the androgen receptor may, therefore, provide an explanation for the apparently higher anabolic/androgenic activity ratios of some synthetic steroids relative to testosterone.

4. CONCLUSIONS

Anabolic steroids have been widely used by athletes in certain sports for a couple of decades. Although the synthetic anabolic agents have some legitimate clinical applications, there is not as yet any clear-cut evidence that these drugs improve athletic performance. In any case, the putative benefits to athletes must be weighed against the potential adverse effects. There are some experimental observations to support the conclusion that the synthetic anabolic agents have higher ratios of anabolic to androgenic activities than the naturally occurring androgens. Nonetheless, all have some androgenic activity. Accordingly, the use of any anabolic steroids is contraindicated in females because of their virilizing effects. Various other adverse effects of the oral anabolic agents should preclude the use of this group of drugs in male athletes as well. Thus, if anabolic steroids are to be used in an attempt to enhance athletic performance, they should be given parenterally as the long-acting ester preparations and only to males.

REFERENCES

1. Hedge GA, Colby HD, Goodman RL (eds): *Clinical Endocrine Physiology*. Philadelphia, W. B. Saunders Co., 1987.
2. Eikelboom FA, van der Vies J (eds): Anabolics in the '80's. *Acta Endocrinol* [Suppl] 271, 1985.
3. Kochakian CD (ed): *Anabolic-Androgenic Steroids*. Handbook of Experimental Pharmacology 43. Berlin, Springer Verlag, 1976.
4. Snyder PJ: Clinical use of androgens. *Annu Rev Med* 35:207–217, 1984.
5. Wilson JD, Griffin JE: The use and misuse of androgens. *Metabolism* 29:1278–1295, 1980.
6. Haupt HA, Rovere GD: Anabolic steroids: a review of the literature. *Am J Sports Med* 12:469–484, 1984.
7. Mainwaring WIP: *The Mechanism of Action of Androgens*. New York, Springer-Verlag, 1977.
8. Dürbeck HW, Büker I: Studies on anabolic steroids. The mass spectra of 17α-methyl-17β-hydroxyl-1,4-androstadien-3-one (Dianabol) and its metabolites. *Biomed Mass Spec* 7:437–445, 1980.
9. MacDonald GS, Sykes PJ, Adhikary PM, et al: The identification of 17α-hydroxy-17-methyl-1,4-androstadien-3-one as a metabolite of the anabolic steroid drug 17β-hydroxy-17-methyl-1,4-androstadien-3-one in man. *Steroids* 18:753–765, 1971.
10. Steele RE, Didato F, Sawyer WK, et al: Evidence that 5α-reduction of Δ^4,3-ketosteroids may be more important for their androgenic than their luteinizing hormone-inhibiting activity. *Endocrinology* 105:1026–1040, 1979.
11. Wignand HP, Bosch AMG, Donker CW: Pharmacokinetic parameters of nandrolone (19-nortestosterone) after intramuscular administration of nandrolone decanoate (Deca-Durabolin) to healthy volunteers. Acta Endocrinol [Suppl] 271:19–30, 1985.
12. Belkien L, Schürmeyer T, Hano R, et al: Pharmacokinetics of 19-nortestosterone esters in normal men. *J Steroid Biochem* 22:623–629, 1985.
13. Massé R, Laliberté C, Tremblay L, et al: Gas chromatographic/mass spectrometric analysis of 19-nortestosterone urinary metabolites in man. *Biomed Mass Spec* 12:115–121, 1985.
14. Bergink EW, Janssen PSL, Turpijn EW, et al: Comparison of the receptor binding properties of nandrolone and testosterone under in vitro and in vivo conditions. *J Steroid Biochem* 22:831–836, 1985.

3

Nutrition, Fluid Balance, and Physical Performance

Richard Cotter

1. INTRODUCTION AND HISTORY

1.1. Development of an Understanding of the Importance of Nutrition and Fluid Balance to Physical Performance

Nutrition, including fluid balance and its effects on physical performance, is not a new concept created in response to the evolution of professional athletics in the twentieth century. Present-day media coverage of this field might lead one to believe that the relationship between nutrition and physical performance is a recent discovery of professional coaching staffs. In truth, professional sports has recently helped expand our knowledge in this area, but our basic knowledge in this field goes back to antiquity and is shrouded in early mythical and religious beliefs. This was followed by the study of nutrition and physical performance under conditions related to some of man's great endeavors—war and industry. In a more recent stage of development, amateur athletics created the proper controlled environment for the study of nutrition and performance during physical activities of varying intensities and comparison of these results to those collected in military and industrial settings. These combined data bases form the foundation for our present understanding of this challenging field, thus allowing us to develop the present nutritional and fluid regimens used by coaches and participants in amateur, collegiate, and professional sports today.

If one is willing to adopt a broad perspective of nutrition and physical performance, its roots can be traced to antiquity. Man's early religious and mystical beliefs postulated that if one consumed the meat of certain animals, one acquired the strength, endurance, and courage of the animal consumed.[1] These beliefs became modified with the civilization of man, so that the ingestion of large meat meals was prescribed for those engaged in heavy muscular work or athletics, the idea being that maintenance and production of muscle mass is achieved by providing muscle as the basic building

Richard Cotter • Clintec Nutrition Company, Affiliated with Baxter Healthcare Corporation, Deerfield, Illinois 60015.

material of the diet.[1–3] This is further illustrated by the prescription of high-fat diets for those performing physical activities in a cold environment.[4,5] In this case, the fat of the diet is believed to provide superior calories for thermal regulation as well as physical performance. Another example is the ingestion of large amounts of fluids to replace sweat lost while working in a hot environment. While these prescriptions are simple and phenomenological in nature, they showed an insight into nutrition and physical performance. The understanding of nutrition and nutritional substrates developed in the twentieth century to the point of realizing that these substrates are basically carbohydrates, lipids, proteins, vitamins, and trace elements. The opportunities to study them and their relation to physical performance in large groups of people occurred as a result of the reinstitution of the Olympic Games in the late eighteen hundreds,[3] the military service of the two world wars,[5] as well as the rapidly developing industrialization of Europe and America.[6] The data collected from these studies provided needed information to improve athletic and military training while industrial studies pointed out the importance of proper nutrition to maintain work output in industrial settings.

Transfer of the above information to the athletic arena was a natural outgrowth of the rapid development of amateur and professional sports in this century. This development required that a sound fundamental knowledge of nutritional requirements and interactions be obtained to maximize athletic performance. This arena also provided the proper controlled environment for the study of nutrition in groups of young healthy children and adults. It is from studies of these subjects engaged in physical performance of varying endurance and intensity that we have obtained our more recent information on the role nutrition plays in physical activity.

The purpose of this chapter will be to summarize the collective knowledge on nutrition and fluid balance and how it relates to physical performance at all levels of athletic endeavor. The reader will be given an updated understanding of the energy, protein, vitamin, mineral, trace element, and fluid balance requirements for physical performance. Lastly, we will review and evaluate the current modulations of nutrition and fluid balance to improve physical performance in modern athletes. For readers who would like to obtain more information on these subjects, several excellent reviews are available.[7–11] For a particularly comprehensive review of this subject, the author would recommend Brotherhood (Ref. 10).

1.2. Present Practices in Athletics in Nutrition and Fluid Balance

The present practices of athletes in this area can be ascertained by reviewing dietary surveys that have been conducted on various groups of athletes. Such surveys have been conducted on athletes participating in the sports of running,[12] cross-country skiing,[13] cycling,[14] swimming,[15] soccer,[16] football,[12] basketball,[12] rowing,[17] and gymnastics,[13,18] and in the Olympics.[18]

From these surveys, the following information may be gleaned. The energy consumption of these athletes varies widely, depending on the sport, the size of the individual, and the motivation for participation. All athletes have high energy consumption; however, this consumption can vary from mildly elevated levels found in swimmers (approximately 38.5 kcal/kg/day) and basketball players (approximately 34.5 kcal/kg/day) through moderately elevated levels in runners (58.8 kcal/kg/day), gymnasts (49.4 kcal/kg/day), cross-country skiers (61.9 kcal/kg/day), soccer players (66.7 kcal/kg/day), and rowers (61.2 kcal/kg/day) to the most highly elevated levels in cyclists (85.9 kcal/kg/day) and football players, whose energy consumption can reach 116 kcal/kg/day. The energy consumption in these various sports is governed by the amount of training time per day, the nature of the sport itself, and the psychological drive of the participants.[10]

Carbohydrate intake provides approximately 30% of calories, but can vary from 20% to more than 40%.[12]

Fat intake also varies greatly among the athletes surveyed, with those in power sports showing higher consumption. The intakes are generally greater than 30% of calories, with an average of approximately 35%.[12]

Protein intake in athletes varies with the sport in which they are involved. Protein intakes of about 15% of calories are common among long-term endurance sport participants (e.g., running), while those in more power-oriented sports (e.g., weight lifting) have intakes more in the area of 20%. Protein intake in athletes is generally in excess of 1.5 g/kg/day.[12,18]

Vitamin and trace element consumption is generally above the recommended daily allowances (RDA). However, there is strong evidence indicating less than optimal intake of iron in female athletes.[19]

Maintaining proper fluid balance during physical performance is of extreme importance to athletes. Fluid losses of approximately 3% of total body water will result in impaired performance.[11] However, athletes in general do not drink adequate volumes of fluids to replace their immediate losses during intense exercise. Instead, they rehydrate over a period of hours after their exercise period, reaching proper fluid balance within approximately a 24-h period.[20]

2. NUTRITION AND FLUID REQUIREMENTS DURING PHYSICAL PERFORMANCE

2.1. Energy Requirements

2.1.1. Carbohydrate and Fat as Fuels

Energy required during exercise is generally obtained from two metabolic sources—carbohydrates and fat. Which substrate is used depends on the intensity and duration of the physical activity performed. A measure of the intensity of the activity is provided by the percentage of the athlete's maximal aerobic capacity (% VO_2 max).[21] In everyday life and activity, the % VO_2 max is less than 30%. At this level of activity, the energy supply is predominantly from fat (75%)[22] that is oxidized within the muscle to produce the high-energy substrate adenosine triphosphate (ATP), which is readily converted to mechanical energy in the muscle. As the athlete steps up the intensity of his activity, carbohydrates contribute more and more to the energy output.[23] At about

50% VO_2 max, there is roughly a 50 : 50 split between fats and carbohydrates as energy substrates. When maximal physical intensity is reached at 75% VO_2 max and greater, the major energy substrate is now carbohydrates (80%).[24] Thus, from the standpoint of sports performance, the intensity and duration of activity determines the fuel and the requirements placed on the body's substrate reserves of fats and carbohydrates. In low-intensity physical activity, fat is the key element. As the physical activity increases, carbohydrate stores become the limiting factor.

The fats and carbohydrates utilized during performance are found in the body in various storage forms. Fats are stored in adipose tissue in the form of triglycerides, which, under hormonal regulation, release on demand free fatty acids into the bloodstream, where they are transported to the muscles for use. Thus, body fat stores provide an adequate energy store in the normal nourished person.[25] Carbohydrates are found stored in limited quantities as glycogen within muscle and liver cells. The liver pool of glycoen is on the order of 90 g or 366 kcal of energy.[26] This pool is used to maintain the blood glucose levels by converting glycogen to glucose on hormonal demand and releasing it into the bloodstream for transport to body tissue for utilization. The muscle glycogen pool, on the other hand, is approximately 300 g or 1200 kcal of energy.[27] The muscle glycogen pool is available only to the muscle cell where it is stored, and is used primarily as an energy source for muscle mechanical work.[23]

During normal activities, the energy required by the muscles is supplied by blood glucose and free fatty acids. However, as the intensity of physical activity increases, the uptake of glucose and fat increases but cannot meet the energy demands of the highly active muscles.[28] The highly active muscle must then turn to its intracellular glycogen stores for its total energy supply at optimal activity output. When muscle fatigue is studied in relation to muscle glycogen levels, a strong correlation is found.[29,30] Fat, on the other hand, appears to be able only to support energy outputs in the range of 50% to 60% VO_2 max. However, when athletes undertake endurance training, they adapt to increased fat utilization and, thus, spare glycogen and increase endurance.[31]

2.1.2. Protein as a Fuel

During physical performance and for some time afterward, protein homeostasis is in dynamic flux. Protein breakdown within the muscle is balanced by subsequent protein synthesis. This occurs with the release of amino acids from the muscle protein during exercise to be used as an energy source for oxidation and gluconeogenesis. Following exercise, a recovery period ensues with the amino acids supplying the building blocks for new protein synthesis.[32] The magnitude of protein breakdown and oxidation will vary with the intensity of the activity. A middle-distance runner who in one hour of training expends 1000 kcal and is using protein to supply 10% of this demand will burn 27 g of protein. Compare this to a marathon runner who can burn about 50 g of protein during a 42.2-km run.[10] Protein degradation and oxidation may be affected by training but the evidence is conflicting.[33,34] One fact that appears certain is that carbohydrates can spare protein during physical activity. It has been shown that glucose taken orally can reduce protein breakdown,[35] and as exercise continues, the protein breakdown increases as the glycogen content of the muscle declines.[36]

2.2. Protein Requirements

Protein requirements of athletes in training have been estimated to be in the range of approximately 1 g protein/kg/day (70 g/day) for endurance athletes and as high as 1.6 g/kg/day (110 g/day) for athletes in training for muscle-building power activities.[10] Protein diets providing large quantities of protein relative to standard diets have not shown any effect on these requirements.[37]

2.3. Vitamin Requirements

There appears at this time to be no strong evidence of increased utilization, destruction, or loss of vitamins associated with physical activity.[38] Therefore, vitamin requirements for physical performance should be met with a normal diet. A word must be said here about two vitamins for which there appears to be an interaction of function with physical performance. B-complex vitamins, especially thiamin, have been shown to be important to energy consumption.[39] Vitamin C has been shown to be involved in tissue repair[39] and, as such, should be considered in physical activities that may induce repeated tissue trauma. However, numerous reviews of the available literature[40–42] indicate that there is no support for a claim that vitamin supplementation of any type improves sports performance or aids in the recovery from trauma.

2.4. Mineral and Trace Element Requirements

Dealing with the requirements for minerals and trace elements in sports performance is difficult as the normal daily requirements for many of these are still undefined. Iron has been the subject of some review.[19] These studies indicate that iron deficiency is often found in athletes in training. This deficiency is found in both male and female performers; however, females, due to menstrual losses, are at greater risk.[19] Deficiencies of potassium, sodium, chloride, and magnesium are associated with fluid balance and sweating and will be discussed in this context in the following section. Little has been reported on deficiencies of calcium, phosphorus, manganese, zinc, or copper in physical performance to indicate that a problem exists with these minerals or elements.[38,43–45]

2.5. Fluid Balance, Thermoregulation, and Nutrition

We have to this point been speaking of providing energy to the muscles during varying degrees of physical performance. This energy is provided by conversion of chemical energy to metabolic and finally to mechanical energy in the muscles. However, the conversion of energy is not very efficient, and the great majority of the energy (80%) is actually given off as heat. This heat must be lost from the body or the core temperature would become lethal within approximately 20 minutes.[46] During physical performance, heat produced in the above manner is controlled by the body thermoregulating by dissipating heat by the evaporation of sweat. Sweating is essential to increased physical performance, and any impairment of sweating will impair the output of the athlete.[47] Sweating, as we have observed, is directly related to the amount of physical performance, and this is directly related to the energy expended to perform. Rates of sweating have been measured at approximately 1.5 liter/h in endurance athletes in normal temperatures, while in hot climates, this rate may exceed 2.5 liter/h.[10,48] To dissipate 100 kcal of heat from the body, approximately 1 liter of sweat must be secreted.[49] Athletes training in temperate climates would have sweat rates not in excess of approximately 3 to 4 liters per day.[10] If training is conducted in hot climates, losses in excess of 5 liters would probably occur. Such losses can easily be handled by the body, as illustrated by rates of up to 10 liters per day reported in hot industrial environments.[50] All these data point to a basic underlying factor in physical performance. Maximal physical performance requires optimal thermoregulation, and optimal thermoregulation requires adequate fluid intake to produce adequate sweating during physical performance.

2.5.1. Fluid Balance and Electrolytes

Electrolyte loss in sweat is considerable. Unlike micronutrients, the loss of electrolytes can affect optimal physical performance. As sweat loss increases with increased activity, the loss of potassium, sodium, chloride, and magnesium also increases. This can lead to increased requirements for these electrolytes during physical activity.[40] Potassium has been observed to be rather constant even after 4 days of heavy activity with a sweat rate of approximately 3 liters per day.[51] There appeared to be a homeostatic balance maintained by a reduction in renal clearance of potassium. Sodium chloride (salt) can be found in significant amounts in sweat, but its concentration in sweat is quite variable (0.5 to approximately 3 g/liter), depending on a large number of factors such as physical activity, heat, sweating, and renal clearance.[10,52] This loss of sodium chloride can be exacerbated by the intake of large volumes of water, which dilute salt concentrations in body fluids.

Magnesium balance during exercise is unique in that during these periods, magnesium appears to temporarily migrate out of serum and into red blood cells and muscle.[48,53] Since this migration is only temporary, true magnesium deficiency does not result, although magnesium determinations during exercise will show low levels.

In conclusion, it may be said that in well-nourished and conditioned athletes, electrolyte deficiency is unlikely.

2.5.2. Fluid Balance and Micronutrients

Sweating, although essential for thermoregulation, creates a flow of essential nutrients from the body, and this must be understood and controlled if optimal performance is to be achieved. Sweat composition is known.[39,52] Sweat contains small amounts of water-soluble constituents such as calcium, vitamins, iron, and various amino acids. These losses are generally considered negligible, and in normal athletes on adequate diets, these losses will not affect performance.[10,43] However, athletes or workers engaged in extremely heavy work producing over 3 liters of sweat per day may exceed the amount of iron absorbed in the diet and develop iron deficiency.[54]

3. NUTRITION AND FLUID BALANCE FOR IMPROVED PHYSICAL PERFORMANCE

3.1. Carbohydrate Loading

Early studies[26,55,56] on the effect of diet on energy substrates in muscles showed a marked ability of the exercised muscle to restore glycogen post-exercise as compared to the nonexercised muscle. This finding was followed by the observation that if an individual was placed on a high-carbohydrate (greater than 50%) diet, the glycogen content of the exercised muscle would rise to twice that of the nonexercised muscle.[56] Further studies of diet manipulation and exercise[30] indicated that when muscle glycogen is depleted by diet manipulation and strenuous exercise, followed by a high-carbohydrate diet, the supply of glycogen in the muscle will be maximized at up to three times normal levels.[30] This was the beginning of the concept of carbohydrate loading.

Carbohydrate loading today is generally conducted by athletes in the following manner. A single period of strenuous exercise followed by a period (3 days) of low-carbohydrate intake with moderate exercise to deplete and maintain low glycogen stores is followed by a period (4 days) of high carbohydrate intake.[30] Such a procedure can extend available energy at high output (>70% VO_2 max) by as much as 2400 kcal.[10] This means of carbohydrate loading is rather severe, and more moderate regimens have been devised. In these,[57,58] the low-carbohydrate intake phase is replaced with a normal diet.

Carbohydrate loading is designed for the endurance athlete, where maximum energy reserves are required for optimal performance. It has not shown to be of benefit in short-duration high-intensity sports where the depletion of glycogen stores is not a limiting factor. This fact should be kept in mind when coaches and athletes consider making carbohydrate loading part of their preparation for competition.

3.2. Fats

Increased fat intake does provide increased energy substrate. However, as we have previously discussed, fat is a poor fuel source for the highly active muscle and, as such, adds nothing to the athlete's diet in quantities above the normal amount provided in nutritiously balanced meals.[22–24]

3.3. Proteins

Diets high in proteins (in excess of 2 g/kg/day) have shown no benefit to the training athlete. Normal protein intake of 1.5 to 2 g/kg/day is adequate as part of any good training diet.[37]

3.4. Vitamins

Vitamin requirements of the training athlete do not appear different from those of the normal individual.[38] Therefore, a normal high-calorie diet will supply adequate vitamins. There has been no evidence of enhanced physical performance with vitamin supplementation.[40–42]

3.5. Minerals and Trace Elements

Supplementation of a normal healthy diet with minerals and electrolytes is of no known advantage to athletes. All requirements are generally provided by a normal diet. Iron is perhaps the one proven exception. As we previously discussed, female and adolescent athletes may be iron deficient, and iron supplementation will be of benefit to these groups.[19,38] Electrolyte balance is maintained by the salt found in the average diet. Athletes who sweat large amounts during their activities may require more electrolyte replacement.

3.6. Fluids

Dehydration is a normal consequence of high levels of physical activity. The more sweating that occurs, the more severe is the dehydration. Supplementation with plain drinking water just prior to training is recommended to offset the dehydration.[27,57]

4. CONCLUSION

We have reviewed the place of nutritional substrates and fluids in the physiology of physical performance. We can see that by understanding basic physiology, biochemistry, and nutrition, we can design optimal diets for athletes and people in physically demanding professions. These diets will not produce superhuman performance, but will allow the physiological conditions to be the most appropriate for optimum human physical performance.

REFERENCES

1. Mayer J, Bullen B: Nutrition and athletic performance. *Physiol Rev* 40:369–397, 1960.
2. Christophe J, Mayer J: Effect of exercise on glucose uptake in rats and men. *J Appl Physiol* 13:269–272, 1958.
3. Novich MN: Research in the physiology of exercise and sports. *J Med Soc NJ* 82:295–299, 1985.
4. Stefanson V: The diets of explorers. *Military Med* 95:1–89, 1944.
5. Johnson RE, Kark RM: Environment and food intake in man. *Science* 106:378–379, 1947.
6. Kraut HA, Muller AE: Calorie intake and industrial output. *Science* 104:495–497, 1946.
7. Passmore R, Darnier VGA: Human energy expenditure. *Physiol Rev* 35:801–840, 1955.
8. Shils ME: Food and nutrition relating to work, exercise and environmental stress, in Goodhart RS, Shils ME (eds): *Modern Nutrition in Health and Disease*, ed 5. Philadelphia, Lea and Febiger, 1980, p 814.

9. Appenzeller O, Atkinson R: Nutrition for physical performance, in Appenzeller O, Atkinson R (eds): *Sports Medicine,* ed 2. Baltimore, Munch, Urban and Schwarzenberg, 1983, p 57..
10. Brotherhood JR: Nutrition and sports performance. *Sports Med* 1:350–389, 1984.
11. Roberts BW: Nutrition and athletic performance. *Nutr Int* 2:1–11, 1986.
12. Short SH, Short WR: Four-year study of university athletes' dietary intake. *J Am Dietetic Assoc* 82:632–645, 1983.
13. Feno-Luzzi A, Venerando A: Aims and results of dietary surveys on athletes, in Parizkova J, Rogozkin VA (eds): *Nutrition, Physical Fitness and Health.* Baltimore, University Park Press, 1978, p 145.
14. Kirsch KA, von Ameln H: Feeding patterns of endurance athletes. *Eur J Appl Physiol* 47:197–208, 1981.
15. Smith MP, Mendez J, Druckenmiller M, et al: Exercise intensity, dietary intake, and high-density lipoprotein cholesterol in young female competitive swimmers. *Am J Clin Nutr* 36:251–255, 1982.
16. Jacobs I, Westlin N, Karlsson J, et al: Muscle glycogen and diet in elite soccer players. *Eur J Appl Physiol* 48:297–302, 1982.
17. DeWign JF, Leusink J, Post GB, et al: Diet, body composition and physical condition of champion rowers during periods of training and out of training. *Biblthca Nutr Dieta* 27:143–148, 1979.
18. Steel JE: A nutritional study of Australian Olympic athletes. *Med J Aust* 2:119–123, 1970.
19. Clement DB, Sawchuk LL: Iron status and sports performance. *Sports Med* 1:65–74, 1984.
20. Brotherhood JR: Aspects of nutrition in endurance sports. *Aust J Sports Med* 14:8–11, 1982.
21. Andersen KL, Masironi R, Rutenfranz J, et al: Grading the intensity of physical activity, in Andersen KL, Masironi R, Rutenfranz J, Seliger V in collaboration with Degre S, Trygg K, Orgim M: *Habitual Physical Activity and Health,* WHO Regional Publications European Series No. 6. Copenhagen, World Health Organization, 1978, pp 18–26.
22. Havel RJ, Pernow B, Jones NL: Uptake and release of free fatty acids and other metabolites in the legs of exercising men. *J Appl Physiol* 23:90–99, 1967.
23. Felig P, Wahren J: Fuel homeostasis in exercise. *N Engl J Med* 293:1078–1084, 1975.
24. Randle PJ: Molecular mechanisms regulating fuel selection in muscle, in Poortmans J, Niset G (eds): *Biochemistry of Exercise IV-A.* Baltimore, University Park Press, 1981, pp 13–28.
25. West JB: Best and Taylor's Physiological Basis of Medical Practice. Baltimore, Williams and Wilkins, 1985, pp 805–817.
26. Hultman E: Liver as a glucose supplying source during rest and exercise with special reference to diet, in Parizkova J, Rogozkin VA (eds): *Nutrition, Physical Fitness and Health.* Baltimore, University Park Press, 1978, pp 9–30.
27. Saltin B: Fluid, electrolyte, and energy losses and their replenishment in prolonged exercise, in Parizkova J, Rogozkin VA (eds): *Nutrition, Physical Fitness and Health.* Baltimore, University Park Press, 1978, pp 76–97.
28. Gollnick PD: Free fatty acid turnover and the availability of substrates as a limiting factor in prolonged exercise. *Ann NY Acad Sci* 301:64–71, 1977.
29. Bergstrom J, Hermansen L, Hultman E, et al: Diet, muscle glycogen and physical performance. *Acta Physiol Scand* 71:140–150, 1967.
30. Saltin B, Hermansen L: Glycogen stores and prolonged severe exercise, in Blix G (ed): *Nutrition and Physical Activity.* Symp Swed Nutr Found V. Uppsala, Almquist and Wiksell, 1967, pp 32–46.
31. Costill DL, Sherman WM, Essig DA: Metabolic responses and adaptations to endurance running, in Poortmans J, Niset G (eds): *Biochemistry of Exercise IV-A.* International Series of Sport Science, vol IIA. Baltimore, University Park Press, 1981, pp 33–45.
32. Goodman MN, Ruderman NB: Influence of muscle use on amino acid metabolism. *Exerc Sports Sci Rev* 10:1–26, 1982.
33. Gontzea I, Sutzescu R, Dumitrache S: The influence of adaptation to physical effort on nitrogen balance in man. *Nutr Rep Int* 11:231–236, 1975.
34. Dohm GL, Hecker AL, Brown WE, et al: Adaptation of protein metabolism to endurance training. *Biochem J* 164:705–708, 1977.
35. Millward DJ, Davies CTM, Halliday D, et al: Effect of exercise on protein metabolism in humans as explored with stable isotopes. *Fed Proc* 41:2686–2691, 1982.

36. Haralambie G, Berg A: Serum urea and amino nitrogen changes with exercise duration. *Eur J Appl Physiol* 36:39–48, 1976.
37. Rasch PJ, Hamby JW, Burns HJ: Protein dietary supplementation and physical performance. *Med Sci Sports* 1:195–199, 1969.
38. Williams HM: Vitamins and mineral supplements to athletes: do they help? *Clin Sports Med* 3:623–637, 1984.
39. Shephard RJ: *Physiology and Biochemistry of Exercise*. New York, Praeger, 1982.
40. Consolazio CF: Nutrition and performance. *Prog Food Nutr Sci* 7(1–2):1–188, 1983.
41. Dwyer T, Brotherhood JR: Long-term dietary considerations in physical training. *Proc Nutr Soc Aust* 6:31–40, 1981.
42. Zanecoskey A: Nutrition for athletes. *Clin Podiatric Med Surg* 3:623–630, 1986.
43. Haralambie G: Changes in electrolytes and trace elements during long-lasting exercise, in Howald H, Poortmans J (eds): *Metabolic Adaptation to Prolonged Physical Exercise*. Basel, Birkhauser Verlag, 1975, pp 340–351.
44. Hecker AL: Nutritional conditioning for athletic competition. *Clin Sports Med* 3:567–582, 1984.
45. Wilmore JH, Freund BJ: Nutritional enhancement of athletic performance. *Curr Concepts Nutr* 15:67–97, 1986.
46. Brotherhood JR: The nutritional stresses consequent to thermoregulation in athletes. *Proc Nutr Soc Aust* 6:123–125, 1981.
47. Greenleaf JE, Castle BL: Exercise temperature regulation in man during hypohydration and hyperhydration. *J Appl Physiol* 30:847–853, 1971.
48. Costill DL: Muscle water and electrolytes during acute and repeated bouts of dehydration, in Parizkova J, Rogozkin VA (eds): *Nutrition, Physical Fitness and Health*. Baltimore, University Park Press, 1978, pp 98–116.
49. Leithead CS, Lind AR: *Heat Stress and Heat Disorders*. London, Cassell, 1964.
50. National Institute for Occupational Safety and Health: Occupational Exposure to Hot Environments—Criteria for a Recommended Standard, Figure 8. National Institute for Occupational Safety and Health, US Department of Health, Education and Welfare, Washington, DC 1972.
51. Costill DL: Sweating: its composition and effects on body fluids. *Ann NY Acad Sci* 301:160–174, 183–188, 1977.
52. Robinson S, Robinson AH: Chemical composition of sweat. *Physiol Rev* 34:202–220, 1954.
53. Stromme SB, Stensvold IC, Meen HD, et al: Magnesium metabolism during prolonged heavy exercise, in Howald H, Poortmans J (eds): *Metabolic Adaptation to Prolonged Physical Exercise*. Basel, Berkhauser Verlag, 1975, pp 361–366.
54. Paulev P-E, Jordal R, Pedersen NS: Dermal excretion of iron in intensely training athletes. *Clin Chim Acta* 127:19–27, 1983.
55. Bergstrom J: Muscle electrolytes in man. *Scand J Clin Lab Invest* 14(Suppl 68):110, 1962.
56. Bergstrom J, Hultman E: Muscle glycogen synthesis after exercise: an enhancing factor localized to the muscle cells in man. *Nature* 210:309–310, 1966.
57. Costill DL, Miller JM: Nutrition for endurance sport: carbohydrate and fluid balance. *Int J Sports Med* 1:2–14, 1980.
58. American Dietetic Association: Nutrition and physical fitness. J Am Dietetic Assoc 76:437–443, 1980.

4

Analgesics and Sports Medicine

Charles R. Craig

1. INTRODUCTION AND A DISCUSSION OF PAIN

Because pain is the most common reason for seeing a physician and because it is often associated with athletic endeavors (the adage "no pain, no gain" is still accepted as dogma by many), a consideration of the properties of analgesic drugs is essential in a publication such as this.

The term "analgesic" or "analgetic" is applied to a variety of chemical entities that have as their only necessary common feature that of being able to alleviate pain. It appears, therefore, that a brief discussion of pain itself is warranted. Pain is a very complex modality, and the processes whereby a painful stimulus is perceived as "pain" in the brain are also complex. Even today, many details of how the brain reacts to pain are poorly understood. It is clear that there are at least two types of pain—acute pain (or sharp pain, fast pain) and slow pain (chronic pain, aching pain) and that different nerve fibers carry the impulses for each type. Acute pain is carried by finely myelinated A delta (Aδ) fibers while slow pain is carried by smaller, unmyelinated type C fibers. The Aδ fibers transmit information much more rapidly than do the C fibers (4 to 30 m/s for Aδ and 2.5 m/s for C fibers). There are other differences as well; for example, pain associated with Aδ fibers is much more localized while pain associated with C fibers is more diffuse and often poorly localized. Additionally, there are differences in the way these two types of fibers carry impulses through the spinal cord to the brain. For the purposes of this discussion, some generalizations will be made. The reader interested in this topic is referred to Williams and Wilson[1] and Willis.[2]

The painful stimulus is detected in specialized tissue known as pain receptors or nociceptors. These receptors respond to a painful stimulus by nervous discharge. Receptors for pain occur in skin (cutaneous nociceptors), muscles, joints, visceral structures (including the heart), and respiratory passages. Nociceptors in certain parts of the body, including the gastrointestinal tract and the brain itself, are poorly defined

Charles R. Craig • Department of Pharmacology and Toxicology, West Virginia University Health Sciences Center, Morgantown, West Virginia 26506.

and may even be absent. The pain fibers (whether Aδ or C) enter the spinal cord through the dorsal root and ascend or descend within one to three segments in an area of the spinal cord known as the *tract of Lissauer*. They then terminate on neurons in the dorsal horn of the gray matter of the cord. Most of the fibers for fast and slow pain cross to the opposite side of the cord and ascend upward to the brain in the lateral division of the anterolateral sensory pathway (in the white matter of the cord). Most pain fibers (75% to 90%) terminate in the reticular formation of the medulla, pons, and mesencephalon. From these areas, other neurons carry the impulses to the thalamus, hypothalamus, and other areas of the brain. A smaller portion of pain fibers do not synapse in the reticular formation, but pass by and synapse directly in the thalamus.

At the level of the thalamus, signals are transmitted to higher brain areas, including the cerebral cortex. A diagrammatic representation of the passage of painful impulses from a nociceptor to the brain is shown in Fig. 1. Several areas of the thalamus are known to be served by pain pathways, but the area best studied in this regard is known as the ventral posterolateral nucleus (VPL nucleus) of the thalamus.

It has been amply demonstrated that every individual can experience pain and, in general, the degree of pain experienced is proportional to the degree of injury. However, it is also clearly established that different individuals may react differently to the same degree of pain. Personality characteristics play an important part in the behavior of individuals in pain and, perhaps, in the intensity of pain experienced. Individuals with anxiety-prone personalities may show the greatest response to painful stimuli.[3]

Another factor in the use of drugs to relieve pain is the placebo effect. The placebo effect is an actual relief of pain that the patient experiences when an inert substance, e.g., lactose, is administered instead of the analgesic drug which the patient believes he/she has received. It has been long known that the administration of a placebo is effective in relieving pain in many individuals; the reasons are just now being understood. In the 1970s, sites in the brain were discovered that avidly bound morphine and other potent analgesics. These sites are known as morphine receptors or opioid receptors. A few years later, a group of peptides were discovered in the brain of humans and other species that also bound to these sites and that produced analgesia. These peptides are called endogenous opioids. Since the original discovery, a variety of analgetic peptides have been shown to occur endogenously: methionine-enkephalin, leucine-enkephalin, beta-endorphin, dynorphin, and others; all are potent analgesics. It is now generally accepted that these substances are normally released from cells into the bloodstream and exert analgesic effects upon binding to opioid receptors. It is possible, therefore, that the "placebo effect" is due in large measure to the release of endogenous opioids as a response to what the individual believes is actually an analgesic. Furthermore, there is evidence that larger than normal amounts of these peptides are released during injury and stress. Appenzeller and coworkers[4] were the first to demonstrate a relationship between exercise and endorphin activity. They measured serum beta-endorphin levels in well-conditioned runners and found a significant rise in levels following a 27.5-mile run. This response has also been shown after other types of exercise such as treadmill running.[5]

It is likely that much of the euphoria experienced by athletes, an example of which

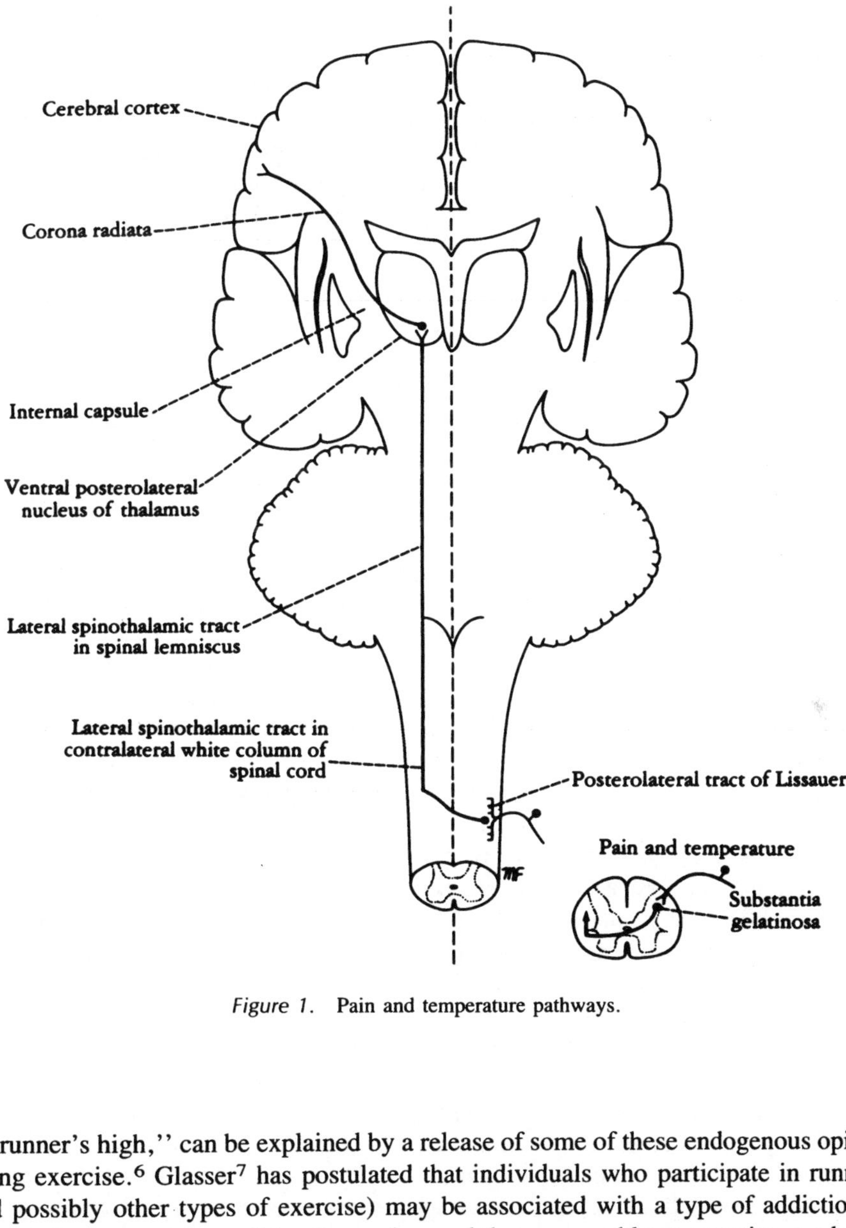

Figure 1. Pain and temperature pathways.

is "runner's high," can be explained by a release of some of these endogenous opiates during exercise.[6] Glasser[7] has postulated that individuals who participate in running (and possibly other types of exercise) may be associated with a type of addiction to these endogenous opiates. It has been observed that many athletes experience a broad range of symptoms if they stop exercising. These can include anxiety, restlessness, irritability, nervousness, guilt, muscle twitching, and sleep disturbances and may constitute a type of "abstinence syndrome."

The ramifications of the role of endogenous analgesic substances are just now being investigated.

2. ANALGESIC DRUGS

Analgesics are broadly categorized as narcotic analgesics (narcotics) and non-narcotic analgesics. Within each of these two classes, further subdivisions are made, based upon chemical and pharmacological characteristics of the various agents. Furthermore, certain analgesics may be used for properties other than the relief of pain: salicylates (aspirin) may be used to relieve pain, to reduce inflammation, and to relieve fever.

2.1. Narcotic Analgesics

When one considers analgesic drugs, the first drugs to come to mind are usually the narcotics, with usually morphine as the specific agent. This is with good reason. The exudate of the opium poppy has been utilized for its analgesic properties since even before the age of recorded history. Opium, or the dried powder of the poppy exudate, contains a number of alkaloids, of which morphine and codeine are the only ones clinically useful as analgesics. Papaverine, another alkaloid found in opium, has limited usefulness as a smooth muscle relaxant.

Morphine and codeine can now be produced synthetically, but due to the cost of this synthesis, their primary source is still extraction from the poppy exudate.

It has long been appreciated that morphine has, in addition to its extremely beneficial analgesic properties, certain distinctly undesirable characteristics. The most important of these are a propensity to cause severe respiratory depression and a serious abuse potential. For many years, organic chemists have been making changes in the structure of morphine in an attempt to produce a compound that maintains analgesic effects without the undesirable side effects of morphine. By making certain modifications to the morphine structure, chemists have discovered agents that are more potent than morphine, but they have yet to be able to clearly separate analgesic activity from all of the undesirable properties. Currently, there are several agents on the market that resemble morphine very closely in analgesic properties, in toxicity, and in abuse potential, and which differ from morphine only in potency and duration of action. In the early investigations, however, certain structural alterations of the morphine molecule led to compounds with pharmacological features not like those of morphine. One important group of compounds was found that was able to antagonize virtually all of the pharmacological features of morphine (and related narcotic analgesics). These narcotic antagonists have proven to be extremely beneficial in the treatment of opiate poisoning, and, in addition, some of these morphine antagonists are useful as analgesics themselves. These agents, known as agonist–antagonists, are discussed later in this chapter.

During World War II, both the Allies and the Axis powers were fearful of being cut off from their sources of opium (primarily Turkey and Asia Minor), and both spent a great deal of effort and money synthesizing potent analgesics that could be easily produced without requiring opium as a starting material. From these efforts, several useful compounds, including meperidine and methadone, resulted.

The search for better and more potent analgesics continues. Currently, the greatest effort is being directed towards compounds chemically related to the endogenous opioid peptides; several peptides are being studied experimentally.

2.1.1. Morphine

Although scores of synthetic and semisynthetic molecules have been tested for their analgetic properties, morphine still remains a widely used drug and, for the relief of severe pain, is not excelled by any other drug. In this chapter, morphine will be considered as the prototype narcotic analgesic and its properties will be discussed in considerable detail. For other agents with morphine-like actions, only differences between that drug and morphine will be considered.

2.1.1a. Pharmacological Properties. Morphine produces a variety of effects; tolerance develops rapidly to most of them. Over time, larger and larger doses of morphine must be given to obtain the same relief of pain. In addition to a profound analgesia, morphine produces drowsiness and may produce nausea and vomiting at therapeutic doses. A major adverse effect seen in cases of morphine overdosage is a respiratory depression that may be very severe. Because of the respiratory depressant effects, morphine and related opioids must be used very carefully in conditions where respiratory function is compromised. In conditions such as emphysema, the imposition of additional respiratory depressant action by narcotics can be fatal.

Morphine also decreases motility of the gastrointestinal tract; this effect is more apparent in the upper part of the small intestine than other locations. Morphine has been used for centuries for the relief of diarrhea, due primarily to this effect. Currently, codeine or other agents are used more commonly than morphine as antidiarrheal agents.

Another effect of morphine is constriction of the pupil. Pinpoint pupils have long been associated with toxic doses of opioids; very little tolerance develops to this effect.

Morphine and related drugs have effects on systems other than the brain and gastrointestinal tract although these are not normally of great importance. Therapeutic doses of morphine produce a peripheral vasodilatation, and when a patient in the supine position rapidly assumes the head-up position, orthostatic hypotension and fainting may occur. Morphine and morphine-like compounds may aggravate hypovolemic shock in patients with decreased blood volume.

2.1.1b. Tolerance, Physical Dependence, and Abuse Liability. The rapid development of tolerance, of habituation, and of physical dependence constitute the greatest deterrence to the use of morphine. Indeed, these are the major reasons pharmaceutical firms spend millions of dollars each year in the search for substitutes for morphine.

Heroin, rather than morphine, is the narcotic usually associated with opiate abuse. Heroin is not legally available in the United States or Canada although it is a legal drug in England. Heroin is more potent than morphine and can easily be chemically synthesized from morphine. Because of its greater potency, it is more profitable for drug dealers to synthesize heroin from morphine than to sell morphine itself. Morphine itself is widely abused, however, as are most of the narcotic analgesics in use today. Some of the newer agonist–antagonist opioids have a lower abuse potential than morphine-like agents.

2.1.1c. Absorption, Distribution, and Fate. While morphine and morphine-like compounds are readily absorbed from the gastrointestinal tract after oral administration, morphine is not normally given by this route because of significant "first-pass" metabolism by the liver following absorption. Morphine is usually administered subcutaneously but may also be given intravenously or intramuscularly. If adjustments are made for the increased rate of metabolism. however, satisfactory analgesia can be provided by oral morphine.

Morphine has a relatively short duration of action (about 2.5 to 3 h) and is excreted in the urine, primarily as the glucuronide conjugate.

2.1.1d. Therapeutic Uses. The primary use of morphine is to relieve moderate to severe pain. Morphine is more effective in relieving dull aching, chronic pain than it is in relieving sharp, acute pain. In addition to relieving the perception of pain, morphine and related drugs are able to decrease the "suffering" of pain by altering the emotional component of the painful experience.

Although morphine possesses a variety of undesirable effects, its ability to relieve moderate to severe pain is unsurpassed by any drug and it continues to be a widely employed agent.

2.1.2. Codeine

Codeine, the other analgesic found in opium, also continues to be widely used. Codeine is not nearly as potent an analgesic as is morphine, and evidence is available that it is impossible to produce the degree of analgesia with codeine that can be achieved with morphine.

Codeine, like morphine, has a pronounced cough suppressant action; this is one of its major uses. As an analgesic, codeine is usually administered as one part of a combination with aspirin or acetaminophen since the combination usually provides additive pain relief. Codeine may be employed alone; it is reasonably effective for mild to moderate pain following oral administration of tablets containing 30 to 60 mg.

2.1.3. Semisynthetic Analgesics

These agents are based on the chemical structure of morphine and have only very slight differences from morphine in pharmacological action.

2.1.3a. Heroin. Diacetylmorphine, or heroin, is 2.5 to 3 times more potent than morphine. Formerly available as a drug in the United States, it is now banned. Heroin does not appear to have any unique therapeutic advantages over any other analgesic.

2.1.3b. Hydromorphine. Hydromorphine (Dilaudid) is up to 10 times more potent than morphine as an analgesic. At an equieffective dose, its capacity to cause respiratory depression is similar to that of morphine.

2.1.3c. Levophanol. Levophanol is about 5 times more effective than morphine as an analgesic and 5 times more effective as a respiratory depressant. It is interesting that the *d*-isomer of the codeine analogue of levophanol, dextromethorphan, retains the antitussive effects of morphine-like compounds but is devoid of analgesic effects, respiratory depressant properties, and addiction liability. Dextromethorphan is widely employed as a cough suppressant.

2.1.4. Synthetic Compounds

2.1.4a. Meperidine (Demerol). Widely employed as a synthetic analgesic drug, meperidine is chemically very dissimilar to morphine, although pharmacologically there are many similarities.

While not as potent as morphine, meperidine is capable of producing relatively the same degree of analgesia, although a higher dose is required. At an equieffective analgesic dose, the degree of respiratory depression is the same as for morphine. The addiction liability for meperidine is similar to that of morphine. Meperidine is not effective for the treatment of cough or diarrhea, but there are some situations in which meperidine is superior to morphine. It is less spasmogenic and may be the analgesic of choice for treatment of biliary colic. Meperidine has a higher incidence of central nervous system (CNS) stimulation than morphine-like agents.

2.1.4b. Methadone. Originally synthesized by the Germans during World War II, methodone has some unique features. It is very effective orally and has an extended duration of action. Methadone may be used as an analgesic, but its greatest use currently is to treat heroin users. Because of its long duration of action and oral efficacy, once-a-day oral administration of methadone is able to prevent the development of abstinence signs in heroin addicts. An earlier method of treating heroin (narcotic) addition was to withdraw the patient totally from the drug. In an individual physically dependent on the drug, this resulted in the appearance of a withdrawal syndrome, or abstinence syndrome, within hours after the last dose. This sterotyped pattern of behavior consists of nausea, vomiting, goose flesh, sweating, and restless sleep which, taken together, constitute a very undesirable period that ordinarily lasts for seven to ten days. At any time, the administration of the original narcotic or any morphine-like narcotic will totally terminate the withdrawal effects. There is typically a high rate of relapse in individuals who are withdrawn from the narcotic in this manner (cold turkey).

Methadone has been used in two ways in treating narcotic addiction. One is to substitute oral methadone during the withdrawal period for the narcotic the patient has been taking. By reducing the amount of methadone a slight amount every day, the withdrawal syndrome is usually very mild. By the tenth day, the patient is drug-free and has experienced only minimal withdrawal effects. This method of "kicking" the narcotic habit is effective, but usually only in highly motivated patients.

Far more narcotic addicts choose to participate in what are known as methadone maintenance programs than in programs in which all narcotics are withdrawn. In methadone maintenance programs, the patient receives methadone once a day, orally. Used in this way, the patient remains dependent on narcotics. However, the drug is generally available at no cost, and the patient does not experience withdrawal effects. Many patients are thus able to carry out a more-or-less normal life, even though they remain dependent on narcotics.

2.1.5. Narcotic-Antagonist Analgesics

In the course of modifying the chemical structure of morphine, the compound nalorphine was synthesized and tested. It was observed that nalorphine was capable of antagonizing the analgesic and the respiratory depressant and other toxic effects of morphine, and that it would precipitate a withdrawal syndrome in an individual physically dependent on narcotics. Further observations revealed, however, that while nalorphine was an antagonist to most of the effects of morphine, it possessed its own analgesic activity. Since it produces dysphoria and an abstinence syndrome (however, different from that of morphine) following withdrawal after chronic use, nalorphine has not become a useful analgesic drug.

More recently, narcotic antagonists have been synthesized that do not have any agonist effects; that is, they do not produce analgesia and there is no abstinence syndrome associated with their withdrawal following chronic use. Two examples are naloxone (Narcan) and naltrexone (Trexan). These agents are used to treat poisoning by narcotics.

A variety of drugs are currently available that have either mixed agonist–antagonist action or act only as partial agonists at narcotic receptors in the brain. Some of these compounds are pentazocine (Talwin), nalbuphine (Nubain), and butorphanol (Stadol).

In general, these agents are effective against moderate pain but are less effective than morphine for severe pain. Most appear to have some liability for abuse, although much less than morphine or heroin.

2.1.6. Peptides

An evaluation of peptides that resemble the endogenous opioids is being carried out with the hope of ultimately finding a compound with potent analgesic effects that does not depress respiration or have a significant abuse liability.

2.2. Non-narcotic Analgesics

Although they are not nearly as effective as the narcotics for moderate or severe pain, the class of compounds known as the non-narcotic analgesics are probably the most widely used of all drugs. Many are available as over-the-counter or nonprescription drugs. The term aspirin-like is used to catagorize these drugs since they are all analgesic and at least have some antipyretic and anti-inflammatory activity. However, the discussion here will center upon the ability of these agents to relieve pain.

The mechanism of pain relief, or analgesia, of aspirin-like agents is thought to be very different from that of the narcotic analgesics. For many years, it was felt that these drugs exerted their effects only peripherally and not in the CNS. There is now evidence that there is a central as well as a peripheral component to their action. It is believed that these agents interfere with pain perception centrally by an action on the hypothalamus in the brain. They appear to alter pain reception peripherally by interfering with the input to peripheral nerve endings. The latter effect is thought to occur as follows. A group of naturally occurring substances, prostaglandins, are always released when cells are damaged. Prostaglandins cause pain when injected and may sensitize nerve endings to pain. All aspirin-like drugs inhibit the biosynthesis and release of prostaglandins in all cells tested, and this is postulated to be the mechanism of their analgesic action. Other classes of drugs do not appear to affect the biosynthesis of prostaglandins.

2.2.2. Agents

There are a large number of aspirin-like drugs; all have analgesic activity. These agents will be discussed separately by chemical class, with aspirin being discussed more completely since it is a prototype drug.

2.2.1a. Salicylates. Aspirin (acetylsalicylic acid) is the most widely used non-narcotic analgesic and it is the standard for comparison and evaluation. Aspirin is effective in relieving pain of low intensity, particularly headache, myalgia, and arthralgia.

Aspirin has several side effects that limit its usefulness, and it is the search for agents with a lower incidence of side effects that has led to the introduction of a large number of non-narcotic analgesics.

Many side effects of aspirin occur at therapeutic doses. At therapeutic doses, aspirin can cause gastrointestinal irritation, including gastric ulceration, erosive gastritis, and exacerbation of peptic ulcer. Ingestion of one or two aspirin tablets causes a definite prolongation of bleeding time. This can adversely affect patients with hypoprothrombinemia, vitamin K deficiency, or hemophilia. Aspirin administration should be discontinued at least one week prior to surgery. On the other hand, there is evidence that aspirin, because of its ability to inhibit platelet aggregation, is of benefit for the prophylaxis of coronary and cerebral arterial thrombosis.[8]

There are other more serious effects that are seen at higher doses, as in the case of accidental overdosage. The accidental ingestion of large amounts of aspirin, particularly by children, can result in very serious toxicity. Early on, salicylate poisoning is characterized by extreme thirst, sweating, blurred vision, tinnitus, nausea, and vomiting. The most serious aspects of salicylate toxicity in children involve changes in acid–base balance. This usually takes the form of a severe acidosis that in extreme cases can be fatal. The introduction of ''child-proof'' caps for aspirin bottles has dramatically decreased the incidence of serious aspirin poisoning.

Another salicyclate, sodium salicylate, is also available for oral use as an analgesic. A newer member of this class is diflunisal (Dolobid). Diflunisal is used most commonly as an analgesic in the treatment of musculoskeletal strains and sprains and in the treatment of osteoarthritis. Two salicylates, salicylic acid and methyl salicylate, are available only for topical use and are not to be taken orally. Salicyclic acid is used to remove warts and corns, while methyl salicyclate, used in ointments and liniments as a counterirritant, is employed for painful muscle or joints. The use of methyl salicylate should be discouraged, however, since absorption can occur through the skin and death has occurred as a result of poisoning.

2.2.1b. para-Aminophenol Derivatives. Several agents in this class have been used as analgesics. The only member of this group that is an official drug today is acetaminophen. Acetaminophen has only weak anti-inflammatory actions but is essentially comparable to aspirin as an analgetic and as an antipyretic agent. Acetaminophen, unlike aspirin, does not cause the prolongation of bleeding time. It also does not have the capacity to cause gastrointestinal irritation, as does aspirin.

The most serious side effect of acute overdosage with acetaminophen is a hepatic necrosis that can be fatal. Acetaminophen is available over the counter as Tylenol and Tempra as well as generic forms. It is also available by prescription in combination with codeine, oxycodone, propoxyphene, or other analgesics.

Agents in this group that are no longer used include acetanilid and phenacetin.

2.2.1c. Arylalkanoic Acids (Propionic Acid Derivatives). Three drugs in this class currently available in the United States are ibuprofen, naproxen, and fenoprofen. Several other agents in this class are marketed in other countries. Ibuprofen, the most widely used agent, has recently been approved for sale in the United States as a nonprescription drug. There are several preparations of ibuprofen including Motrin, Rufen, Nuprin, and Advil. This class of compounds appear to share all the properties of aspirin, including analgesia, antipyresis, and anti-inflammatory action; they also prolong bleeding time and may cause gastrointestinal irritation. The incidence of adverse effects of these drugs after overdosage appears to be less than that of either aspirin or acetaminophen. They appear particularly useful for relief of pain associated with dysmenorrhea.

2.2.1d. Other Agents. There are large numbers of aspirin-like agents that could be used for relief of pain but that are employed clinically for their anti-inflammatory effects. These include such agents as phenylbutazone (Butazolidin), indomethacin (Indocin), sulindac (Clinoril), mefenamic acid (Punstel), tolmetin (Tolectin), and piroxican (Feldene).

REFERENCES

1. Williams NE, Wilson H (eds.): Pain and its management. *International Encyclopedia of Pharmacology and Therapeutics,* Section 112. New York, Pergamon Press, 1983.

2. Willis WD: *The Pain System. The Neural Basis of Nociceptive Transmission in the Mammalian Nervous System. Vol. 8. Pain and Headache* (PL Gildenberg, series editor). Basel, Karger, 1985.
3. Schalling D, Levander S: Ratings of anxiety proneness and responses to electrical pain stimulation. *Scand J Psychol* 5:1–9, 1964.
4. Appenzeller O, Standefer J, Appenzeller J, et al: Neurology of endurance training. V. Endorphins. *Neurology (NY)* 30:418–419, 1980.
5. Gambert SR, Garthwaite TL, Hagen TC, et al: Exercise increases plasma beta-endorphin (EP) in untrained human subjects. *Clin Res* 29:429A, 1981.
6. Mellion MB: Exercise therapy for anxiety and depression. *Postgrad Med* 77:91–98, 1985.
7. Glasser W: *Positive Addiction*. New York, Harper & Row, 1976.
8. Marcus AJ: Aspirin as an anti-thrombotic medication. *N Engl J Med* 309:1515–1516, 1983.

5

Calcium

Michael J. Glade and Paula H. Stern

1. DIETARY CALCIUM REQUIREMENTS

Calcium plays an esssential role in the regulation of many metabolic processes. It is also necessary for the development and maintenance of the skeletal framework which supports and allows strenous physical activity. In general, the overall calcium status of the athlete will reflect the net balance between calcium losses and calcium gains.

Calcium is added to the body by its absorption from the diet in the digestive tract, while it is lost in sweating and urine formation and excretion. The rate of new bone formation during growth or injury repair (fracture healing) and the net balance of bone turnover (the differences between the rates of local bone loss and its replacement) further modulate the basal metabolic and physiological requirements for calcium.

Nutritional "requirements" for humans are usually expressed as "recommended dietary allowances" (RDA), which are typically somewhat higher than the "minimum essential requirements" (MER) to meet physiological needs. The RDA are estimated from scientific data concerning actual physiological requirements, and therefore include the MER. The RDA also include various "fudge factors" which are intended to account for variations among individuals and their actual diets, as well as to provide safety margins for scientific uncertainties. Current RDA for calcium in the U.S. are given in Table 1.

The calcium recommendations for juveniles reflect both increasing body mass and skeletal growth. Peak calcium needs occur during adolescence, after which recommended calcium intakes decrease to those recommended for prepubescent children (800 mg/day). No further changes are recommended during adulthood, for either men or women, with the exception of pregnant and lactating women. For the latter group, it is recommended that calcium intake be increased by 50% (1200 mg/day), in order to supply the estimated 30 g of calcium accumulated by the fetus during the last trimester[1,2] and the 250 mg secreted each day in breast milk.[3] Any similar adjustments mandated by physiological changes (exercise, diet, etc.) have been assumed to be covered by the "safety margins" included in the recommended intakes.

Michael J. Glade and Paula H. Stern • Department of Pharmacology, Northwestern University, Chicago, Illinois 60611.

Table 1. Current US Recommended Daily Allowances for Calcium[a]

Group	Age (years)	Calcium (mg)
Infants	0–0.5	360
	0.5–1	540
Children	1–10	800
Adolescents	11–18	1200
Adults	19+	800
Pregnant women		+400
Lactating women		+400

[a]Ref. 3.

Despite the existence of such a table, no consensus exists concerning the calcium needs of either adults or children. The recommendations of several national/international organizations vary by as much as 100% (Table 2). These recommendations have been based on the traditional nutritional concept of "balance", i.e., daily dietary calcium intake should equal the total of calcium losses in the urine and feces, plus any deposited in new bone or fetal development and any secreted in breast milk. However, nutritionists have become increasingly concerned that "balance" is not a sufficiently sensitive or even physiologically relevant indicator of dietary calcium adequacy. A number of investigators have attempted to utilize directly various skeletal characteristics in efforts to reevaluate the calcium needs of humans. While debate continues, several issues have been placed into clearer focus.

Table 2. Comparison of US, UK, and FAO/WHO Recommended Daily Allowances for Calcium

Group	Age (years)	Calcium (mg)		
		US[a]	UK[b]	FAO/WHO[c]
Infants	0–1	360–540	600	500–600
Children	1–10	800		
	1–8		700	
	1–9			400–500
Adolescents	9–15		700	
	10–15			600–700
	11–18	1200		
	16–18		600	500–600
Adults	19+	800	500	400–500
Pregnant women		1200	1200	1000–1200
Lactating women		1200	1200	1000–1200

[a]Ref. 3.
[b]Ref. 226.
[c]Ref. 227.

Adolescence may well be the most critical period in terms of calcium status. Approximately 45% of adult skeletal mass is formed during adolescence[4]; during this time, calcium requirements may actually be two to three times higher than during adulthood.[5–8] Bone mineral density has been shown to be proportional to calcium intake in a group of 13- to 16-year-old children[9] and in a group of 31 matched 14-year-old girls.[10] Children have been reported to maximize their retention of dietary calcium when ingestion averaged between 1000 and 1500 mg/day.[3]

Several studies have indicated that calcium intakes below 1200 mg/day are inadequate for either adult men or women.[11,12] In adult women ranging from 18 to 72 years of age, metacarpal thickness,[13,14] mandibular density,[15] and alveolar density[16] have been shown to be proportional to daily calcium intake. In addition, it is well known that the efficiency of calcium absorption decreases during aging,[17–22] probably from impairment of vitamin D function,[18,23,24] although decreased stomach acid production may also be involved.[25] Women over 50 years of age may require 1500 mg calcium/day.[26,27] Consequently, a National Institutes of Health Consensus Panel in 1984 suggested increases in dietary calcium recommendations for adult women, to 1000 mg/day premenopausally and to 1500 mg/day after menopause.[28]

A controversial complication in the discussion of basic adult calcium requirements involves the possibility that dietary calcium may be able to ameliorate either essential hypertension or that secondary to high sodium intakes. Several studies have gathered data suggesting that the incidence of hypertension among adult humans is inversely related to their dietary calcium intakes.[29–38] Elevated blood pressure, whether primary or secondary to high sodium intakes, has been reduced in experimental rats whose diets have been supplemented with additional calcium,[31,39,40] while reductions in calcium intakes have been observed to enhance the development of hypertension in young rats.[39] Human hypertensives have exhibited decreased blood pressures during calcium supplementation.[41,42] This effect required two to four times the current RDA.[31,39,41] However, the mechanism by which calcium confers protection against hypertension remains unknown; it apparently does not involve elevated sodium excretion or alterations in the physiological handling of sodium by the renin–angiotensin system.[31,32] It may be that inadequate calcium intakes directly affect peripheral vascular tone.[43] Alternatively, elevated parathyroid hormone (PTH) concentrations, which tend to accompany human hypertension,[44,45] may elevate blood pressure.[45]

2. RELATIONSHIP OF EXERCISE TO CALCIUM NEEDS

A plethora of cross-sectional studies of various human populations have reported increases in bone mineral density[46–54] or bone mass[55–64] to be associated with physical activity or exercise compared to sedentary behavior. However, the mixed natures of the populations that have been studied, the variation in types of exercise activity reported (i.e., general athletics,[55] cross-country running,[56] ballet,[65] and weight lifting[65]), and the methods used have limited the reliability of any conclusions drawn from these investigations.[66,67] For example, bone mass is apparently locally dependent on muscle mass[68] as well as the type of exercise performed. For example, the dominant arms of men and women professional tennis players exhibited 35% and 28% greater humoral cortical thickness, respectively, than did their nondominant arms.[60]

In experimental female rats and yearling pigs, running, swimming, and weight lifting have been shown to increase femoral and humoral cortical thickness.[69,70] Increases in serum concentrations of 1,25-dihydroxyvitamin D and intestinal calcium absorption may accompany these phenomena.[71,72] Regular exercise regimens have resulted in increased rates of bone turnover, by increasing both local formation and removal, in birds,[73,74] horses,[75,76] and adult humans.[77,78] This combination of findings suggests that exercise, by increasing local mechanical loading, stimulates the reorganization of bony architecture into structures of greater mechanical efficiency. Such an effect first requires the removal of inappropriate tissue, and hence accelerated resorption, followed by the formation of new tissue. In concert, the efficiency of intestinal absorption of calcium increases, providing more material for newly formed bone. The net result would then be increased bone mass, mechanical strength, and capacity.

A basic requirement of the exercising individual is thermoregulation, accomplished in man largely by sweating. While few measures of the calcium lost in sweat are available, some data suggest that 1 to 2 mg Ca per kg body weight are excreted per hour of sweating.[79–83] Although the loss of 70 to 140 mg of calcium in one hour may not be of physiological significance to the health-conscious exerciser, the daily loss of 140 to 420 mg by a serious athlete may carry dire consequences, particularly if calcium intake is at or below the recommended 800 mg/day. In such individuals, exercise induction of bone resorption unaccompanied by enhanced bone formation (because dietary calcium is actually physiologically deficient) could lead eventually to "spontaneous" mechanical failure of the loaded skeleton.

Physical exercise is also typically accompanied by increased water intake to replenish fluids lost as sweat. Imbibed water, once it exceeds the minimum demands for rehydration, increases renal blood flow and renal glomerular filtration. More rapid throughput of plasma decreases the efficiency of renal mineral reabsorption, encouraging accelerated sequestration of minerals (including calcium) into the urinary bladder. Salt pills may be taken to restore electrolytes believed lost in sweat. Sodium intakes over 2000 mg/day (one tablespoon of salt) may stimulate PTH secretion and increase the acute loss of calcium from bone.[84] In concert, these mechanisms may account, at least in part, for the increased urinary excretion of calcium reported to accompany acute exercise.[71]

3. CHANGES IN CALCIUM REQUIREMENTS SECONDARY TO OTHER DIETARY COMPONENTS

Athletic individuals tend to consume diets that share several common characteristics. These include relatively large intakes of protein and carbohydrates. Such diets are intended to improve athletic potential and enhance fitness and performance, but they can also impact on skeletal health and calcium requirements.

Perhaps the most controversial aspect of athletic diets during the past decade has been that of high protein intakes, largely through the ingestion of meat and liquefied protein supplements. High levels of protein intake were found to be associated with increased urinary excretion of calcium, regardless of amount (or lack of) physical activity.[85,86] The calcium losses often resulted in decreased or even negative calcium balances.[85–88] It has been estimated that for every gram of protein intake above the RDA of 56 g/day, 1 mg of additional calcium is lost through the urine.[89] Because of the relative inefficiency of calcium absorption as intake increases,[90] a typical 10-fold increase in protein intake by an athlete[91] could increase dietary calcium requirements by as much as 1000 to 2000 mg/day. Unfortunately, calcium losses accompanying high protein intakes have been found to be only partially reversible when concurrent calcium ingestion has been increased.[88,92,93]

Increased calcium excretion secondary to high protein intakes has been attributed to decreased efficiency of renal recycling of calcium via tubular reabsorption.[94] It has been suggested that the calciuric effect of dietary protein is triggered by the sulfur-containing amino acids such as methonine.[94–96] Sulfurous amino acids result in the acidification of renal tubular fluid as the amino acids are oxidized and sulfuric acid is formed.[97,98] Decreased pH of renal filtrate may interfere with renal reabsorptive functions, increasing urinary losses of minerals.[94,98,99] Experimental studies in horses suggest that the ingestion of methonine in excess of threshold amounts is followed by renal filtration of sulfur in excess of local buffering capacity, resulting in a transient impairment of calcium reabsorbing ability.[94]

Obviously, it is not desirable for athletes to induce nutritionally the net loss of calcium from their mechanical support structures. Unfortunately, additional calcium intake may be of dubious protective value, any increment in absorbed calcium also being lost through continued inefficiency in renal retention.[92,93] However, it has been suggested that concurrent dietary reinforcement of renal buffering capacity might be of some benefit,[94] in much the same way as nutritional supplementation with bicarbonates has been successfully used to raise urinary pH in children suffering from renal tubular acidosis.[100]

When meat is a primary source of dietary protein, there is also the danger of unbalanced phosphorus intake as a result of the low Ca : P ratio in meat. It has been suggested that the optimal dietary Ca : P ratio for adults is 1 : 1[101]; below that, intestinal absorption of calcium decreases.[101–103] However, apparently there is no decrease in net body calcium balance,[5,89,103,104] probably because decreasing absorption of calcium coupled with large amounts of ingested and absorbed phosphorus tends to depress serum calcium concentrations, stimulating secretion of PTH by the parathyroid glands. A secondary effect of PTH is to reduce calcium excretion by the kidney, thereby helping to preserve calcium balance.[105] This protective effect of PTH may prevent acute calcium losses, but the primary action of PTH to mobilize calcium from bone by inducing the local dissolution of bone tissue may well be detrimental to the skeletal integrity of the chronic ingester of large amounts of meat.

Increased ingestion of carbohydrates may be able to partially offset the deleterious effects of high-protein diets. Increasing glucose[106–108] or lactose[109,110] intakes can increase the efficiency of intestinal absorption of calcium by humans. Whether these effects can quantitatively overcome the negative effects of high phosphorus intakes has not yet been demonstrated. However, care must be taken in the choice of carbohydrate sources; some, such as corn and bran, themselves contain 10 to 100 times as much phosphorus as calcium.[111] Others, such as broad leafy vegetables (most notably, spinach), contain large amounts of oxalic acid; in the digestive tract, oxalates complex with ionic calcium, preventing its absorption.[112,113] The oxalates in tea may also bind calcium.[114] Dietary fiber from unrefined cereals, whole wheat, and some vegetables and fruits also decreases the efficiency of the intestinal absorption of calcium,[115–120] by directly binding calcium to the uronic acids in hemicellulose macromolecules.[115,121] However, uronic acids are fermented in the human colon, perhaps releasing bound calcium.[121] Nonetheless, according to one estimate, every ounce of dietary fiber increases an adult's calcium requirement by 16 mg.[122] Few other components of the athlete's diet will affect calcium nutrition.[123] It does appear that ascorbic acid, commonly taken as part of large-scale vitamin supplementation by athletes, may improve the efficiency of calcium absorption.[124,125] It has been reported that medium-chain triglycerides fed to neonates may have similar effects on calcium absorption,[125] but whether this occurs in adults is unknown.

4. CHANGES IN CALCIUM REQUIREMENTS SECONDARY TO DRUGS USED BY ATHLETES

Medications have become a routine part of athletic conditioning and performance. Some, such as antibiotics, have genuine medicinal value. Others are used to relieve pain (analgesics) and for short-term acceleration of recovery after injury (anti-inflammatory agents). Still others are used for their putative abilities to stimulate muscle development (anabolic steroids, growth hormones). None of these drugs are without systemic side effects, and most affect calcium status.

At one time, glucocorticoids were the anti-inflammatory agents of choice in the treatment of athletic injuries. Their use has diminished considerably since the elucidation of their locally destructive effects on bone and cartilage[126–128] and their inhibitory effects on calcium absorption.[129–132] Nonetheless, their use is still frequently prescribed for the treatment of connective tissue diseases affecting ligaments and tendons.[133] Several reports suggest that doubling or tripling calcium intake during glucocorticoid treatment can maintain bone structure,[133,134] although cartilage damage will not be prevented.[135]

Glucocorticoids have largely been replaced by a family of more benign nonsteroidal anti-inflammatory drugs (NSAIDs).[136–138] (See Chapter 8.) This class of compounds includes the commonly used aspirins, aspirin substitutes, and phenylbutazone and its derivatives. Although commonly believed to be free from harmful side effects, these agents have been implicated in cases of gastroenteric bleeding, nephrotic syndrome. acute interstitial nephritis, acute tubular necrosis, papillary necrosis, renal failure, acute glomerulitis, and vasculitis.[139–142] In addition, NSAIDs as well as glucocorticoids may encourage the persistence of underlying connective tissue disease.[143] Furthermore, these agents in very low doses have recently been associated with paradoxical increases in prostaglandin PGE_2 secretion by bone itself[144]; PGE_2 can stimulate local resorption (destruction) of bone tissue. While NSAIDs inhibit PGE_2 secretion at therapeutic dosages, they may transiently disrupt healthy supportive skeletal architecture when their serum concentrations decrease overnight or during withdrawal of therapy.

Intestinal absorption of calcium is also inhibited by a number of antibiotics and other pharmacological agents.[145,146] Among these are neomycin, which binds to calcium and prevents its absorption.[147] Laxatives and aluminum-containing antacids decrease calcium absorption by both complex formation and accelerated passage through the gut.[148] Aluminum-containing antacids trigger secondary urinary calcium loss by complexing with phosphorus in the gut, decreasing phosphorus absorption.[148,149] Diuretics directly stimulate urinary calcium excretion, decreasing calcium balance.[146,150] The anticonvulsants phenobarbital, phenytoin, primidone, and ritalin interfere with vitamin D metabolism and action, thereby inhibiting calcium absorption.[151,152] The cardiac glycosides, strophanthin and digoxin, stimulate urinary excretion of calcium.[153] Interestingly, thiazides inhibit urinary calcium excretion,[154] potentially protecting against bone loss from other causes.

Emphasis on muscle development among athletes of both sexes has resulted, perhaps predictably, in widespread use of anabolic steroids. In addition to building muscle mass, size, and strength under certain conditions,[155–157] these compounds may also stimulate local bone formation at loci of mechanical stress, as well as increasing total skeletal mass.[158–160] In one study, stanozolol at 6 mg/day for 30 months resulted in a 4% increase in total body calcium (and presumably total bone mass).[160] Caution should be exercised when interpreting these results as being indicative of a "positive" effect of anabolic steroids on bone; the incorporation of increased amounts of calcium into certain portions of certain bones, dictated by loading stresses, may require excessive resorption at other skeletal locations in order to maintain the serum calcium concentrations necessary for proper neuronal and muscular electrical activity.

The use of growth hormone to stimulate muscle mass development, previously impractical because of limited availability, may become more common with the commercial production of synthetic human growth hormone. (See Chapter 13.) However, in a clinical trial of such a product, 50 or 100 μg per kg body weight administered intramuscularly stimulated both increase in muscle mass and generalized resorption of bone in otherwise healthy and well-fed adult men, while lower doses had neither effect.[161] In light of the increases in growth hormone secretion[162–170] and bone mass (see above) which accompany intensive exercise, it may be suggested that dosages of exogenous growth hormone sufficient to promote muscular hypertrophy exert secondary destructive effects on bone. By the same token, large amounts of supplemental arginine, taken for its potent ability to stimulate endogenous growth hormone secretion, may also impair skeletal function.

Stimulants are occasionally used by some athletes. The most common and pervasive of these is caffeine. (See Chapter 14.) Preliminary reports have indicated that adult women ingesting over 6 mg of caffeine per kg of lean body mass (LBM) per day (about 4 cups of coffee per day[111]) exhibited decreased renal tubular calcium reabsorption and, consequently, increased urinary calcium losses and bone resorption.[171,172] Lower caffeine intakes were without effect on calcium balance, unless calcium intake fell below 600 mg/day. Apparently, caffeine impairs the retention of calcium, but if the dietary supply of calcium is not limiting, enhanced intestinal absorption can counterbalance this effect.

5. CHANGES IN CALCIUM REQUIREMENTS SECONDARY TO MAJOR PHYSIOLOGICAL CHANGES

The effects on calcium needs of growth, aging, pregnancy, and lactation have been described above. Two additional conditions of special interest to female athletes merit further discussion.

A clinical condition that appears to have become both common and fashionable among serious female athletes has become known as "exercise-induced amenorrhea." (See Chapter 12.) Menstrual irregularity and amenorrhea occur in 20% of female athletes, compared to 5% of the general female population.[173] Furthermore, chronic strenuous exercise by prepubescent girls is frequently associated with delayed menarche.[174–177] Through vaguely understood mechanisms, chronic hard exercise,[48–50,178–181] intentional weight restriction,[173,182,183] and the emotional stress of competition itself,[181,184] either individually or in concert, induce a reduction in pituitary follicle-stimulating hormone (FSH) secretion,[185] eventually preventing follicle development and therefore ovarian estrogen secretion. Failure of follicular maturation also results in decreased progesterone production.[186] Altered endocrine status results in "premenopausal osteopenia," characterized by a steadily decreasing total bone mass.[187–189] The loss of skeletal support persists even if calcium intake meets or even exceeds 800 mg/day.[182] Furthermore, the bone-enhancing effects of exercise *per se* are inadequate to compensate for the effects of estrogenic endocrine imbalance.[48,187] Most discouragingly, successful therapeutic restoration of menses (usually simply via the reduction of exercise intensity) only partially reverses the previous skeletal loss.[48,56,190]

A related syndrome, postmenopausal osteoporosis, afflicts a large segment of the general female population.[191] The hallmark of this syndrome is an acceleration of the normal adulthood reduction in skeletal mass, commencing with the onset of menopause. This accelerated reduction in bone mass affects 15 to 20 million people in the United States[28] and increases their risk of disabling and potentially fatal fractures.[192] It has been estimated that about 35% of all American women over 50 years of age will suffer hip, wrist, or vertebral fractures,[193] perhaps accounting for 1.2 to 1.3 million fractures annually.[28,194]

Unfortunately, the physiological causes of this progressive skeletal dissolution remain unknown,[194,195] although a number of risk factors have been identified, including alcoholism, cigarrette smoking, use of corticosteroids, bilateral oophorectomy, rheumatoid arthritis, and especially the lack of physical activity during adulthood[196–198]. Strenuous physical activity, such as athletics, may result in a paradoxical increased fracture incidence among the mature and elderly.[199] This possibility arises when severe mechanical loading stresses are inflicted upon increasingly porotic bone.[199] The potential for dietary calcium supplementation to decrease the fracture risks attendant upon exercise by older adults has become an attractive possibility and has received considerable attention among those attempting to ensure healthy and active longevity.

Such studies have yielded mixed results.[195,200] Several have led to the conclusion that calcium supplements may retard the progression of bone loss in postmenopausal women. Apparently effective daily dosages have included 1200 mg/day,[201–203] 1500 mg/day,[204,205] 2000 mg/day,[206] and 2500 mg/day.[207] In some cases, additional supplementation with 40 to 80 mg/day of sodium fluoride has been required for maximal beneficial effect.[208] One retrospective dietary survey has also demonstrated that the rate of "age-related bone loss" was inversely proportional to postmenopausal dietary calcium intake.[13] It has been proposed that the mechanism of this putative effect of calcium supplementation is the reduction of bone resorption, preserving skeletal mass.[204,209]

There have also been reports that increasing calcium intake in adolescence[210] or during the perimenopausal period[204,206,208,210,211] may decrease the postmenopausal loss of bone and risk of fracture. This might occur by maximization of the bone mass of mid-adulthood, when skeletal mass peaks around age 35.[212] Larger skeletal reserves of both mineral and total mass would then be available for the mechanisms of osteoporosis to draw upon, possibly postponing the time at which the skeleton would be reduced to a threshold of high fracture risk.

Contradictory reports describing a relative ineffectiveness of dietary calcium supplementation in the prevention of osteoporotic bone loss are also numerous.[47,202,203,211,213–216] Attempts to reconcile these contradictions have focused on methodological and study population differences.[194,195] Nonetheless, no definitive conclusions can be drawn at this time. This unsatisfactory situation illustrates the difficulties of studying complex physiological disease processes which occur over several decades and emphasizes the dangers inherent in attempting to recommend training and nutritional regimes on the basis of little clear knowledge and understanding.

6. DIETARY SOURCES OF CALCIUM

A variety of foods contain substantial amounts of calcium (Table 3). In addition to the traditionally recognized dairy products, fish and some vegetables can also boost calcium intake. However, the bioavailability of calcium from the latter sources may be limited by oxalates or phytates (see above).

7. CALCIUM SUPPLEMENTS

A large number of calcium supplements have become available to the consumer. These vary in their actual calcium content, and this must be taken into account when calculating dosage or ingestion rate. Among generally available supplements, the one containing the greatest proportion of calcium by weight is calcium carbonate, which

Table 3. Calcium Content of Some Foods[a]

Food	Serving size	Calcium provided (mg)
Alligator meat	3 ½ oz	1231
Skim milk	1 qt	1212
Whole milk	1 qt	1152
Ice cream	1 qt	666
Reindeer milk	1 cup	508
Dried almonds	1 cup	380
Chocolate milk shake	8 oz	363
Sardines in oil	8 medium	354
Low fat yogurt	1 cup	345
Goat milk	1 cup	315
Chick peas	1 cup	300
Buttermilk	8 oz	298
Wheat flour	1 cup	298
Lobster thermidor	1	290
Dandelion greens	1 cup	280
Roasted cashews	1 cup	267
Cooked turnip greens	½ cup	246
Eggnog	6 oz	242
Cheddar cheese	1 oz	211
Creamed cottage cheese	1 cup	211
Dried figs	1 cup	189
New England clam chowder	1 cup	180
Spinach	1 cup	166
Scalloped oysters	6	158
Oatmeal	¾ cup	153
Fried oysters	4 oz	152
Raw shrimp	8 medium	126
Cooked spinach	½ cup	113
Artichoke	1 bud	100
Chocolate fudge	3 ½ oz	100

[a]Ref. 111.

contains 40% calcium. Other relatively potent sources are calcium chloride (36% calcium) and dibasic calcium phosphate (31% calcium). Popular but less potent forms include organically chelated calcium (usually about 20% calcium), calcium lactate (13% calcium), and calcium gluconate (9% calcium). Consequently, in order to increase calcium intake by 500 mg/day, 1250 mg of calcium carbonate must be ingested, compared to 2500 mg of chelated calcium. While potentially trivial, this difference can significantly affect the number of pills that must be taken daily and hence the willingness of an individual to continue supplementation.

The bioavailability and physiological effects of these calcium sources may not be uniform. For example, the percentage of the calcium that is absorbed may differ among calcium chloride, calcium carbonate, and chelated calcium citrate.[217,218] Some forms of calcium may stimulate greater urinary excretion of calcium than do others.[219] Therefore, the net benefits to be obtained may vary considerably.

8. TOXICITY OF EXCESS CALCIUM INTAKE

Prolonged calcium intakes of over 2000 mg/day may be associated with urolithiasis (the formation of kidney stones).[220] Males appear more susceptible to this hazard.[220] However, hypercalciuria usually requires calcium intakes of over 3000 mg/day,[221,222] decreasing the potential for urinary calculi formation.[220]

Calcium is a potent stimulator of gastrin secretion, which triggers release of hydrochloric acid into the stomach. Chronic excessive gastric acid secretion could feasibly cause gastric ulceration.[223,224]

In the past, a condition known as "milk–alkali syndrome" was recognized among peptic ulcer patients.[225] Hypercalcemia and nephrocalcinosis commonly resulted when these patients combined calcium intakes of over 2000 to 5000 mg/day (usually from milk) with large amounts of absorbable alkali (usually from sodium bicarbonate). This syndrome could experience a resurgence if large numbers of people begin ingesting 2000 mg or more of calcium as calcium carbonate daily. Experimental intakes of 8000 or 12,000 mg of calcium carbonate have triggered hypercalcemia in humans.[25] However, no side effects were observed when calcium ingestion was limited to 1600 mg (4000 mg calcium carbonate). As with all nutritional supplements, there is a beneficial range for calcium supplementation, beyond which clinical complications and compromised health are invited.

REFERENCES

1. Pitkin RM: Calcium metabolism in pregnancy: a review. *Am J Obstet Gynecol* 121:724–737, 1975.
2. Duggin GG, Lyneham RC, Dale NE, et al: Calcium balance in pregnancy. *Lancet* 2:926–927, 1974.
3. National Research Council: *Recommended Dietary Allowances*, ed 9. Washington, DC, National Academy of Sciences, 1980.
4. Dunger DB, Preece MA: Growth and nutrient requirements of adolescence, in: *Pediatric Nutrition: Theory and Practice*. Boston, Butterworth, 1987, pp 357–371.
5. Heaney RP, Gallagher JC, Johnston CC: Calcium nutrition and bone health in the elderly. *Am J Clin Nutr* 36:986–1013, 1982.
6. Trotter M, Hixon BB: Sequential changes in weight, density and percentage ash weight of human skeletons from an early fetal period through old age. *Anat Rec* 179:1–18, 1974.
7. Mazess RB: On aging bone loss. *Clin Orthop Relat Res* 165:239–252, 1982.
8. Leitch I, Aitken FC: The estimation of calcium requirements: a reexamination. *Nutr Abstr Rev* 29:393, 1959.
9. Eyberg CJ, Pettifor JM, Moodley G: Dietary calcium intake in rural black South African children. *Hum Nutr Clin Nutr* 40:69–74, 1986.
10. Matkovic V, Fontana D, Tominac C, et al: Influence of calcium on peak bone mass: a pilot study. *J Bone Min Res* 1:(Abstr 168), 1986.
11. Heaney RP, Recker RR, Saville PD: Calcium balance and calcium requirements in middle-aged women. *Am J Clin Nutr* 30:1603–1611, 1977.
12. Spencer H, Kramer L, Lesniak M, et al: Calcium requirements in humans. *Clin Orthop Rel Res* 184:270–280, 1984.
13. Matkovic V, Kostial K, Simonovic I, et al: Bone status and fracture rates in two regions in Yugoslavia. *Am J Clin Nutr* 32:540–549, 1979.
14. Garn SM, Solomon MA, Friedl J: Calcium intake and bone quality in the elderly. *Ecol Food Nutr* 10:131–133, 1981.
15. Kribbs PJ, Smith DE, Chesnut CH: Oral findings in osteoporosis. Part II: relationship between residual

ridge and alveolar bone resorption and generalized skeletal osteopenia. *J Prost Dent* 50:719–724, 1983.
16. Wical KE, Swoope CC: Studies of residual ridge resorption. Part II. The relationship of dietary calcium and phosphorus to residual ridge resorption. *J Prost Dent* 32:13–22, 1974.
17. Bullamore JR, Gallagher JC, Wilkinson R, et al: The effect of age on calcium absorption. *Lancet* 2:535–537, 1970.
18. Gallagher JC, Riggs BL, Eisman J, et al: Intestinal calcium absorption and serum vitamin D metabolites in normal subjects and osteoporotic patients: effect of age and dietary calcium. *J Clin Invest* 64:729–736, 1979.
19. Avioli LV, McDonald JE, Lee SW: The influence of age on the intestinal absorption of ^{47}Ca in women and its relation to ^{47}Ca absorption in postmenopausal osteoporosis. *J Clin Invest* 44:1960–1967, 1965.
20. Alevizaki CC, Ikkos DC, Singhelakis PJ: Progressive decrease of true intestinal calcium absorption with age in normal man. *Nucl Med* 14:760–762, 1973.
21. Nordin BEC, Williams R, Marshall DH, et al: Calcium absorption in the elderly. *Calcif Tissue Res* 21:422–451, 1975.
22. Ireland P, Fordtran JS: Effect of dietary calcium and age on jejunal calcium absorption in humans studied by intestinal perfusion. *J Clin Invest* 52:2672–2681, 1973.
23. Manolagas SC, Culler FL, Howard JE, et al: The cytoreceptor assay for 1,25-dihydroxyvitamin D and its application to clinical studies. *J Clin Endocrinol Metab* 56:751–760, 1983.
24. Tsai K-S, Heath H, Kumar R, et al: Impaired vitamin D metabolism with aging in women: possible role in pathogenesis of senile osteoporosis. *J Clin Invest* 73:1668–1672, 1984.
25. Ivanovich P, Fellows H, Rich C: The absorption of calcium carbonate. *Ann Intern Med* 66:917–923, 1967.
26. Heaney RP, Recker RR, Saville PD: Menopausal changes in calcium balance performance. *J Lab Clin Med* 92:953–963, 1978.
27. Heaney RP, Recker RR: Distribution of calcium absorption in middle-aged women. *Am J Clin Nutr* 43:299–305, 1986.
28. Anonymous: Consensus Conference: Osteoporosis. *JAMA* 252:799–802, 1984.
29. Weinsier RL, Norris D: Recent developments in the etiology and treatment of hypertension: dietary calcium, fat and magnesium. *Am J Clin Nutr* 42:1331–1338, 1985.
30. Kok FJ, Vandenbroucke JP, vander Heide-Wessel C, et al: Dietary sodium, calcium, potassium, and blood pressure. *Am J Epidemiol* 123:1043–1048, 1986.
31. Jones MR, Ghaffari F, Tomerson BW, et al: Hypotensive effect of a high calcium diet in the Wistar rat. *Min Electrol Metab* 12:85–91, 1986.
32. Luft FC, Aronoff GR, Sloan RS, et al: Short-term augmental calcium intake has no effect on sodium homeostasis. *Clin Pharmacol Ther* 39:414–419, 1985.
33. McCarron DA, Morris CD, Henry HJ, et al: Blood pressure and nutrient intake in the United States. *Science* 224:1392–1398, 1984.
34. McCarron DA, Morris CD, Cole C: Dietary calcium in human hypertension. *Science* 217:267–269, 1982.
35. Ackley S, Barrett-Connor E, Suarez L: Dairy products, calcium and blood pressure. *Am J Clin Nutr* 38:457–461, 1983.
36. Stitt FW, Crawford MD, Clayton DG, et al: Clinical and biochemical indicators of cardiovascular disease among men living in hard and soft water areas. *Lancet* 1:122–126, 1973.
37. Schroeder HA: Relation between morality from cardiovascular disease and treated water supplies: variations in states and 163 largest municipalities of the United States. *JAMA* 172:1902–1908, 1960.
38. McCarron DA, Stanton J, Henry HJ, et al: Assessment of nutritional correlates of blood pressure. *Ann Intern Med* 98:715–719, 1983.
39. Pernot F, Schleiffer R, Bertelot A, et al: Dietary calcium and arterial hypertension in the rat. *Arch Mal Coeur* 78:1725–1729, 1985.
40. Doris PA: Sodium and hypertension: effect of dietary calcium supplementation on blood pressure. *Clin Exp Hypertens* 71:1441–1456, 1985.
41. McCarron DA, Morris CO: Blood pressure response to oral calcium in persons with mild to moderate hypertension: a randomized, double-blind, placebo-controlled crossover trial. *Ann Intern Med* 103:825–831, 1985.

42. Belzian JM, Villar J, Pineda O, et al: Reduction of blood pressure with calcium supplementation in young adults. *JAMA* 249:1161–1165, 1983.
43. Hollaway ET, Bohr DF: Reactivity of vascular smooth muscle in hypertensive rats. *Circ Res* 33:678–685, 1973.
44. McCarron DA, Pingree PA, Rubin RS, et al: Enhanced parathyroid function in essential hypertension: a homeostatic response to a urinary calcium leak. *Hypertension* 2:162–168, 1980.
45. Rosenthal FD, Ray S: Hypertension and hyperparathyroidism. *Br Med J* 4:396–397, 1972.
46. Aloia JF, Cohn SH, Ostuni JA, et al: Prevention of involutional bone loss by exercise. *Ann Intern Med* 89:356–358, 1978.
47. Smith EL Jr, Reddan W, Smith PE: Physical activity and calcium modalities for bone mineral increase in aged women. *Med Sci Sports Exerc* 13:60–64, 1981.
48. Drinkwater BL, Nilson K, Chestnut CH, et al: Bone mineral content of amenorrheic and eumenorrheic athletes. *N Engl J Med* 311:277–281, 1984.
49. Marcus R, Cann C, Madvig P, et al: Menstrual function and bone mass in elite women distance runners. *Ann Intern Med* 102:158–163, 1985.
50. Lindberg JS, Fears WB, Hunt MM, et al: Exercise-induced amenorrhea and bone density. *Ann Intern Med* 101:647–648, 1984.
51. Rigotti NA, Nussbaum SR, Herzog OB, et al: Osteogenesis in women with anorexia nervosa. *N Engl J Med* 311:1601–1606, 1984.
52. Stillman RJ, Lohman TG, Slaughter MH, et al: Physical activity and bone mineral content in women aged 30 to 85 years. *Med Sci Sports Exerc* 18:576–580, 1986.
53. Krolner B, Toft B, Nielsen SP, et al: Physical exercise as prophylaxis against involutional vertebrae bone loss: a controlled trial. *Clin Sci* 64:541–546, 1983.
54. Lane NE, Block DA, Jones HH, et al: Long distance running, bone density and osteoarthritis. *JAMA* 255:1147–1151, 1986.
55. Nilsson BE, Westlin NE: Bone density in athletes. *Clin Orthop Relat Res* 77:179–182, 1971.
56. Dalen N, Olsson KE: Bone mineral content and physical activity. *Acta Orthop Scand* 45:170–174, 1974.
57. Aloia JF, Cohn SH, Babu T, et al: Skeletal mass and body composition in marathon runners. *Metabolism* 27:1793–1796, 1978.
58. Smith EL Jr, Smith PE, Ensign CJ, et al: Bone involution decrease in exercising middle-aged women. *Calcif Tissue Int* 36:S129–S138, 1984.
59. Williams JA, Wagner J, Wasnich R, et al: The effect of long distance running upon appendicular bone mineral content. *Med Sci Sports Exerc* 3:223–227, 1984.
60. Jones HH, Priest JD, Hayes WC, et al: Humeral hypertrophy in response to exercise. *J Bone Jt Surg* 59A:204–208, 1977.
61. Brewer V, Meyer BM, Keele MS, et al: Role of exercise in prevention of involutional bone loss. *Med Sci Sports Exerc* 15:445–449, 1983.
62. Chow E, Harrison JE, Brown CF, et al: Physical fitness effect on bone mass in postmenopausal women. *Arch Phys Med Rehabil* 67:231–234, 1986.
63. Smith RT, Sunde ML, Smith EL: The influence of dietary calcium and exercise on the mechanical properties of bone. *Med Sci Sports Exerc* 16:164, 1984.
64. Pocock NA, Eisman JA, Yeates MG, et al: Physical fitness is a major determinant of femoral neck and lumbar spine bone mineral density. *J Clin Invest* 78:618–621, 1986.
65. Nilsson BE, Anderson SM, Havdrup T, et al: *Am J Roentgenol* 131:539, 1978.
66. Drinkwater BL: Exercise and bone mass, in: *Exercise and Bone Mass*. Indianapolis, American Society for Bone and Mineral Research, 1987, pp 11–21.
67. Heaney RP: Calcium, bone health and osteoporosis, in Peck WA (ed): *Bone and Mineral Research IV*. Amsterdam, Elsevier Science Publishers, 1986, pp 255–301.
68. Crilly RG, Richardson LFO, Anderson C: Anthropometry and bone mass in postmenopausal women. *J Bone Min Res* 2:Suppl 1 (Abstr 342), 1987.
69. Woo SLY, Kuei SC, Amiel D, et al: The effect of prolonged physical training on the properties of long bone: a study of Wolff's law. *J Bone Jt Surg* 63A:780–787, 1980.
70. Chavapil M, Bartos D, Bartos F: Effect of long-term physical stress on collagen growth in the lung, heart and femur of young and adult rats. *Gerontologia* 19:263–270, 1973.

71. Yeh JK, Aloia JF: Effect of physical activity on absorption and excretion of calcium in the rat. *J Bone Min Res* 1(Abstr 237), 1986.
72. Yeh JK, Aloia JF: Effects of physical activity on intestinal active and passive transport of calcium in the rat. *J Bone Min Res* 2(Suppl 1) (Abstr 459), 1987.
73. Lanyon LE, Bourn S: The influence of mechanical function on the development and remodeling of the tibia. *J Bone Jt Surg* 61A:263–273, 1979.
74. Rubin CT, Lanyon LE: Regulation of bone formation by applied dynamic loads. *J Bone Jt Surg* 66A:397–402, 1984.
75. Schryver HF, Hintz HF, Lowe JE: Calcium metabolism, body composition and sweat losses of exercised horses. *Am J Vet Res* 39:245–248, 1978.
76. Raub RH, Jackson SG, Baker JP: The effect of exercise on bone development and growth and the circulating level of cortisol, insulin and thyroxine in weanling horses. *Proc Eq Nutr Physiol Symp* 10:409–414, 1987.
77. Emiola L, O'Shea JP: Effects of physical activity and nutrition on bone density measured by radiographic techniques. *Nutr Rep Intern* 6:669–681, 1978.
78. Ragan C, Briscoe AM: Effect of exercise on the metabolism of ^{40}calcium and ^{47}calcium in man. *J Clin Endocrinol Metab* 24:385–392, 1964.
79. Consolazio CF, Matoush LD, Nelson RA, et al: Relationship between calcium in sweat, calcium balance and calcium requirements. *J Nutr* 78:78–88, 1962.
80. Robinson S, Robinson AH: Chemical composition of sweat. *Physiol Rev* 34:202–220, 1954.
81. Costill DL: Sweating: its composition and effects on body fluids. *Ann NY Acad Sci* 301:160–174, 1977.
82. Talbert GA, Haugen C, Carpenter R, et al: Simultaneous study of the constituents of the sweat, urine and blood; also gastric acidity and other manifestations resulting from sweating. X. Basic Methods. *Am J Physiol* 104:441–442, 1933.
83. Mitchell HH, Hamilson TS: The dermal excretion under controlled environmental conditions of nitrogen and minerals in human subjects, with particular reference to calcium and iron. *J Biol Chem* 178:345–361, 1949.
84. Goulding A: Effects of dietary NaCl supplements on parathyroid function, bone turnover and bone composition in rats taking restricted amounts of calcium. *Min Electrol Metab* 4:203–208, 1980.
85. Johnson N, Alcantara E, Linkswiler H: Effect of level of protein intake on urinary and feed calcium and calcium retention of young adult males. *J Nutr* 100:1425–1430, 1970.
86. Walker R, Linkswiler HM: Calcium retention in the adult human male as affected by protein intake. *J Nutr* 102:1297–1302, 1972.
87. Allen CH, Oddoye EA, Margen S: Protein-induced hypercalciuria: a longer term study. *Am J Clin Nutr* 32:741–749, 1979.
88. Kim Y, Linkswiler HM: Effect of level of protein intake on calcium metabolism and on parathyroid and renal function in the adult human male. *J Nutr* 109:1399–1404, 1979.
89. Heaney RP, Recker RR: Effects of nitrogen, phosphorus and caffeine on calcium balance in women. *J Lah Clin Med* 99:46–55, 1982.
90. Heaney RP, Skillman TG: Secretion and excretion of calcium by the human gastrointestinal tract. *J Lab Clin Med* 64:29–41, 1964.
91. Notelovitz M: Interrelations of exercise and diet on bone metabolism and osteoporosis, in Winick M (ed): *Nutrition and Exercise.* New York, John Wiley and Sons, 1986, pp 203–228.
92. Anand CR, Linkswiler H: Effect of protein intake on calcium balance of young men given 500 mg calcium daily. *J Nutr* 104:695–700, 1974.
93. Margen S, Chu JY, Kaufman NA, et al: Studies in calcium metabolism. I. The calciuretic effect of dietary protein. *Am J Clin Nutr* 27:584–589, 1974.
94. Glade MJ, Beller D, Bergen J, et al: Dietary protein in excess of requirements inhibits renal calcium and phosphorus reabsorption in young horses. *Nutr Rep Intern* 31:649–659, 1985.
95. Schuette SA, Zemel MB, Linkswiler HM: Studies on the mechanism of protein-induced hypercalciuria in older men and women. *J Nutr* 110:305–315, 1980.
96. Block GD, Wood RJ, Allen CH: A comparison of the effects of feeding sulfur amino acids and protein on urine calcium in man. *Am J Clin Nutr* 3:2128–2136, 1980.

97. Goulding A, Malthus RS: Effects of the protein content of the diet on the development of nephrocalcinosis in rats. *Aust J Exp Biol Med Sci* 48:313–320, 1970.
98. Whiting SJ, Draper HH: The role of sulfate in the calciuria of high protein diets in adult rats. *J Nutr* 110:212–222, 1980.
99. Jacob M, Smith JC Jr, Chan JCM: Effects of metabolic acidosis on zinc and calcium metabolism in rats. *Ann Nutr Metab* 27:380–385, 1983.
100. McSherry E, Morris RC Jr: Attainment and maintenance of normal stature with alkali therapy in infants and children with classic renal tubular acidosis. *J Clin Invest* 61:509–527, 1978.
101. Life Sciences Research Office: Evaluation of the Health Aspects of Phosphates as Food Ingredients. SCOGS-32. Bethesda, MD, FASEB, 1975.
102. Bell RR, Draper HH, Tzeng DYM, et al: Physiological responses of human adults to foods containing phosphate additives. *J Nutr* 107:42–50, 1977.
103. Spencer H, Kramer L, Osis D, et al: Effect of phosphorus on the absorption of calcium and on the calcium balance in man. *J Nutr* 108:447–457, 1978.
104. Goldsmith RS, Jowsey J, Dube WJ, et al: Effects of phosphorus supplementation on serum parathyroid hormone and bone morphology in osteoporosis. *J Clin Endocrinol Metab* 43:523–532, 1976.
105. Spencer H, Kramer L, DeBartolo M, et al: Further studies of the effect of a high protein diet as meat on calcium metabolism. *Am J Clin Nutr* 37:924–929, 1983.
106. Wood RJ: Glucose polymer enhancement of calcium bioavailability, in Gussler JD (ed): *Osteoporosis: Current Concepts*. Columbus, OH, Ross Laboratories, 1987, pp 66–68.
107. Norman DA, Morawski SG, Fortran JS: Influence of glucose, fructose and water movement on calcium absorption in the jejunum. *Gastroenterology* 78:22–25, 1980.
108. Monnier L, Colette C, Acquirre L, et al: Intestinal and renal handling of calcium in human diabetes mellitus: influence of acute glucose loading and diabetic control. *Eur J Clin Invest* 8:225–231, 1978.
109. Kabayashi A, Kawai S, Ohbeard Y, et al: Effects of dietary lactose and lactase preparation on the intestinal absorption of calcium and magnesium in normal infants. *Am J Clin Nutr* 28:681–683, 1975.
110. Kocian J, Skala I, Bakos K: Calcium absorption from milk and lactose-free milk in healthy subjects and patients with lactose intolerance. *Digestion* 9:311–324, 1973.
111. Church CF, Church HN: *Food Values of Portions Commonly Used*, ed 12. Philadelphia, JB Lippincott Co, 1975.
112. Jeaghers H, Murphy R: Practical aspects of oxalate metabolism. *N Engl J Med* 233:208–215, 1945.
113. Pingle U, Ramasastri BV: Absorption of calcium from a leafy vegetable rich in oxalates. *Br J Nutr* 39:119–125, 1978.
114. Zarembski PM, Hodkinson A: The oxalic acid content of English diets. *Br J Nutr* 16:627–634, 1962.
115. Kelsay JL, Behall KM, Prather ES: Effect of fiber from fruits and vegetables on metabolic responses of human subjects, II. Calcium, magnesium, iron and silicon balances. *Am J Clin Nutr* 32:1876–1880, 1979.
116. Ismail-Beigi F, Reinhold JG, Faradji B, et al: Effects of cellulose added to diets of low and high fiber content upon the metabolism of calcium, magnesium, zinc and phosphorus by man. *J Nutr* 107:510–518, 1977.
117. Reinhold JG, Faradji B, Abadi P, et al: Decreased absorption of calcium, magnesium, zinc and phosphorus by humans due to increased fiber and phosphorus consumption as wheat bread. *J Nutr* 106:493–503, 1976.
118. McCance RA, Widdowson EM: Mineral metabolism of healthy adults on white and brown bread intakes. *J Physiol* 101:44–85, 1942.
119. Cummings JH, Hill MJ, Houston H, et al: The effect of meat protein and dietary fiber on colonic function and metabolism. I. Changes in bowel habit, bile acid excretion and calcium absorption. *Am J Clin Nutr* 32:2086–2093, 1979.
120. Rheinhold JG, Nasr K, Lahimgarzadel A, et al: Effects of purified phytate and phytate-rich bread upon metabolism of zinc, calcium, phosphorus and nitrogen in man. *Lancet* 1:283–288, 1973.
121. James WPT, Branch WJ, Southgate DAT: Calcium binding by dietary fiber. *Lancet* 1:638–639, 1978.
122. Sandstead HH, Klevay LM, Jacob RA, et al: Effects of dietary fiber and protein level on mineral element metabolism, in Inglett GE, Falkhaged SI (eds): *Dietary Fibers, Chemistry and Nutrition*. New York, Academic Press, 1979, pp 147–156.

123. Allen LH: Calcium bioavailability and absorption: a review. *Am J Clin Nutr* 35:783–808, 1982.
124. Leichsenring JM, Norris LM, Halbert ML: Effect of ascorbic acid and of orange juice on calcium and phosphorus metabolism of women. *J Nutr* 63:425–435, 1957.
125. Tantibhedhyangkul P, Hashim SA: Medium-chain triglyceride feeding in premature infants: effects on calcium and magnesium absorption. *Pediatrics* 61:537–545, 1978.
126. Glade MJ, Krook L: Glucocorticoid-induced inhibition of osteolysis and the development of osteopetrosis, osteonecrosis and osteoporosis. *Cornell Vet* 72:76–91, 1982.
127. Meunier PJ, Dempster DW, Edouard C, et al: Bone histomorphometry in corticosteroid-induced osteoporosis and Cushing's syndrome. *Adv Exp Med Biol* 171:191–200, 1984.
128. Jowsey J, Riggs BL: Bone formation in hypercortisonism. *Acta Endocrinol* 63:21–28, 1970.
129. Glade MJ, Krook L, Schryver HF, et al: Calcium metabolism in glucocorticoid-treated foals. *J Nutr* 112:67–76, 1982.
130. Klein RG, Arnaud SB, Gallagher JC, et al: Intestinal calcium absorption in exogenous hypercortisonism. *J Clin Invest* 60:253–259, 1977.
131. Hahn TJ, Halstead LR, Baran DT: Effects of short-term glucocorticoid administration on intestinal calcium absorption and circulating vitamin D metabolite concentrations in man. *J Clin Endocrinol Metab* 52:111–115, 1981.
132. Nordin BEC, Marshall DH, Francis RM, et al: The effects of sex steroid and corticosteroid hormones on bone. *J Steroid Biochem* 15:171–174, 1981.
133. Reid IR, Ibbertson HK: Calcium supplements in the prevention of steroid-induced osteoporosis. *Am J Clin Nutr* 44:287–290, 1986.
134. Wilkinson R: Absorption of calcium, phosphorus and magnesium, in Nordin BEC (ed): *Calcium, Phosphate and Magnesium Metabolism.* Edinburgh, Churchill Livingstone, 1975, p 37.
135. Glade MJ, Krook L, Schryver HF, et al: Morphologic and biochemical changes in cartilage of foals treated with dexamethasone. *Cornell Vet* 73:170–192, 1983.
136. Wolf RE: Nonsteroidal anti-inflammatory drugs. *Arch Intern Med* 144:1658–1660, 1984.
137. Hess EV: Nonsteroidal anti-inflammatory drugs: new perspectives in the inflammatory process and immunologic function. *Am J Med* 77(4B):1–2, 1984.
138. Mills JA: Nonsteroidal anti-inflammatory drugs. *N Engl J Med* 290:781–784, 1974.
139. Carmichael J, Shankel SW: Effects of nonsteroidal anti-inflammatory drugs on prostaglandins and renal function. *Am J Med* 78:992–1000, 1985.
140. Garella S, Matarese RA: Renal effects of prostaglandins and clinical adverse effects of nonsteroidal anti-inflammatory agents. *Medicine* 63:165–181, 1984.
141. Clive DM, Stoff JS: Renal syndromes associated with nonsteroidal anti-inflammatory drugs. *N Engl J Med* 310:563–572, 1984.
142. Patmas MA, Wilborn SL, Shankel SW: Acute multisystem toxicity associated with the use of nonsteroidal anti-inflammatory drugs. *Arch Intern Med* 144:519–521, 1984.
143. Bjarnason I, So A, Levi AJ, et al: Intestinal permeability and inflammation in rheumatoid arthritis: effects of nonsteroidal anti-inflammatory drugs. *Lancet* 2:1171–1173, 1984.
144. Simmons HA, Raisz LG: Biphasic effects of cyclo-oxygenase inhibitors on prostaglandin production by cultural neonatal rat calvaria. *J Bone Min Res* 2(Suppl 1) (Abstr 27), 1987.
145. Walker WA, Hendricks KM: *Manual of Pediatric Nutrition.* Philadelphia, W.B. Saunders Co., 1985.
146. Roe DA: *Drug-Induced Nutritional Deficiency,* ed 2. Westport, CT, A.V.I. Publishing Co., Inc., 1985.
147. Faloon WW, Fisher CJ, Duggan KC: Occurrence of a sprue-like syndrome during neomycin therapy. *J Clin Invest* 37:893, 1958.
148. Spencer H, Kramer L, Norris C, et al: Effect of small doses of aluminum-containing antacids on calcium and phosphorus metabolism. *Am J Clin Nutr* 36:32–40, 1982.
149. Spencer H, Lender M: Adverse effects of aluminum-containing antacid on mineral metabolism. *Gastroenterology* 76:603–606, 1979.
150. Spencer H, Derler J, Osis D: Calcium requirement, bioavailability and loss. *Fed Proc* 46:631 (Abstr 1834), 1987.
151. Hahn TJ, Birge SJ, Scharp CR, et al: Phenobarbital-induced alterations in vitamin D metabolism. *J Clin Invest* 51:741–748, 1972.

152. Hahn TJ, Hendin BA, Scharp CR, et al: Effect of chronic anticonvulsant therapy on serum 25-hydroxycalciferol levels in adults. *N Engl J Med* 287:900–909, 1972.
153. Kupfer S, Kosovsky JD: Effects of cardiac glycosides on renal tubular transport of calcium, magnesium, inorganic phosphate and glucose in the dog. *J Clin Invest* 44:1132–1143, 1965.
154. Wasnich RD, Benfante RJ, Yano K, et al: Thiazide effect on the mineral content of bone. *N Engl J Med* 309:344–347, 1983.
155. American College of Sports Medicine: Position statement on the use and abuse of anabolic-androgenic steroids in sports. *Med Sci Sports* 9:xi–xii, 1977.
156. Lamb DR: Androgens and exercise. *Med Sci Sports* 7:1–5, 1975.
157. Ryan AJ: Athletics, in Kochakian CD (ed): *Anabolic-Androgenic Steroids*. Berlin, Springer-Verlag, 1976, pp 515–536.
158. Chestnut CH: Synthetic salmon calcitonin, diphosphonates and anabolic steroids in the treatment of post-menopausal osteoporosis, in Christiansen C, Arnaund CP, Nordin BEC, et al (eds): *Osteoporosis: Proceedings of the Copenhagen International Symposium on Osteoporosis*. Copenhagen Aalborg Stiftsbogtrykkeri, 1984, pp 549–555.
159. Chesnut CH: Treatment of post-menopausal osteoporosis. *Compr Ther* 10:41–47, 1984.
160. Chesnut CH, Ivey JL, Gruber HE, et al: Stanozolol in postmenopausal osteoporosis: therapeutic efficacy and possible mechanisms of action. *Metabolism* 32:571–580, 1983.
161. Peacock M, Henry DP, Johnson CC Jr., et al: The effect of Humatrope (biosynthetic human growth hormone) on bone biochemistry in men. *J Bone Min Res* 2(Suppl 1) (Abstr 340), 1987.
162. Buckler JMH: Exercise as a screening test for growth hormone release. *Acta Endocr (Copenhagen)* 69:219–229, 1972.
163. Berchtold P, Berger M, Cuppers HJ, et al: Non-glucoregulatory hormones during physical exercise in juvenile-type diabetes. *Horm Metab Res* 10:269–273, 1978.
164. Schwarz F, TerHaar DJ, van Riet HG, et al: Response of growth hormone, FFA, blood sugar and insulin to exercise in obese patients and normal subjects. *Metabolism* 18:1013–1020, 1969.
165. Sutton JR, Young JD, Lazarus L: The hormonal response to physical exercise. *Aust Ann Med* 18:84–90, 1969.
166. Schlach DS: The influence of physical stress and exercise on growth hormone and insulin secretion in man. *J Lab Clin Med* 69:256–269, 1967.
167. Kuoppasalmi K: Plasma testosterone and sex-hormone-binding globulin capacity in physical exercise. *Scand J Clin Lab Invest* 40:411–418, 1980.
168. Nilsson KO, Heding LG, Hokfelt B: The influence of short-term submaximal work on the plasma concentrations of catecholamines, pancreatic glucagon and growth hormone in man. *Acta Endocr (Copenhagen)* 79:286–294, 1975.
169. Hansen AP: The effect of adrenergic receptor blockade on the exercise-induced serum growth hormone rise in normals and juvenile diabetics. *J Clin Endocrinol Metab* 33:807–812, 1971.
170. Blackard W, Hubbell GL: Stimulatory effect of exogenous catecholamines on plasma HGH concentrations in presence of beta adrenergic blockade. *Metabolism* 19:547–552, 1970.
171. Bergman EA, Sherrard DJ, Massey LK: Effects of dietary caffeine on calcium metabolism and bone turnover in adult women. *Fed Proc* 46:632 (Abstr 1840), 1987.
172. Massey LK, Sherrard DJ, Bergman EA: Dietary caffeine lowers ultrafiltrable calcium levels in women consuming low dietary calcium. *J Bone Min Res* 2(Suppl 1) (Abstr 479), 1987.
173. Shangold MM, Levine HS: The effect of marathon training upon menstrual function. *Am J Obstet Gynecol* 143:862–869, 1982.
174. Malina RM, Harper AB, AVent HH, et al: Age at menarche in athletes and non-athletes. *Med Sci Sports* 5:11–13, 1973.
175. Warren M: The effects of exercise on pubertal progression and reproductive function in girls. *J Clin Endocrinol Metab* 51:1150–1157, 1980.
176. Frisch RE, Gotz-Welbergen AV, McArthur JW, et al: Delayed menarche and amenorrhea of college athletes in relation to age of onset of training. *JAMA* 246:1559–1563, 1981.
177. Baker ER, Mathur RS, Kirk RF, et al: Female runners and secondary amenorrhea: correlation with age, parity, mileage and plasma hormonal and sex-hormone-binding globulin concentrations. *Fertil Steril* 36:183–187, 1981.

178. Jurkowski JE, Jones NL, Walker WC, et al: Ovarian hormonal responses to exercise. *J Appl Physiol Respirat Environ Exercise Physiol* 44:109–114, 1978.
179. Bonen A, Ling WY, MacIntyre KP, et al: Effects of exercise on the serum concentrations of FSH, LH, progesterone and estradiol. *Eur J Appl Physiol* 42:15–25, 1979.
180. Keizer HA, Portman J, Bunnik GSJ: Influence of physical exercise on sex hormone metabolism. *J Appl Physiol Respirat Environ Exercise Physiol* 48:765–769, 1980.
181. Tylavsky FA, Halioua L, Doherty A: The effects of menstrual status on radial bone parameters of premenopausal women. IXth International Congress on Calcium Regulating Hormones and Bone Metabolism, Nice, France, 1966.
182. Nelson ME, Fisher EL, Catsos PD, et al: Diet and bone status in amenorrheic runners. *Am J Clin Nutr* 43:910–916, 1986.
183. Wentz AC: Body weight and amenorrhea. *Obstet Gynecol* 56:482–487, 1980.
184. Schwartz B, Cumming DC, Riordan E, et al: Exercise-associated amenorrhea: a distinct entity? *Am J Obstet Gynecol* 141:662–670, 1981.
185. Bonen A, Belcastro AN: Effect of exercise and training on menstrual cycle hormones. *Austr J Sports Med* 10:39–43, 1978.
186. Shangold M, Freeman R, Thysen B, et al: The relationship between long-distance running, plasma progesterone and luteal phase length. *Fertil Steril* 31:130–133, 1979.
187. Cann CE, Martin MC, Genant HK, et al: Decreased spinal mineral content in amenorrhetic women. *JAMA* 251:626–629, 1984.
188. Koppelman MCS, Kurtz DW, Morrish KA, et al: Vertebral body bone mineral content in hyperprolactinemic women. *J Clin Endocrinol Metab* 59:1050–1053, 1984.
189. Meema J, Meema HE: Menopausal bone loss and estrogen replacement. *Isr J Med Sci* 12:601–606, 1976.
190. Drinkwater BL, Nilson K, Ott S, et al: Bone mineral density following resumption of menses in amenorrheic athletes. *JAMA* 256:380–382, 1986.
191. Albright F, Smith PH, Richardson AM: Postmenopausal osteoporosis; its clinical features. *JAMA* 116:2465–2474, 1941.
192. Cummings SR: Epidemiology of osteoporotic fractures: selected topics, in Gussler JD (ed): *Osteoporosis: Current Concepts*. Columbus, OH, Ross Laboratories, 1987, pp 3–8.
193. Cummings SR, Kelsey JL, Nevitt MC: Epidemiology of osteoporosis and osteoporotic fractures. *Epidemiol Rev* 7:178, 1985.
194. Riggs BL, Melton LJ: Involutional osteoporosis. *N Engl J Med* 314:1676–1686, 1986.
195. Heaney RP, Gallagher JC, Johnston CC, et al: Calcium nutrition and bone health in the elderly. *Am J Clin Nutr* 36:986–1013, 1982.
196. Paganini-Hill A, Ross RK, Gerkins VR, et al: Menopausal estrogen therapy and hip fractures. *Ann Intern Med* 95:28–31, 1981.
197. Williams AR, Weiss NS, Ure CL, et al: Effect of weight, smoking, and estrogen use on the risk of hip and forearm fractures in postmenopausal women. *Obstet Gynecol* 60:695–699, 1982.
198. Hutchinson TA, Polansky SM, Feinstein AR: Postmenopausal estrogens protect against fractures of hip and distal radius. *Lancet* 2:705–709, 1979.
199. Sinaki M, Mikkelsen BA: Evaluation of therapeutic exercise programs in postmenopausal spinal osteoporosis: flexion vs. extension exercises. IXth International Congress on Calcium Regulating Hormones and Bone Metabolism, Nice, France, 1986.
200. Martin AD, Houston CS: Osteoporosis, calcium and physical activity. *Can Med Assoc J* 136:587–593, 1987.
201. Lee CJ, Lawler GS, Johnson GH: Effects of supplementation of the diets with calcium and calcium-rich foods on bone density of elderly females with osteoporosis. *Am J Clin Nutr* 34:819–823, 1981.
202. Albanese AA, Edelson AH, Lorenze EJ Jr., et al: Problems of bone health in elderly; a 3-year study. *NY State J Med* 75:326–336, 1975.
203. Nordin BEC, Horsman A, Crilly RG, et al: Treatment of spinal osteoporosis in postmenopausal women. *Br Med J* 280:451–454, 1980.
204. Recker RR, Saville PD, Heaney RP: The effect of estrogens and calcium carbonate on bone loss in postmenopausal women. *Ann Intern Med* 87:649–655, 1977.

205. Horsman A, Gallagher JC, Simpson M, et al: Prospective trial of estrogen and calcium in postmenopausal women. *Br Med J* 2:789–792, 1977.
206. Riis B, Thomsen K, Christiansen C: Does calcium supplementation prevent postmenopausal bone loss? *N Engl J Med* 316:173–177, 1987.
207. Thalassinos NC, Gutteridge DH, Joplin GF, et al: Calcium balance in osteoporotic patients on long-term oral calcium therapy with and without sex hormones. *Clin Sci* 62:221–226, 1982.
208. Riggs BL, Seeman F, Hodgson SF, et al: Effect of the fluoride/calcium regimen on vertebral fracture occurrence in postmenopausal osteoporosis: comparison with conventional therapy. *N Engl J Med* 306:446–450, 1982.
209. Riggs BL, Jowsey J, Kelly PJ, et al: Effects of oral therapy with calcium and vitamin D in primary osteoporosis. *J Clin Endocrinol Metab* 42:1139–1144, 1976.
210. Sandler RB, Slemenda CW, LaPorte RE, et al: Postmenopausal bone density and milk consumption in childhood and adolescence. *Am J Clin Nutr* 42:270–274, 1985.
211. Nilas L, Christiansen S, Rodbro P: Calcium supplementation and postmenopausal bone loss. *Br J Med* 289:1103–1106, 1984.
212. Walker ARP: The human requirement of calcium—should low intakes be supplemented? *Am J Clin Nutr* 25:518–530, 1972.
213. Garn SM: *The Earlier Gain and the Later Loss of Cortical Bone in Nutritional Perspective*. Springfield, IL, Charles C. Thomas, 1970.
214. Garn SM, Rohmann CG, Wagner B, et al: Population similarities in the onset and rate of adult endosteal bone loss. *Clin Orthop* 65:51–60, 1969.
215. Riggs BL, Wahner HW, Melton LJ, et al: In women dietary calcium intake and rates of bone loss from midradius and lumbar spine are not related. *J Bone Min Res* 1(Abstr. 96), 1986.
216. Lamke B, Sjoberg HE, Sylven M: Bone mineral content in women with Colles' fracture: effect of calcium supplementation. *Acta Orthop Scand* 49:143–146, 1978.
217. Weaver CM, Heaney RP, Martin BR: Oxalic acid inhibits calcium absorption. *Fed Proc* 46:631 (Abstr 1836), 1987.
218. Miller JZ, Jiang X, Smith DL, et al: Calcium absorption from calcium carbonate and calcium carbonate citrate-malate in healthy male and female adolescents. *Fed Proc* 46:631 (Abstr 1838), 1987.
219. Lewis NM, Marcus MS, Behling AR, et al: Calcium and chloride interactions in humans. *Fed Proc* 46:887 (Abstr 3328), 1987.
220. Robertson WG, Peacock M, Hodgkinson A: Dietary changes and the incidence of urinary calculi in the UK between 1958 and 1976. *J Chronic Dis* 32:469–476, 1979.
221. Gallagher JC, Aaron J, Horsman A, et al: The crush fracture syndrome in postmenopausal women. *Clin Endocrinol Metab* 2:293–315, 1973.
222. Heaney RP, Saville PD, Recker RR: Calcium absorption as a function of calcium intake. *J Lab Clin Med* 85:881–889, 1975.
223. Austin LA, Heath H, Go VL: Regulation of calcitonin secretion in normal man by changes of serum calcium within the physiologic range. *J Clin Invest* 64:1721–1724, 1979.
224. Barreras RF: Acid secretion after calcium carbonate in patients with duodenal ulcer. *N Engl J Med* 282:1402–1405, 1970.
225. Burnett CH, Commons RR, Albright F, et al: Hypercalcemia without hypercalciuria or hypophosphatemia, calcinosis and renal insufficiency: a syndrome following prolonged intake of milk and alkali. *N Engl J Med* 240:787–794, 1949.
226. Department of Health and Social Security: Recommended Intakes of Nutrients for the United Kingdom. Reports on Public Health and Medical Subjects, No. 120. London, HMSO, 1969.
227. FAO/WHO Joint Expert Committee on Nutrition: Food and Nutrition Strategies in National Development. Technical Report Series 584. Geneva, World Health Organization, 1976.

6

Muscle Relaxants

Donald B. Hoover

The vast majority of drugs that are used to produce relaxation of skeletal muscle achieve this effect by an action at some point in the neuronal pathways involved in muscle regulation. Although the skeletal muscles are under voluntary control, there is an abundance of neuronal circuitry which participates in the generation of smooth, coordinated movement. All of the neural information is ultimately channeled through the alpha motoneurons which are responsible for causing contraction of skeletal muscle cells. To fully appreciate the actions of muscle relaxants, it will be necessary to briefly review certain aspects of the neuroregulation of skeletal muscles.

1. NEUROREGULATION OF SKELETAL MUSCLE

1.1. Alpha Motoneurons and Neuromuscular Transmission

Alpha motoneurons are large neurons which have their cell body located in the anterior gray matter of the spinal cord or in the brainstem. Motoneurons in the spinal cord control skeletal muscles in the neck, trunk, and limbs, while brainstem motoneurons are predominantly involved in the control of muscles in the head. Skeletal muscles used in breathing are controlled by motoneurons found at spinal and supraspinal levels. Each of these motoneurons has a single axon which carries electrical impulses to skeletal muscle. The alpha motoneurons are the final common pathway in the neuroregulation of skeletal muscle contraction. They receive input from various sites within the central nervous system and from peripheral sensory nerves. The output of the motoneuron (i.e., the frequency of electrical impulses) is determined by the relative amounts of excitatory and inhibitory input which it receives.

The axon of a motoneuron may have numerous terminal branches and thereby affect several muscle fibers (i.e., muscle cells), or it may have only a few branches and consequently have a more discrete effect. The motoneuron and all the muscle fibers which it affects are called the motor unit. Small motor units are found in muscles which

Donald B. Hoover • Department of Pharmacology, Quillen-Dishner College of Medicine, East Tennessee State University, Johnson City, Tennessee 37601.

perform intricate movements (e.g., muscles of the hands), while large motor units are typically found in muscles responsible for relatively gross movement (e.g., muscles of the thigh).

1.2. Neuromuscular Junction

The site where a nerve ending acts to stimulate a skeletal muscle fiber is the neuromuscular junction (Fig. 1). The nerve ending and muscle fiber are separated by a very narrow space called the junctional gap. Signal transfer from nerve to muscle is not by direct electrical stimulation but requires a chemical mediator, acetylcholine. Acetylcholine is synthesized in the nerve endings of motoneurons and is stored in vesicles. When an electrical impulse reaches the nerve endings, it causes the vesicles to fuse with the nerve membrane and release their acetylcholine into the junctional gap. The acetylcholine diffuses across the gap and combines with specific acetylcholine receptor molecules in the muscle cell membrane. The relationship between acetylcholine and its receptor is analogous to that of a key and lock. The structure of acetylcholine is complementary to a specific region of the receptor. The combination of acetylcholine with its receptor results in the opening of ion channels in the muscle cell membrane. Flow of specific ions through these channels produces an electrical potential (i.e., depolarization) at the muscle membrane. If enough channels are opened, an electrical impulse is generated and causes release of calcium from storage sites inside the muscle cell into the muscle cytoplasm. Calcium is then able to trigger the process of contrac-

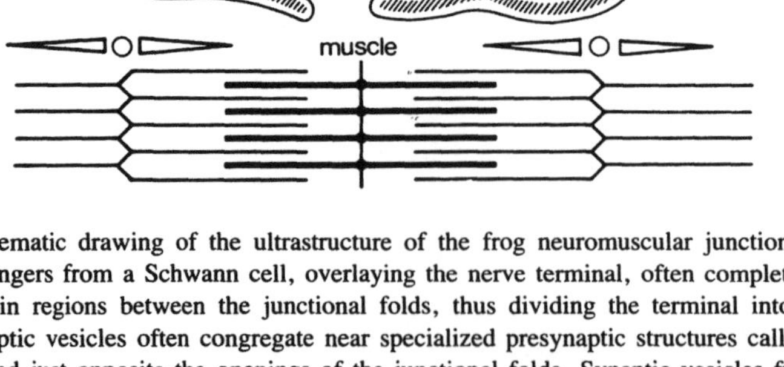

Figure 1. Schematic drawing of the ultrastructure of the frog neuromuscular junction in longitudinal section. Thin fingers from a Schwann cell, overlaying the nerve terminal, often completely embrace the nerve terminal in regions between the junctional folds, thus dividing the terminal into compartments. Numerous synaptic vesicles often congregate near specialized presynaptic structures called active zones. These are located just opposite the openings of the junctional folds. Synaptic vesicles fuse at the active zones. Acetylcholine (ACh) receptors are located in a high density mainly at the crests of the junctional folds. The distance between the folds is about 1 μm. The same structures are found in mammalian motor end plates, but their arrangement is not as regular as in the frog neuromuscular junction. (From Dreyer F: Acetylcholine receptor. *Br J Anaesth* 54:115–130, 1982.)

tion. Relaxation occurs when calcium is removed from the cytoplasm and sequestered in the storage sites.

Attachment of acetylcholine to its receptor is brief and is followed by rapid enzymatic inactivation or diffusion of the chemical from the junctional gap. Acetylcholinesterase, the enzyme which inactivates acetylcholine, is concentrated in the muscle membrane at the neuromuscular junction. The muscle membrane returns to its prestimulation state (i.e., repolarizes) well in advance of muscle relaxation.

The neuromuscular junction is a specific example of a synapse. The synapse is defined as the anatomical site of chemically mediated communication between a neuron and another cell (e.g., neurons, cardiac muscle cells, smooth muscle cells).

1.3. Spinal Reflexes

Spinal reflexes are one mechanism by which sensory input affects skeletal muscles.[1] They are important factors in controlling muscle tone, maintaining posture, and generating smooth, rhythmic movement. They also serve to protect skeletal muscles from damage due to stretch or excessive load.

Monosynaptic stretch reflexes are the simplest reflexes (Fig. 2). The basic circuitry mediating the stretch reflex consists of a sensory nerve and an alpha motoneuron. The reflex is initiated by stretch-induced activation of sensory nerve endings located in structures called muscle spindles. (Sensory nerve endings are located in the central, nuclear bag region of the muscle spindle.) These spindles are strategically placed for sensing muscle stretch, being oriented parallel to the muscle fibers and having one end anchored to connective tissue surrounding muscle fibers and the other to muscle connective tissue as well or to tendon. An electrical impulse produced at the sensory nerve ending is carried into the spinal cord by the sensory nerve. One branch of this sensory nerve forms a synapse with an alpha motoneuron. Chemical transmitter is released from the sensory nerve and excites (i.e., depolarizes) the motoneuron. If the stimulation is of sufficient intensity, the motoneuron causes contraction of the muscle fiber it innervates and thereby opposes the stretch. Muscle spindles also contain their own muscle fibers (intrafusal fibers), located between the nuclear bag region and the muscle spindle anchor sites. Intrafusal muscle is controlled by gamma motoneurons, which are located in the same regions as the larger alpha motoneurons. Contraction of intrafusal muscle fibers does not contribute to the force generated by the main body of muscle fibers (extrafusal fibers). However, contraction of intrafusal muscle fibers causes stimulation of sensory nerve endings in the muscle spindle by stretching the nuclear bag region. In contrast, contraction of extrafusal fibers removes tension from the muscle spindle an terminates the stimulation of the sensory endings. Gamma motoneurons have an important physiological role in the regulation of muscle tone.

Most reflexes involve more than two neurons (Fig. 2) and are referred to as polysynaptic reflexes (i.e., having more than one synapse). The withdrawal reflex is an example of a polysynaptic relfex. It can be triggered by activation of sensory nerve endings in the skin which are sensitive to painful stimuli (e.g., pinching or heat). Pain fibers carry an electrical impulse to the spinal cord but do not form a synapse with motoneurons. Instead, the sensory nerve forms a synapse with a small neuron called an

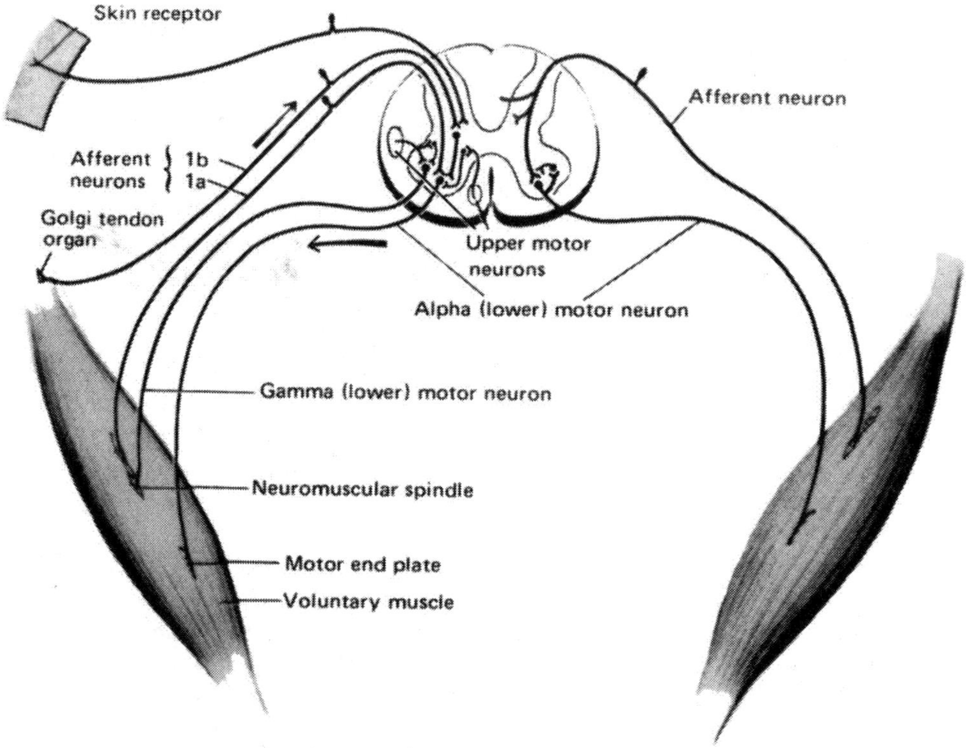

Figure 2. The stretch reflex (monosynaptic) is represented on the right and left. The withdrawal reflex and the Golgi tendon reflex (polysynaptic) are diagramed on the left. A neuromuscular spindle is an elongated, encapsulated sensory receptor composed of 2 to 10 thin, striated muscles (called intrafusal muscle fibers) two afferent nerve endings (called primary and secondary sensory endings), and a gamma motor nerve innervating the intrafusal muscle fibers. Each muscle spindle is oriented with its long axis parallel to the voluntary muscle fibers, called extrafusal fibers. The spindle acts as a strain gauge that constantly monitors the tension in the muscle. (From Noback CR, Demarest RJ: *The Nervous System: Introduction and Review*. New York, McGraw-Hill, 1972.)

interneuron, and the interneuron forms a synapse with the motoneuron. Therefore, the circuitry for this reflex has two synapses in the spinal cord. Transmission at both of these synapses is excitatory. Excitation of motoneurons by this reflex causes contraction of the flexor muscle, which pulls the limb away from the painful stimulus. Another branch of the sensory nerve forms a synapse with another interneuron which simultaneously inhibits the motoneuron to the corresponding extensor muscle and causes it to relax. Therefore, relfexes can cause contraction or relaxation.

1.4. Regulation of Skeletal Muscle by the Brain

The neurons which initiate movements (i.e., upper motoneurons) are located in the motor cortex of the cerebrum. Axons of these neurons project to the regions of brainstem and spinal cord where alpha motoneurons are found, but only a small percent form synapses with the lower motoneurons.[1] Usually an interneuron receives the input from upper motoneurons, and the interneuron forms a synapse with the motoneuron. Other brain regions involved in regulation of the skeletal muscles include the basal ganglia, reticular formation, and cerebellum (Fig. 3). Information from sensory nerves is also sent to the brain through the spinal cord (Fig. 4) and has a major impact on motor control. Thus, an extremely elaborate system of neuronal circuits is involved in maintaining and adjusting posture and executing smooth, coordinated movements.

1.5. Skeletal Muscle Spasm

Skeletal muscle spasm is an involuntary muscle contraction. It can be precipitated by local injury to the musculoskeletal system, musculoskeletal inflammation, or emotional stress. Injuries which may cause spasm include strains, sprains, and muscle, ligament, or tendon tears. All of these conditions result in marked stimulation of sensory nerve fibers (especially those mediating pain) and bombardment of the central nervous system with nerve impulses. Spinal reflexes will result in stimulation of alpha motoneurons and increased muscle tone. Sensory input also acts at supraspinal centers to cause a facilitation of gamma motoneurons. Contraction of intrafusal fibers activates

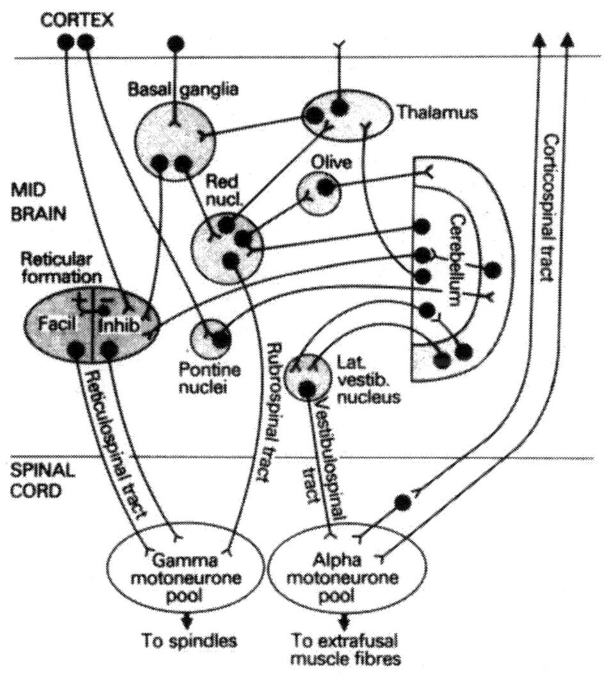

Figure 3. The main motor output from the central nervous system involved in the control of posture and movement. (From Bowman WC, Rand MJ: *Textbook of Pharmacology*, ed 2. London, Blackwell Scientific Publications, 1980.)

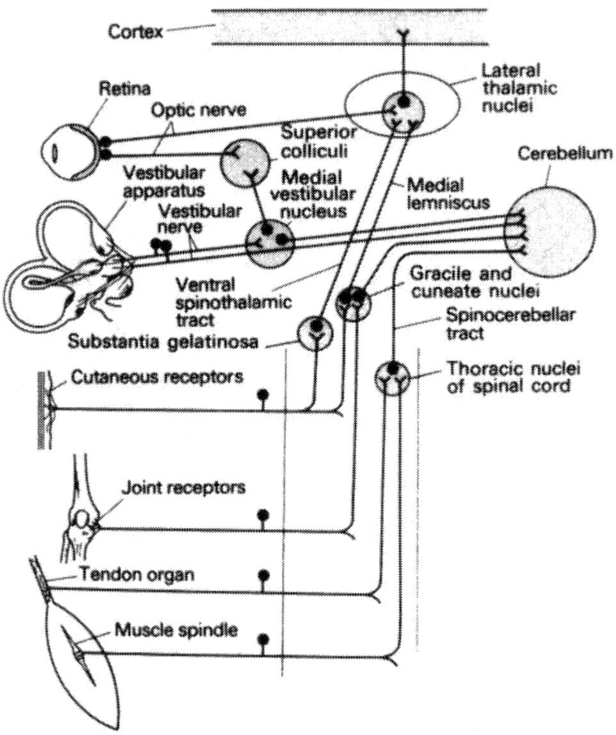

Figure 4. The main sensory input to the central nervous system involved in the control of posture and movement. (From Bowman WC, Rand MJ: *Textbook of Pharmacology*, ed 2. London, Blackwell Scientific Publications, 1980.)

sensory fibers in the muscle spindles and thereby provokes even greater activity of alpha motoneurons. The perception of pain by the brain and the consequent anxiety may also lead to activation of neural pathways which enhance firing of alpha motoneurons. Severe spasm may fuel itself by creating additional pain. Chronic inflammatory disorders (e.g., osteoarthritis) can generate muscle spasm by similar mechanisms.

Acute muscle spasm resulting from localized injury is usually self-limiting, having a duration of about two weeks. The tautness of the muscle can often be felt on physical examination. Pain is the most frequent complaint associated with muscle spasm and results in reduced range of movement and decreased mobility. Physical therapy is the primary treatment, but muscle relaxants and analgesics can be useful adjuncts in cases of moderate or severe spasm.

2. GENERAL MECHANISMS OF MUSCLE RELAXANTS

There are clearly several sites at which a drug could act to produce relaxation of skeletal muscle. Many of the drugs in clinical use cause muscle relaxation by effects within the central nervous system. The complexity of the neural pathways and the numerous neurotransmitters involved in the central regulation of skeletal muscles has made detailed analysis of mechanisms of drug action difficult, but the centrally acting muscle relaxants all produce changes that are reflected in a reduction in the activity of lower motoneurons. Another target for drug action to produce muscle relaxation is the neuromuscular junction. Drugs acting at this site block the chemical transmission which is mediated by acetylcholine. Agents used clinically work by blocking the action of acetylcholine after it is released from the nerve terminal of the motoneuron. There are also drugs which cause muscle relaxation by inhibiting synthesis of acetylcholine or by blocking its release from the nerve terminal. Although the latter drugs are not used clinically, they have been valuable tools in the study of chemical transmission at the neuromuscular junction. Finally, muscle relaxation can occur by drug action inside muscle cells. Dantrolene works at this inside location by inhibiting the release of stored calcium, which is required to trigger the contractile process.

3. DRUGS ACTING AT THE NEUROMUSCULAR JUNCTION

There are two major categories of drugs which produce muscle relaxation by blocking the action of acetylcholine at the neuromuscular junction. (+)-Tubocurarine is the prototype of the competitive, nondepolarizing class of neuromuscular blocking drugs and will be the agent from this category to be emphasized here. Several newer agents and their advantages will also be mentioned. The other category consists of drugs referred to as depolarizing neuromuscular blockers. Succinylcholine is the only agent from this group that is used clinically. The primary clinical application of the neuromuscular blocking drugs is as adjuncts to general anesthesia.

3.1. Competitive, Nondepolarizing Neuromuscular Blockers

3.1.1. Tubocurarine

Tubocurarine is the major active component of the South American arrow poisons referred to as curare. Indians prepared curare from specific plants and used it to kill animals for food. Animals impaled by an arrow or dart that had been dipped into curare would die from respiratory paralysis. Although tubocurarine could readily enter the bloodstream from the site of the arrow or dart tip, it was not well absorbed from the stomach or intestine. Consequently, the meat from animals killed with curare was safe for the Indians to eat.

Tubocurarine and other curare-like drugs produce skeletal muscle relaxation by an action at the neuromuscular junction. In the middle of the nineteenth century, the famous French physiologist Claude Bernard demonstrated that curare blocked nerve-stimulated muscle contractions when it was applied to the muscle but not when applied to the nerve. This observation was made many decades before the process of chemical transmission of nerve impulses was established. Today, we know that curare-like drugs bind to acetylcholine receptors on muscle fibers but do not cause opening of ion channels.[2] When tubocurarine is bound to the receptors at the neuromuscular junction, acetylcholine binding is blocked. Tubocurarine actually competes with acetylcholine for receptors and is therefore classified as a competitive antagonist of acetylcholine. Tubocurarine normally has an advantage in the competition because it is not metabolized by acetylcholinesterase whereas this enzyme rapidly destroys acetylcholine. The advantage can be shifted in favor of acetylcholine by administering a drug which inhibits acetylcholinesterase (e.g., neostigmine). This will allow the concentration of acetylcholine to build up in the junctional gap and, consequently, increases the probability of acetylcholine interacting with its receptors. Although curare-like drugs block skeletal muscle contractions caused by nerve stimulation or local injection of acetylcholine, contractions can still be produced by direct electrical stimulation of the muscle (Fig. 5). The latter method bypasses the acetylcholine receptor.

Tubocurarine is not well absorbed when taken orally, so it must be given by injection. The onset of neuromuscular blockade occurs promptly after intravenous admininstration of the drug. Initial muscle weakness is followed by flaccid paralysis of skeletal muscles. Muscles do not all relax at once, but rather a characteristic sequence is followed. Muscles of the fingers and eyes relax first, followed by muscles of the limbs, neck, and trunk. Muscles required for breathing (i.e., intercostals and diaphragm) are the last to be affected. As the drug effect wears off because of its metabolism and excretion, muscles recover in the reverse order (i.e., respiratory muscles recover first). A single dose of tubocurarine can produce clinically useful muscle relaxation of about 30 minutes duration, but a smaller magnitude of blockade persists for several hours. A smaller second dose of tubocurarine is capable of producing the same degree of blockade achieved with the first dose because of residual effects from the initial dose.

Prolonged neuromuscular blockade can result from administration of large amounts of tubocurarine. Under these circumstances, an inhibitor of acetylcholinesterase can be given to reverse the blockade. Adverse effects can also result from binding of tubocurarine to acetylcholine receptors in other tissues and from tubocurarine-stimulated release of histamine from mast cells.[3,4] Acetylcholine receptors on skeletal muscles, in ganglia of the autonomic nervous system, and in the adrenal medulla all belong to a subgroup called nicotinic receptors. Acetylcholine is the neurotransmitter at all of these sites, but nicotine will likewise cause stimulation by binding to these

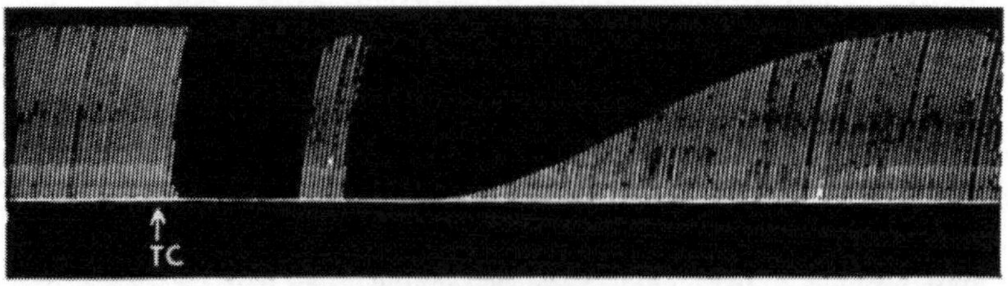

Figure 5. Effect of tubocurarine on contractions of the cat tibialis muscle evoked by motor nerve stimulation. At TC, 0.5 mg/kg of tubocurarine was injected intravenously. The contractions evoked by nerve stimulation were blocked but those elicited by direct stimulation of the muscle during the period marked by the horizontal bar were unaffected. (From Bowman WC: Chapter 16, in Laurence DR, Bacharach AL, (ed): *Evaluation of Drug Activities: Pharmacometrics,* vol 1. London, Academic Press, 1964.)

acetylcholine receptors. Skeletal muscle nicotinic receptors, however, have a different sensitivity to blocking drugs. Therapeutic doses of tubocurarine cause total blockade of skeletal nicotinic receptors but only a partial blockade of nicotinic receptors at autonomic ganglia and the adrenal medulla. Partial blockade of acetylcholine binding at these sites can reduce blood pressure and heart rate by decreasing the number of neuronal impulses (sympathetic nervous system) to the blood vessels and heart and by reducing release of epinephrine from the adrenal glands. Histamine released by tubocurarine may contribute to the decrease in blood pressure by dilating blood vessels. Although histamine can cause constriction of the airways, the amount released by tubocurarine does not appear to cause significant impairment of breathing in patients with normal respiratory function.[5] Tubocurarine is, however, contraindicated in patients with asthma.

3.1.2. Other Curare-like Drugs

Several other competitive, nondepolarizing neuromuscular blocking drugs have been developed in an effort to eliminate the adverse effects which are sometimes produced by tubocurarine. Atacurium and vercuronium are the newest neuromuscular blockers, and neither drug appears to produce cardiovascular side effects. At doses which produce muscle relaxation, these drugs do not block nicotinic receptors at sites other than the neuromuscular junction and usually do not cause release of histamine from mast cells. Gallamine and pancuronium are less prone to cause histamine release compared to tubocurarine and do not cause significant blockade of nicotinic receptors in autonomic ganglia at clinical doses. However, these drugs can increase heart rate by blocking muscarinic acetylcholine receptors in the heart. The increase in heart rate can, in some cases, cause an elevation of blood pressure. Metacurine has a similar chemical structure to tubocurarine, but clinical doses of this drug have little or no effect on histamine release and no blocking activity at autonomic ganglia.

3.2. Succinylcholine

Succinylcholine[6–8] is the only depolarizing neuromuscular blocker that is still used clinically. It causes neuromuscular blockade by binding to nicotinic receptors on skeletal muscle fibers, but the characteristics of the binding and its effects are different from those of curare-like drugs. The initial binding of succinylcholine to nicotinic receptors causes opening of ion channels and depolarization of the muscle membrane. These effects result in a brief period of unsynchronized muscle contractions, which are called fasciculations. After this initial stimulation, the muscle membrane stays depolarized and, consequently, is unresponsive to nerve stimulation. With prolonged exposure to succinylcholine or with high doses, the nature of the blockade can change. The muscle cell membrane repolarizes in spite of the continued presence of succinylcholine, but sensitivity to acetylcholine does not return. It has been suggested that blockade at this time may be due to temporary inability of receptors to mediate responses. This is referred to as desensitization.

Succinylcholine is administered by intravenous injection and has a very rapid onset of action. Muscle relaxation reaches a maximum within about 2 minutes and lasts for about 5 minutes. This short duration of action is the sole advantage of succinylcholine with respect to the curare-like drugs and is the result of rapid metabolic inactivation of the compound in the blood. Succinylcholine is not metabolized by acetylcholinesterase at the neuromuscular junction but is inactivated by a related enzyme called pseudocholinesterase (also called plasma cholinesterase). Pseudocholinesterase is made by the liver, and large amounts of this enzyme are found in the blood. Some individuals will experience very prolonged neuromuscular blockade after receiving succinylcholine because they have a deficiency of pseudocholinesterase or have an atypical enzyme that does not metabolize the drug. Both of these abnormalities have a genetic basis. Although only 1 in 100,000 patients will lack pseudocholinesterase, approximately 1 in 2500 patients will have a deficiency of pseudocholinesterase that is sufficient to caused increased sensitivity to succinylcholine.[6] A disadvantage of succinylcholine is the lack of a reliable drug for reversing its neuromuscular blocking action.

Several of the adverse effects associated with succinylcholine have been attributed to the depolarization and contraction of muscle fibers. Loss of potassium ions from depolarized muscle fibers elevates potassium ion concentration in the serum (hyperkalemia). This effect is negligible in most patients but can be quite substantial in burn patients and patients with motor nerve damage who develop an increased sensitivity to succinylcholine. Large increases in serum potassium can cause cardiac arrhythmias or cardiac arrest. Postoperative muscle pain occurs in a significant number of patients treated with succinylcholine. Several explanations have been proposed for this effect but all are based on the stimulant effect of the drug on skeletal muscles. The incidence of postoperative muscle pain is greater for ambulatory patients (70%) than it is for patients who remain in bed (10%).[5] Some patients will require analgesics for relief of this pain. Contracture of extraocular muscles is produced by succinylcholine and causes an increase of intraocular pressure which lasts for 5 to 10 minutes. Because of this effect, succinylcholine should not be used while the eye is opened surgically or from a wound.

Malignant hyperthermia is a rare adverse reaction (1 in 100,000 patients) which can result from effects of succinylcholine at skeletal muscle. It is most commonly seen in patients anesthetized with halothane and appears to have a genetic basis. Muscle rigidity is usually but not always present. The condition progresses rapidly and can be fatal. Dantrolene is effective in treating malignant hyperthermia.

Succinylcholine does not block autonomic ganglia as tubocurarine does, but it can cause some stimulation at these sites. Increases or decreases in heart rate can occur, depending on which specific autonomic ganglia are primarily affected.

3.3. Clinical Uses of the Neuromuscular Blocking Drugs

Neuromuscular blocking drugs are primarily used as adjuncts to general anesthesia. Relaxation of skeletal muscles is an important component of general anesthesia because it facilitates surgical manipulations. In orthopedic medicine, this effect aids in the repair of dislocations and fractures. The ideal gaseous anesthetic would be able to cause unconsciousness, amnesia, analgesia, and muscle relaxation needed for surgery, but good muscle relaxation cannot usually be obtained safely by using only anesthetic gas. The use of neuromuscular blockers along with gaseous anesthetics reduces the amount of gas required and, therefore, increases the safety of general anesthesia. Anesthetics also increase the effectiveness of neuromuscular blockers and can decrease the severity of fasciculations produced by succinylcholine. The choice of neuromuscular blocker for use during surgery depends on the duration of the procedure and patient pathology which might predispose to adverse effects with a specific drug. Succinylcholine is used for brief procedures such as placement of an endotracheal tube. Curare-like drugs are used for longer procedures because they have fewer adverse effects and can be reversed with drugs which inhibit cholinesterases. Succinylcholine should not be used for long procedures because of increased potential for adverse effects, variable characteristics of blockade, and lack of a reliable drug for reversing the blockade. Ventilation must be controlled by the anesthetist when neuromuscular blockers are used because skeletal muscles used in breathing are also paralyzed by these drugs.

Neuromuscular blockers are used with general anesthetics during electroconvulsive shock therapy to prevent fractures and dislocations. These agents may also be used to inhibit the muscle spasms associated with tetanus.

4. CENTRALLY ACTING SKELETAL MUSCLE RELAXANTS

Numerous centrally active drugs are available for use in the treatment of skeletal muscle spasm. Three of these drugs (diazepam, cyclobenzaprine, and chlorzoxazone w/acetaminophen) are included in a recent listing of the 200 most prescribed drugs.[9] Centrally acting muscle relaxants have many dissimilarities in chemical structure but have many similar pharmacological properties. Most of them disrupt polysynaptic reflexes and can cause sedation. Some authorities believe that sedation is the basis for their effectiveness as muscle relaxants. Potential side effects are likewise similar, with drowsiness being most common. Most of the centrally acting muscle relaxants are central nervous system depressants, and an enhanced depression of central function can result if taken in combination with other depressants such as alcohol. Finally, some of these agents can cause physical and psychological dependence with prolonged use.

4.1. Diazepam

Diazepam (Valium) is a widely prescribed drug which belongs to the benzodiazepine chemical family. Benzodiazepines are most commonly used in the treatment of anxiety and insomnia. Diazepam is also approved for use as a skeletal muscle relaxant.

The actions of diazepam and other benzodiazepines are closely linked to one central nervous system neurotransmitter, gamma-aminobutyric acid (GABA). GABA is a neurotransmitter which is frequently used by interneurons in the spinal cord and brain. These GABAergic neurons release GABA in the same fashion that lower motoneurons release acetylcholine. Binding of GABA to specific GABA receptors on neurons which receive input from GABAergic nerons produces an inhibitory effect (i.e., decreased neuronal excitability). Benzodiazepine receptors have recently been found to exist in close association with GABA receptors.[10] Binding of diazepam to benzodiazepine receptors enhances the effectiness of GABA (i.e., GABA causes greater inhibition). Naturally, the benzodiazepine receptors are not present in the brain for the purpose of mediating the effect of drugs. It is postulated that the nervous system makes some chemical which utilizes these receptors in producing its effects and that diazepam binds to these sites because of a structural resemblence to the endogenous chemical.[11]

Animal experiments have demonstrated that diazepam inhibits polysynaptic spinal reflexes. However, inhibition of polysynaptic pathways located in the reticular formation of the brainstem may be more important in producing relaxation of skeletal muscles.[12] It has also been shown that neurons in the reticular formation are more easily inhibited by diazepam than are spinal interneurons. In addition, the antianxiety effect of diazepam has been suggested to contribute to the patient response in conditions that are thought to have a psychological component (e.g., lower-back pain).

Diazepam is marketed in tablets and time-release capsules for oral use. An injectable formulation is available for intramuscular or intravenous administration of the drug. The liver has a major role in the fate of diazepam in the body. The drug undergoes extensive metabolism at this site. Some active metabolites are formed and contribute significantly to the duration of response. Eventually, metabolites of diazepam are eliminated by the kidneys. These can be readily detected in drug screens of the urine.

At doses used for relaxation of skeletal muscle, diazepam can cause drowsiness and some impairment of motor and intellectual function. Overdoses cause depression of the central nervous system and can necessitate support of respiratory and cardiovascular function. Fatal overdose from diazepam alone is reportedly uncommon.[13] However, diazepam overdose in combination with other central nervous system depressants (e.g., alcohol) has frequently resulted in death.

Diazepam and other benzodiazepines are capable of causing physical and psychological dependence, but their abuse potential is relatively low.[13] Development of physical dependence on the benzodiazepines is most likely to occur with long-term therapy (two months or more). Diazepam would generally be used on a short-term basis for treatment of muscle spasm resulting from injury. The withdrawal syndrome which occurs following long-term use of benzodiazepines is generally mild if normal doses were taken. The patient might experience symptoms such as anxiety, tension, difficulty concentrating, and sensory disturbances. In contrast, severe reactions have been reported to occur during withdrawal from high doses of benzodiazepines. Such withdrawal reactions can generally be avoided by gradual dose reduction.

4.2. Chemical Congeners of Mephenesin

Chlorphenesin carbamate (Maolate) and methocarbamol (Robaxin) are chemical analogues of mephenesin. Mephenesin was the first centrally acting compound to be studied extensively for its ability to cause relaxation of skeletal muscles.[1,14] Its effects in animals can range from decreased muscle tone at low doses to unconsciousness, respiratory depression, and death at much higher doses. Its overall effects appear similar to those of barbiturates with the distinction that greater muscle relaxation occurs at doses causing equivalent levels of sedation.[14] Experimental data indicate that mephenesin can block polysynaptic reflexes at lower doses than required for blocking monosynaptic reflexes (Fig. 6), but the exact mechanism by which it produces skeletal muscle relaxation has still not been firmly established. Mephenesin is no longer used clinically because it has a short duration of action and produces more adverse effects than newer drugs. It is still used, however, as a standard for comparison in some basic studies. Recent experiments have demonstrated that chlorphenesin carbamate blocks polysynaptic pathways at both spinal and supraspinal levels.[15] It has also been shown that this drug decreases the excitability of lower motoneurons. Methocarbamol presumably has similar actions.

Chlorphenesin carbamate and methocarbamol are available in tablet form for oral administration. Methocarbamol is also marketed in a formulation for intravenous or intramuscular injection. Both drugs are inactivated in the liver, and metabolites are eliminated in the urine. Methocarbamol has a shorter half-life than chlorphenesin carbamate. Drowsiness and dizziness are the most frequent side effects caused by these drugs. Decreases in heart rate and blood pressure can occur with intravenous administration of methocarbamol.

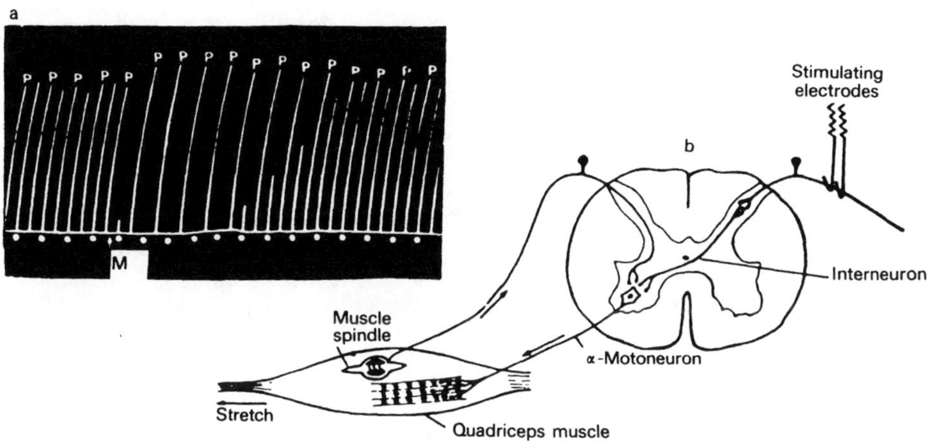

Figure 6. Effects of mephenesin on spinal reflexes. (a) Kymograph recording of contractions of the quadriceps femoris muscle of an anesthetized cat elicited every 30 s, alternatively by tapping the patellar tendon (monosynaptic stretch reflex; contractions labeled P) and by stimulating the central end of the cut contralateral sciatic nerve (polysynaptic crossed-extensor reflex; contractions unlabeled). At M, 15 mg/kg of mephenesin was injected intravenously. Mephenesin blocked the crossed-extensor reflex but slightly potentiated the patellar reflex, probably because it blocked inhibitory interneurons that normally exert a suppressant action on the monosynaptic pathway. (b) Neuronal pathways involved in the experiment illustrated in (a). (From Bowman WC, Rand MJ: *Textbook of Pharmacology,* ed. 2. London, Blackwell Scientific Publications, 1980.)

4.3. Chlorzoxazone

Chlorzoxazone (Paraflex) has a distinct chemical structure from mephenesin but has the same or a very similar mechanism for causing skeletal muscle relaxation. Animal studies have shown that it inhibits brainstem and spinal polysynaptic pathways that facilitate motoneuron activity. Chlorzoxazone is taken orally and metabolized by the liver. Its primary side effects are gastrointestinal disturbances and drowsiness. Liver damage has occurred in a very small number of patients who received chlorzoxazone, but it has not been established whether this pathology was caused by the drug.

4.4. Cyclobenzaprine

Cyclobenzaprine (Flexeril) is similar in chemical structure to the tricyclic antidepressants and has some side effects typical for that group of drugs. Its effects have been examined in a number of animal experimental models used for screening of potential muscle relaxants.[16] In particular, cyclobenzaprine has been shown to alleviate muscle hyperactivity that occurs in decerebrate cat preparations. Muscle relaxation is produced with doses of drug which do not produce ataxia or obvious behavioral depression. Although cyclobenzaprine has both spinal and supraspinal actions, the latter appear to be more important.[16–18] The brainstem has been implicated as a major target site for cyclobenzaprine, and it has been suggested that its effect may be the removal of a reticulospinal input that facilitates motoneuron activity (see Fig. 3). Recent evidence has implicated the locus coeruleus in the actions of cyclobenzaprine.[19] The locus coeruleus is a major nucleus of noradrenergic neurons in the brainstem, and its projections to the spinal cord enhance monosynaptic reflexes. Cyclobenzaprine depresses monosynaptic reflex responses in experimental animals and also inhibits the activity of neurons in the locus coeruleus. Phenoxybenzamine, a drug which blocks responses at alpha adrenergic receptors, also depresses monosynaptic reflex responses, and cyclobenzaprine is unable to cause significant additional suppression after adrenergic receptor blockade. The implication of these observations is that cyclobenzaprine suppresses monosynaptic reflexes by inhibiting the noradrenergic neurons which normally facilitate the response. The contribution of central noradrenergic neurons to the muscle relaxant effects of cyclobenzaprine have not been studied in man.

Cyclobenzaprine is taken orally and is well absorbed. It is highly bound to plasma proteins and has a long elimination half-life (1 to 3 days). In spite of this long half-life, the drug is generally taken three times daily. Hepatic metabolism of cyclobenzaprine is extensive, and metabolites are eliminated in the urine.

Drowsiness, dry mouth, and dizziness are the most frequently reported adverse effects. Premarketing trials found a 40% incidence of drowsiness, but the incidence was less in postmarketing surveillance.[20] Dry mouth results from the blocking action of cyclobenzaprine at muscarinic acetylcholine receptors. Other less common side effects which can occur because of muscarinic receptor blockade include blurred vision, increased heart rate, constipation, and urinary retention. Cyclobenzaprine will enhance the effects of muscarinic receptor blocking drugs and central nervous system depressants. Adverse effects can also result if cyclobenzaprine is given to patients being treated for depression with monoamine oxidase inhibitors. Potential for this interaction persists for about 14 days after monoamine oxidase inhibitors are discontinued.

4.5. Orphenadrine

Orphenadrine (Norflex) is structurally related to the antihistamine diphenhydramine (Benadryl). It has activity as an antihistamine, muscarinic receptor blocker, and local anesthetic. The drug is sometimes used in treating parkinsonism, the basis for its effectiveness being the blockade of muscarinic receptors in the striatum. The mechanism for its effect as a centrally acting muscle relaxant has not been determined but may be related to the blockade of central muscarinic receptors.

Orphenadrine is usually taken orally. Its primary side effects are due to blockade of peripheral muscarinic receptors (e.g., dry mouth).

4.6. Carisoprodol

Carisoprodol is structurally related to the sedative–hypnotic drug meprobamate (Miltown) and is sold by a number of pharmaceutical companies (under the trade name Rela, Soma, and Soprodol). The drug inhibits brainstem and spinal polysynaptic pathways and has sedation as a primary side effect. Because of its similarity to meprobamate, it might be anticipated that long-term use of carisoprodol could produce physical and psychological dependence.

4.7. Clinical Use of Centrally Acting Muscle Relaxants

Centrally acting muscle relaxants are approved for use as adjuncts to rest and physical therapy in the treatment of acute musculoskeletal conditions. Analgesics and anti-inflammatory drugs can also be used in the treatment of these conditions. Numerous clinical studies have examined the effectiveness of muscle relaxants in relieving the muscle spasm and pain that is associated with trauma (e.g., strains, sprains, and contusions) or inflammation. Elenbaas[21] has reviewed much of the literature on this topic and has noted that many studies have been flawed by not defining patient selection criteria, by not controlling for factors such as physical therapy and other medications, and by use of improper statistical methods. She also noted the lack of objective methods for the evaluation of muscle spasm and the self-limiting nature of the condition. Taking these factors into consideration, she concluded that none of the centrally acting muscle relaxants could be singled out as superior to others when given orally. Most centrally acting muscle relaxants are usually judged superior to placebo on the basis of subjective evaluation. It should be noted that placebo responses are often quite high in these studies. Elenbaas was unable to conclude whether the muscle relaxants are better than analgesics or physical therapy. There have been no landmark studies since this review which would alter its conclusions.

Parenteral preparations of diazepam and methocarbamol are available and can be

Table 1. Muscle Relaxant–Analgesic Combinations

Trade name	Components
Norgesic	25 mg orphenadrine citrate 385 mg aspirin 30 mg caffeine
Norgesic Forte	50 mg orphenadrine 770 mg aspirin 60 mg caffeine
Parafon Forte	250 mg chlorzoxazone 300 mg acetaminophen
Robaxisal	400 mg methocarbamol 325 mg aspirin
Soma Compound	200 mg carisoprodol 325 mg aspirin
Soma Compound with Codeine	200 mg carisoprodol 325 mg aspirin 16 mg codeine phosphate

very useful in the initial management of moderate to severe muscle spasm. If muscle relaxants are continued, an oral preparation would be used.

The adverse effects of individual muscle relaxants have already been noted. Sedation can be produced by all of these drugs, and some authorities believe that this is the basis of their effectiveness. Sedation could impair both intellectual and motor performance. The self-limiting nature of acute musculoskeletal disorders and the occurrence of side effects with the oral muscle relaxants provide a strong rationale for keeping the duration of therapy as brief as possible.

Many of the centrally acting muscle relaxants are also marketed in combination with an analgesic (Table 1). The rationale behind these preparations is the inclusion of ingredients for both muscle spasm and pain. There have been fewer clinical investigations of these preparations, and the FDA has classified them as "possibly" effective. Although the use of an analgesic and a muscle relaxant may seem logical based on the symptoms, use of separate preparations would allow more flexibility in dosing.

It should be noted that none of the drugs reviewed in this section, with the exception of diazepam, are effective in the treatment of spasticity caused by neurological disorders. Diazepam can also be used for treating the muscle spasm of tetanus.

REFERENCES

1. Bowman WC, Rand MJ: *Textbook of Pharmacology*, ed 2. London, Blackwell Scientific Publications, 1980.
2. Colquhoun D: On the principles of postsynaptic action of neuromuscular blocking agents, in Kharkevich DA (ed): *New Neuromuscular Blocking Agents*. Berlin, Springer-Verlag, 1986, p 59.

3. Bowman WC: Non-relaxant properties of neuromuscular blocking drugs. *Br J Anaesth* 54:147–160, 1982.
4. Kharkevich DA, Shorr VA: Antimuscarinic and ganglion-blocking activity of neuromuscular blocking agents, in Kharkevich DA (ed): *New Neuromuscular Blocking Agents*. Berlin, Springer-Verlag, 1986, p 191.
5. AMA Drug Evaluations, ed 5. Chicago, American Medical Association, 1983.
6. Durant NN, Katz RL: Suxamethonium. *Br J Anaesth* 54:195–208, 1982.
7. Smith SE: Neuromuscular blocking drugs in man, in Zaimis E (ed): *Neuromuscular Junction*. Berlin, Springer-Verlag, 1976, p 593.
8. Zamis E, Head S: Depolarizing neuromuscular blocking drugs, in Zaimis E (ed): *Neuromuscular Junction*. Berlin, Springer-Verlag, 1976, p 365.
9. The top 200 Rx drugs of 1986. *Am Druggist,* February 1987, pp 19–32.
10. Martin IL: The benzodiazepine receptor: functional complexity. *TIPS* 5:343–347, 1984.
11. Guidotti A, Forchetti CM, Corda MG, et al: Isolation, characterization, and purification to homogeneity of an endogenous polypeptide with agonistic action on benzodiazepine receptors. *Proc Natl Acad Sci USA* 80:3531–3535, 1983.
12. Tseng T-C, Wang SC: Locus of action of centrally acting muscle relaxants, diazepam and tybamate. *J Pharmacol Exp Ther* 178:350–360, 1971.
13. Hyman SE, Arana GW: *Handbook of Psychiatric Drug Therapy*. Boston, Little, Brown, 1987.
14. Smith CM: Relaxants of skeletal muscle, in Roots WS, Hofmann FG (eds): *Physiological Pharmacology*. New York, Academic Press, vol 2, 1965, p 1.
15. Kurachi M, Aihara H: Effect of a muscle relaxant, chlorphenesin carbamate, on spinal neurons of rats. *Japan J Pharmacol* 36:7–13, 1984.
16. Share NN, McFarlane CS: Cyclobenzaprine: a novel centrally acting skeletal muscle relaxant. *Neuropharmacology* 14:675–684, 1975.
17. Share NN: Cyclobenzaprine: effect on segmental monosynaptic and tonic vibration reflexes in the cat. *Neuropharmacology* 17:721–727, 1978.
18. Barnes CD, Adams WL: Effects of cyclobenzaprine on interneurones of the spinal cord. *Neuropharmacology* 17:445–450, 1978.
19. Barnes CD, Fung SJ, Gintautas J: Brainstem noradrenergic system depression by cyclobenzaprine. *Neuropharmacology* 19:221–224, 1980.
20. Nibbelink DW, Strickland SC: Cyclobenzaprine (Flexeril): report of a postmarketing surveillance program. *Curr Therap Res* 28:894–903, 1980.
21. Elenbaas JK: Centrally acting oral skeletal muscle relaxants. *Am J Hosp Pharm* 37:1313–1323, 1980.

7

Anabolic and Androgenic Steroids

Edward J. Keenan

Androgens are steroid hormones that possess virilizing (androgenic) actions and, consequently, serve to stimulate differentiation and maintenance of the androgen-dependent tissues of the male reproductive system. These hormones also play an important role in facilitating protein synthesis (anabolic actions) in androgen-sensitive tissues such as skeletal muscle, the kidneys, and bone. The fact that testosterone and related hormones produce both androgenic and anabolic actions has been recognized since the 1930s. Not surprisingly, much effort has been devoted since then to the development of androgens that are devoid of virilizing actions. To a certain extent, this has been accomplished with the synthesis of 19-nortestosterone derivatives of the natural androgen, testosterone.

The stimulatory effects of androgens on protein synthesis have been of therapeutic interest and since the 1950s have been exploited by some athletes to enhance performance. The use of androgens by athletes has never been condoned by either physicians or athletic officials, nor has the effectiveness of these drugs in enhancing athletic performance or muscle strength been conclusively demonstrated. Furthermore, the androgens are capable of producing significant undesirable effects. Hence, the use of androgenic and anabolic steroids by athletes for nontherapeutic purposes should be considered unethical, trivial, and potentially harmful.

1. PHYSIOLOGY OF THE ANDROGENS

The physiologically important androgens in the male are synthesized and secreted by the Leydig cells of the testes. In women, androgens are produced by the ovaries, the adrenal cortex, and the placenta. Testosterone is the principal biologically active androgen in the blood of both men and women, and it is characterized as a 19-carbon steroid derived from cholesterol (Fig. 1). The presence of angular methyl groups at positions 18 and 19 is the fundamental structural characteristic of the androgenic

Edward J. Keenan • Departments of Pharmacology, Surgery, and Medicine, School of Medicine, The Oregon Health Sciences University, Portland, Oregon 97201.

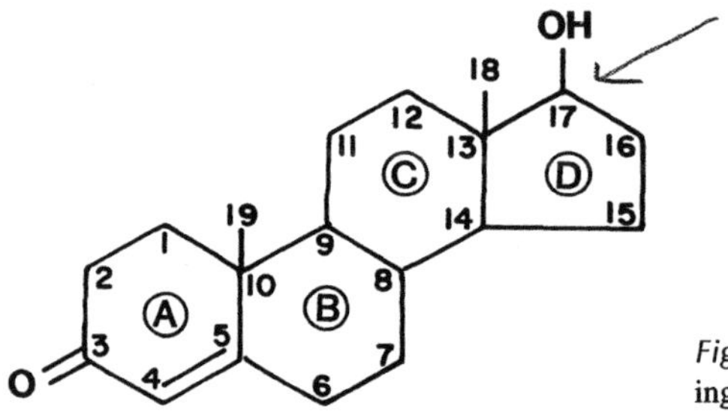

Figure 1. Molecular structure of testosterone, showing the numbering of the carbon atoms.

steroids. Substitution of a hydrogen atom at position 5 yields the more potent series of androgens, the androstanes, of which 5α-dihydrotestosterone (DHT) is a significant member. Like most steroid hormones, the androgens are highly lipid soluble, a property that markedly influences their pharmacological use. Because of its chemical characteristics, testosterone is poorly absorbed from the gastrointestinal tract. The testosterone that is absorbed is readily inactivated by hepatic oxidative enzyme systems. Chemical modifications of the testosterone molecule have increased the therapeutic usefulness of the androgenic steroids. For example, alkylation at the C-17 position confers significant oral efficacy due to reduced susceptibility to hepatic metabolism. As will be discussed later, additional molecular alterations result in androgens that exhibit predominantly anabolic effects as compared to virilizing androgenic effects (i.e., the 19-nortestosterone derivatives).

Regulation of testicular androgen biosynthesis involves an intricate balance among the hypothalamus, the adenohypophysis, and the testes. Gonadotropin-releasing hormone (GnRH) is released by the hypothalamus and traverses the hypothalamic–adenohypophyseal portal vasculature to interact with specific receptor sites incorporated in the plasma membranes of pituitary gonadotrophs. GnRH stimulates the release of luteinizing hormone (LH) and follicle-stimulating hormone (FSH) from the anterior pituitary gland into the systemic circulation. Subsequently, LH stimulates the biosynthesis of testosterone by the testicular Leydig cells. FSH is responsible for regulating Sertoli cell function and spermatogenesis, which are further dependent on androgens. Circulating androgens, principally testosterone, exert negative feedback effects on the adenohypophysis and the hypothalamus, suppressing LH and GnRH release and thereby modulating peripheral levels of androgens (Fig. 2). Administration of exogenous androgen also causes negative feedback inhibition of the testicular function.

In men, total plasma levels of testosterone change very little with age. Although the rate of secretion of testosterone declines after the fifth decade of life, a commensurate reduction in clearance of the androgens occurs, resulting in relatively stable blood levels of testosterone throughout adulthood. It does appear that the concentration of unbound (i.e., free) testosterone declines with age.

In men and women, approximately 98% of peripheral testosterone is bound to plasma proteins. These proteins consist primarily of sex hormone-binding globulin

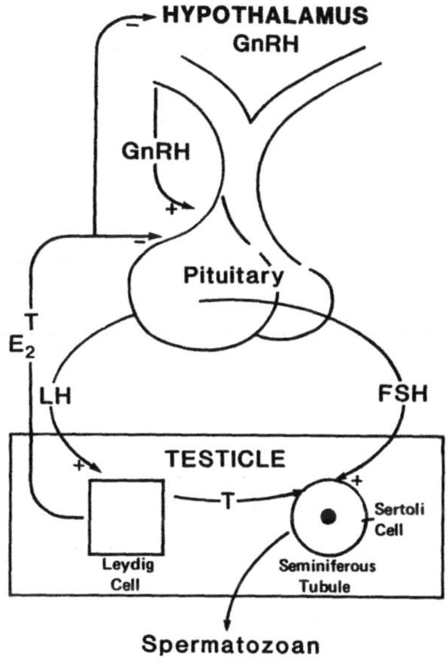

Figure 2. Regulation of testicular androgen biosynthesis. E_2, estradiol; FSH, follicle-stimulating hormone; GnRH, gonadotropin-releasing hormone; LH, luteinizing hormone; T, testosterone.

(SHBG) and albumin (Fig. 3). The binding to albumin is relatively nonspecific, demonstrates low affinity, and is of high capacity. In contrast, the association of testosterone with SHBG is specific, demonstrates high affinity, and is of limited capacity. Approximately 58% of plasma testosterone is bound to SHBG, 40% is bound to albumin, and the remaining 2% is unbound (free). Only the free testosterone is available for assimilation by peripheral target and nontarget tissues. Therefore, exogenous androgens are generally available for distribution to peripheral tissues.

The unbound testosterone or related analogues are available either for oxidative metabolism by the liver and subsequent renal excretion or for assimilation by androgen-dependent tissues (e.g., prostate, seminal vesicles, epididymis) and by androgen-sensitive tissues (e.g., kidney, skeletal muscle, bone, hypothalamus). Reductive metabolism of testosterone predominates in androgen-dependent tissues. Testosterone is reduced to 5α-DHT and subsequently to androstanediol. The plasma half-life of testosterone is approximately 10 to 20 min; its short half-life largely limits the therapeutic use of this natural androgen.

The hepatic metabolism of testosterone involves the production of the primary metabolites etiocholanolone and androsterone, as well as small amounts of testosterone glucuronides and sulfates that are eliminated via the kidney. Only 6% of the testosterone is excreted unchanged, usually via the bile (Fig. 3). The result of hepatic metabolism of testosterone is increased solubility relative to testosterone, and an increased urinary elimination of testosterone metabolites.

Free testosterone entering androgen-dependent tissues such as the prostate gland and related male accessory organs is readily metabolized to the 5α-DHT derivative. DHT is about 1.5 to 2.5 times more potent than testosterone as an androgenic steroid.

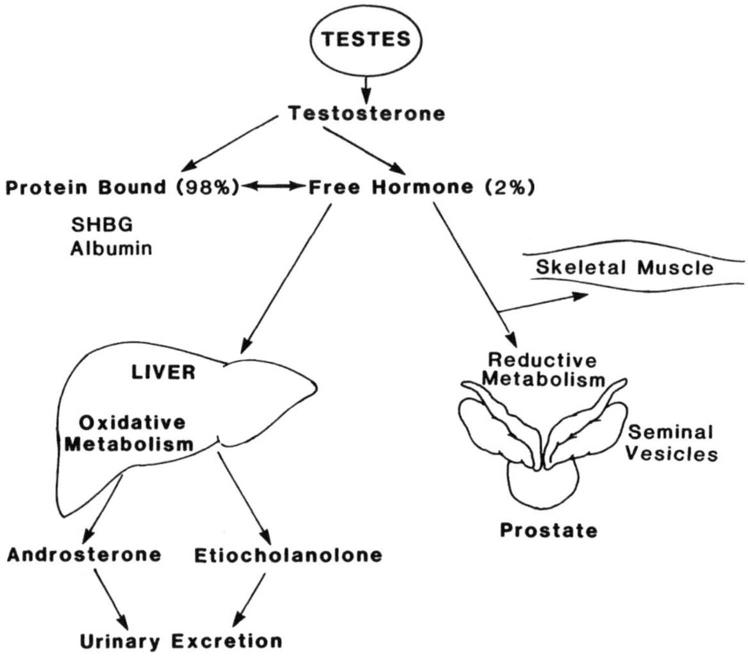

Figure 3. Dynamics of androgen assimilation. SHBG, sex-hormone-binding globulin.

Androgen-sensitive tissues such as the kidneys and skeletal muscles are organs that do not grow in response to testosterone but are otherwise influenced by testosterone. In general, these tissues do not readily convert testosterone to 5α-reduced metabolites, and testosterone itself represents the active androgen.

Androgens, like all steroid hormones, produce their effects in target cells by associating with specific receptor proteins that exhibit both a high degree of specificity and a high affinity for androgenic steroids and related derivatives (Fig. 4). Androgen-dependent and -sensitive tissues contain cytosolic and nuclear receptor proteins that recognize both testosterone and dihydrotestosterone. Little is known concerning the actual activation process for androgen receptors or the precise nature of the molecular events that mediate androgen effects. However, the importance of androgen receptors in mediating the actions of androgens is well recognized and is supported by the existence of complete or partial androgen insensitivity syndromes in humans that result from androgen receptor absence or the presence of abnormal androgen receptor proteins.

Normally, the majority (70–80%) of androgen receptors are localized in the nuclear compartment. The predominance of androgen receptors in the nucleus is a reflection of the relatively stable circulating levels of testosterone and of the significant availability of DHT in target tissues. In the nucleus, the androgen–receptor complexes associate with select sites on DNA, resulting in the stimulation of RNA synthesis and

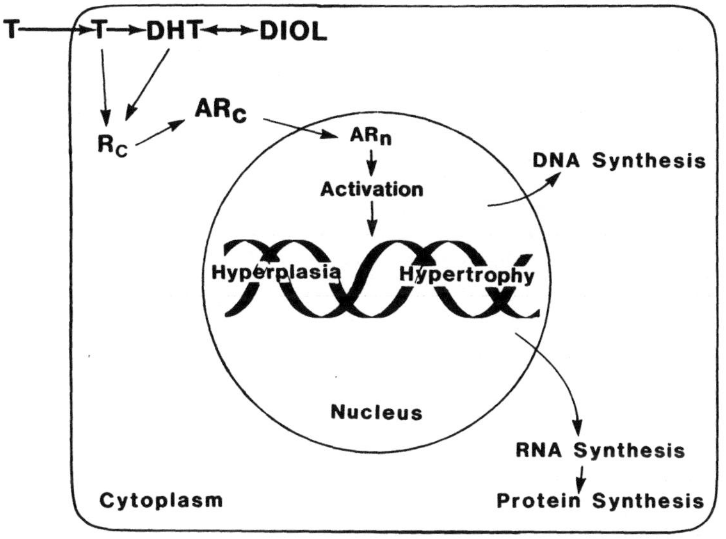

Figure 4. Schematic representation of the mechanism of androgen action. AR_c, androgen–cytosolic receptor complex; AR_n, androgen–nuclear receptor complex; DHT, dihydrotesterone; Diol, androstanediol; R_c, cytoplasmic receptor; T, testosterone.

protein synthesis and, at the appropriate periods of development, the proliferation of androgen-dependent target cells (Fig. 4).

2. PHYSIOLOGICAL AND PHARMACOLOGICAL ACTIONS OF THE ANDROGENS

The androgens in males are responsible for the development and maintenance of the secondary sexual characteristics, normal reproductive function, and sexual performance. Androgens also stimulate growth and development of the skeleton and skeletal muscles during puberty (Table 1). These hormones induce increases in long bone growth and subsequently terminate growth by initiating closure of the epiphyseal plates. Consequently, exposure of prepubertal males to excessive doses of androgens can interrupt skeletal development due to premature closing of the growth plates.

Growth of pubic hair and probably stimulation of libido are functions of androgens in women. Excessive production of androgens in women results in virilization characterized by acne, hirsutism, hoarseness, baldness, clitoromegaly, and menstrual irregularities.

The role of androgens in mediating aggressive male behavior is poorly understood, probably due to the complexity of factors influencing expression of behavior. It is likely that not only peripheral levels of androgens but also the androgen-mediated imprinting of behavior combine to constitute the male behavioral pattern. Additional

Table 1. Physiological and Pharmacological Actions of the Androgens

Androgenic actions
Stimulate development of male reproductive tract *in utero*
Stimulate growth of male accessory sex organs, penis, and scrotum at puberty
Stimulate long bone growth and subsequent induction of epiphyseal plate closure at puberty
Maintain male secondary sex characteristics
Increase libido
Aggravate aggressive behavior in males (?)
Anabolic actions
Stimulate muscle development
Stimulate erythropoiesis

factors are no doubt involved. In athletes, androgens are believed by some to enhance the motivation to train and thereby to lead to better physical development.

The physiological and pharmacological actions of androgens can be further classified as either morphogenic or excitatory, i.e., maintenance activity. The morphogenic actions occur during embryogenesis and involve differentiation of the central nervous system and male reproductive system. The excitatory or maintenance actions consist of the pubertal and postpubertal effects of androgens on the male reproductive system and skeletal muscles. These effects are generally reversible, while the *in utero* effects of androgens are irreversible. Androgens are not involved in gonadal differentiation, but they do stimulate differentiation of the Wolffian ducts into seminal vesicles, epididymis, and vas deferens. Androgens also stimulate the development of the labioscrotal swellings into the scrotum, the genital tubercle into the penis, and the urogenital sinus into the prostate gland. In addition to the protein anabolic actions of androgens on skeletal muscle, these steroids stimulate erythropoiesis by increasing renal production of erythropoietin and by exerting direct effects on bone marrow stem cell division.

3. ANDROGENIC AND ANABOLIC STEROID DRUGS

The androgens are classified broadly as either androgenic or anabolic in terms of biological activity. It should be emphasized that no androgen exhibits solely androgenic or anabolic effects. The androgenic steroid drugs are listed in Table 2. These agents are further delineated as either natural and esterified androgens or as 17α-alkylated derivatives (Fig. 5). Esterification of testosterone extends its duration of action by delaying systemic absorption from intramuscular sites. In general, the longer the carbon chain of the ester substituent, the slower is the release of the hormone into the circulation from intramuscular depot sites. Testosterone propionate is administered intramuscularly two to three times per week, while the longer-acting cypionate and

Table 2. The Androgenic Steroid Drugs

Drug	Trade name
Natural and esterified derivatives	
Testosterone	Oreton, Neo-Hombreol
Testosterone propionate	Oreton Propionate
Testosterone cypionate	Andro-Cyp, Depo-Testosterone, T-Ionate-PA
Testosterone enanthate	Andryl, Delatestryl, generic
17α-Alkylated derivatives	
Methyltestosterone	Metandren, Oreton Methyl, Testred
Fluoxymesterone	Halotestin

enanthate derivatives are injected at two- to four-week intervals. Alkylation at the 17α-position retards the hepatic oxidative metabolism of testosterone. Therefore, methyltestosterone and fluoxymesterone are orally active androgenic steroid drugs. In contrast to the esterified derivatives, these androgenic hormones must be administered daily. The half-lives of the orally active androgenic steroids are brief, 10 hr for fluoxymesterone and 2.5 h for methyltestosterone. Alkylation of the 17α-position confers the potential for inducing hepatotoxicity.

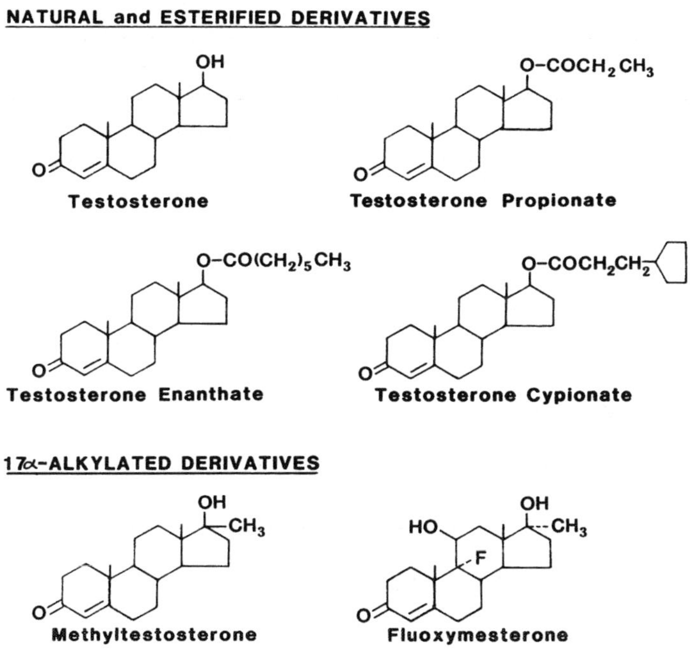

Figure 5. Chemical structure of the androgenic steroid drugs.

The androgens that predominantly produce anabolic activity are listed in Table 3, and their molecular structures are depicted in Fig. 6. It can be seen that some of these drugs are 19-nortestosterone derivatives, i.e., they lack the C-19 methyl group. Anabolic androgens can be administered either orally or parenterally (Table 3). Ethylestrenol, methandrostenolone, oxandrolone, oxymetholone, and stanozolol are orally active as a result of aklylation at C-17 of the androgen steroid nucleus. The anabolic steroids suitable for intramuscular injection are nandrolone phenpropionate, nandrolone decanoate, and methandriol. Among this group of anabolic drugs, only methandriol contains a 17α-alkyl group (Fig. 6). The anabolic actions of these steroid drugs are largely a reflection of dose. When administered in high doses, even the anabolic androgens will produce virilizing side effects.

4. THERAPEUTIC USES OF THE ANDROGENS

4.1. Androgenic Steroid Drugs

The androgenic steroids are used primarily for the induction of puberty in hypogonadism and in replacement or maintenance therapy in hypogonadism resulting from pre- or postpubertal failure of the testes (Table 4). The longer-acting esterified derivatives of testosterone, the cypionate and enanthate esters, are preferred for induction of full sexual development when normal pubertal development fails. Administration of 100 to 200 mg every two weeks will establish normal adult male plasma levels of testosterone. The use of the long-acting esters is convenient and also avoids the potential hepatotoxicity associated with the 17α-alkylated derivatives.

Testosterone propionate, the short-acting ester form, must be administered parenterally several times a week and is therefore not convenient for long-term replacement therapy. In older patients requiring androgenic steroids, the initial administration of a

Table 3. The Anabolic Steroid Drugs

Drug	Trade name
Oral administration	
Ethylestrenol	Maxibolin
Methandrostenolone	Dianabol
Oxandrolone	Anavar
Oxymetholone	Anadrol-50
Stanozolol	Winstrol
Parenteral administration	
Nandrolone phenpropionate	Androlone, Durabolin, Nandrolin
Nandrolone decanoate	Androlone-D, Deca-Durabolin
Methandriol	Anabol, Durabolic, Methabolic, Methyldiol, Steribolic

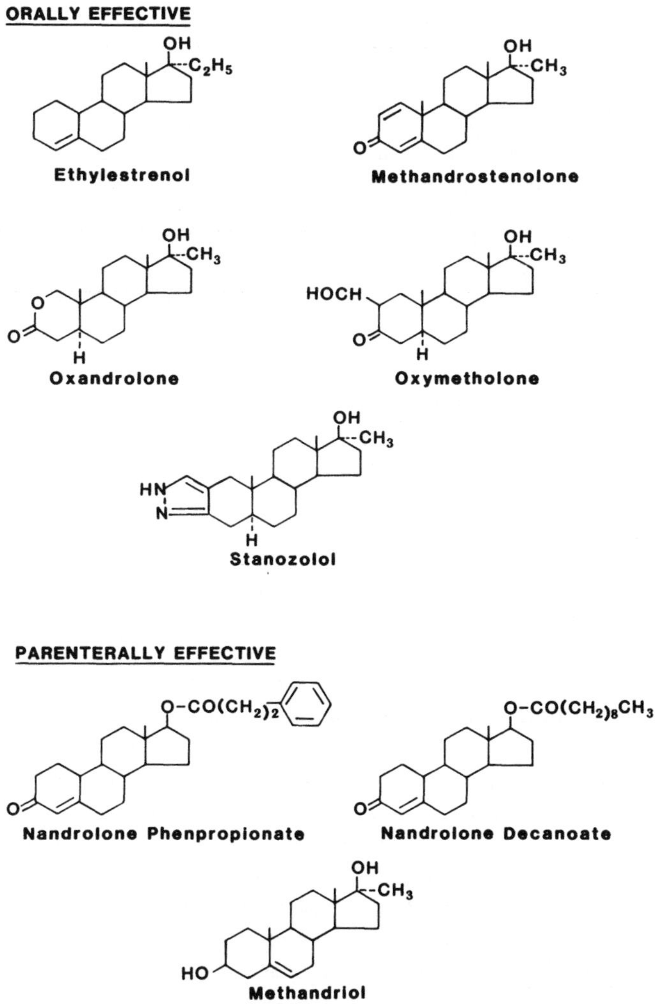

Figure 6. Chemical structure of the anabolic steroid drugs.

short-acting androgenic steroid is sometimes beneficial. If such therapy induces hypertrophy of the prostate gland and urethral obstruction, these adverse effects can be readily reversed by cessation of therapy.

The short-acting orally active androgenic steroids with 17α-alkyl substitutions, such as fluoxymesterone and methyltestosterone, are generally less effective in the induction of puberty than are the testosterone esters. However, they are useful in maintenance therapy when hypogonadism occurs in adulthood or after the development of secondary sexual characteristics. Doses ranging from 10 to 40 mg/day are usually employed in the management of androgen deficiency.

Table 4. Therapeutic Uses of the Androgenic and Anabolic Steroids

Induction of puberty in males
Replacement therapy in hypogonadism in males
Maintenance of secondary sex characteristics in males
Stimulation of libido in females
Stimulation of erythropoiesis (severe anemia)
Reverse negative nitrogen balance (catabolic states)

4.2. Anabolic Steroid Drugs

Anabolic steroids are usually utilized to reverse the negative nitrogen balance associated with certain catabolic states and to stimulate erythropoiesis in severe anemias (Table 4). These drugs are sometimes used controversially for stimulation of growth in children. An anabolic steroid with a favorable anabolic/androgenic ratio is usually chosen for promoting growth. The objective is to stimulate long bone growth without initiating premature closure of the epiphyseal plates and thereby limiting adult height.

Refractory anemias are sometimes managed with anabolic steroids. However, fewer than 50% of patients usually respond to this therapeutic approach. Three months of therapy are required. Anabolic steroids with low androgenic potency are usually used in women and children to minimize masculinzation. Only esterified androgenic steroids are utilized for long-term, high-dose therapy in order to avoid hepatic dysfunction.

Administration of high doses of glucocorticosteroids produces a negative nitrogen balance, which can be reversed by anabolic steroids. The use of anabolic steroids prevents corticosteroid side effects such as muscle wasting and demineralization of bone. Patients with chronic debilitating illnesses and those recovering from severe infections, surgery, burns, trauma, irradiation, or cytotoxic drug therapy often demonstrate defective protein synthesis, resulting in a negative nitrogen balance. Anabolic steroids are effective in alleviating or reversing this clinical condition, but their efficacy is contingent on adequate protein and caloric intake.

Athletes will occasionally use anabolic steroids to improve athletic performance, particularly in those events requiring acute muscular exertion. Such use of anabolic steroids is trivial and in most instances ineffective. In well-conditioned males, there is little evidence to support the efficacy of these drugs. Androgens also do not improve performance in activities requiring energy derived from aerobic metabolism. The weight gain associated with the use of anabolic steroids by these individuals is most likely related to fluid retention. Furthermore, large doses of anabolic steroids with 17α-alkyl groups may produce altered hepatic function, reduced serum gonadotropin and testosterone levels, and azoospermia (see Table 5). Greater stimulatory effects of anabolic steroids on skeletal muscular development are observed in female athletes.

However, the virilizing actions of these drugs and the menstrual irregularities associated with their use underscore the inappropriateness of such use of the anabolic steroids. Small doses of androgens are sometimes useful in increasing libido in women.

4.3. Adverse Effects of Androgen Therapy

In contrast to other classes of steroid hormones, particularly the estrogens and glucocorticoids, the androgens are seldom capable of producing serious toxic side effects. The untoward effects associated with androgen therapy usually result from chronic administration and excessive dose (Table 5). An excessive degree of virilization can occur in children and in women. In children, this will be evidenced by signs of precocious puberty; in women, signs of hirsutism, deepening of the voice, acne, alopecia, clitoral enlargement, and menstrual irregularities will indicate excessive androgenic stimulation. Acne and facial hair will usually be the earliest signs indicating excessive dosing. Bone growth in prepubertal children may also be impaired by inappropriate use of androgens.

Androgens may stimulate benign enlargement of the prostate gland in men, particularly older individuals, resulting in urethral obstruction. It is presently unknown if the use of androgens by young males (e.g., athletes) enhances the incidence of benign prostatic hyperplasia or carcinoma. Both of these prostatic diseases exhibit androgen dependence and their incidence increases markedly with advancing age. Paradoxically, androgens may cause gynecomastia (breast enlargement) in men and in boys as a result of the peripheral conversion of testosterone to estrogenic substances. This is more likely to occur after prolonged high-dose therapy or in men with liver disease. Androgenic and anabolic steroids will also suppress gonadotropin secretion in males. The fall in FSH impairs spermatogenesis (azoospermia), which may lead to sterility, and the decline in LH levels reduces the rate of testicular androgen synthesis, resulting in decreased plasma levels of testosterone. These effects of androgens are generally reversible.

The alkylated androgenic and anabolic steroids have also been noted to produce

Table 5. Adverse Effects of the Androgenic and Anabolic Steroid Drugs

Excessive virilization in children and women
Stimulation of prostatic hyperplasia and aggravation of prostatic carcinoma
Azoospermia
Gynecomastia
Salt and water retention
Jaundice (17α-alkylated derivatives)
Hepatic peliosis (blood-filled cysts)
Hepatocellular malignancy
Masculinization of the female fetus

hepatic dysfunction. Clinical jaundice occurs rarely, but the incidence suggests caution in the use of these drugs by patients with preexisting liver disease. Long-term, high-dose therapy with 17α-alkylated derivatives has been associated with the development of hepatic cysts and hepatocellular malignancy. Intrahepatic hemorrhage can occur following the rupture of these cystic lesions. The testosterone esters and other parenteral androgens lacking the 17α-alkyl substitution do not produce hepatic pathology.

Androgens may produce fluid and salt retention, resulting in significant weight gain. This is not usually a serious problem except for elderly patients with congestive heart failure. These steroids may also contribute to the development of atherosclerosis by reducing plasma levels of high-density lipoproteins (HDL) and raising the circulating concentrations of low-density lipoproteins (LDL).

Pregnant women should not be treated with androgenic or anabolic steroids, since these agents can potentially masculinize the female fetus. Likewise, the androgens should not be administered to patients with prostatic carcinoma, since these cancers often exhibit androgen dependence and administration of the androgens may exacerbate the disease.

Androgens can also interact with other drugs. The risk of hemorrhage in patients receiving coumarin and indandione anticoagulants is increased when 17α-alkylated androgens are administered. The androgens appear to enhance the potency of the anticoagulants. Methandrostenolone may inhibit the metabolism of oxyphenbutazone, producing a longer and more variable degree of anti-inflammatory activity. Anabolic steroid use may require decreasing dosage of antidiabetic medication.

SUGGESTED READINGS

Physiology of the Androgens

Kochakian CD: The protein anabolic effects of steroid hormones. *Vitam Horm* 4:255–264, 1956.

Brooks RV: Androgens. *Clin Endocrinol Metab* 4:503–520, 1975.

deGroat WC, Booth AM: Physiology of male sexual function. *Ann Int Med* 92:329–331, 1980.

Lipsett MB: Physiology and pathology of the Leydig cell. *N Engl J Med* 303:682–688, 1980.

Grody WW, Schrader WT, O'Malley BW: Activation, transformation and subunit structure of steroid hormone receptors. *Endocr Rev* 3:141–163, 1982.

Wilson JD, George FW, Griffin JE: The hormonal control of sexual development. *Science* 211:1278–1284, 1981.

Rubin RT, Reinisch JM, Haskett RF: Postnatal gonadal steroid effects on human behavior. *Science* 211:1318–1324, 1981.

Mooradian AD, Morley JE, Korenman SG: Biological actions of androgens. *Endocr Rev* 8:1–28, 1987.

Pharmacology of the Androgens

Kelley VC, Ruvalcaba RHA: Use of anabolic agents in treatment of short children. *Clin Endocrinol Metab* 11:25–41, 1982.

Lipsett MB: Use and abuse of androgens. *Consultant* 20:146–151, 1980.

Ryan AJ: Anabolic steroids are fool's gold. *Fed Proc* 40:2682–2688, 1981.

Snyder PJ: Clinical use of androgens. *Annu Rev Med* 35:207–219, 1984.

Wilson JD, Griffin JE: Use and misuse of androgens. *Metabolism* 29:1278–1295, 1980.

Payne AH: Anabolic steroids in athletics. *Br J Sports Med* 9:83–88, 1975.
Wright JE: Anabolic steroids and athletics. *Exerc Sport Sci Rev* 8:149–202, 1980.
Kopera H: The history of anabolic steroids and a review of clinical experience with anabolic steroids. *Acta Endocrinol* 271(suppl):11–18, 1985.
Haupt HA, Rovere GD: Anabolic steroids: a review of the literature. *Am J Sports Med* 12:469–484, 1984.
Mellion MB: Anabolic steroids in athletics. *Ann Family Prac* 30:113–119, 1984.
Lamb DR: Anabolic steroids in athletics: how well do they work and how dangerous are they? *Am J Sports Med* 12:31–38, 1984.
MacDougall D: Anabolic steroids. *Physician Sports Med* 11:95–100, 1983.
Strauss RH, Wright JE, Finerman GAM, Catlin DH: Side effects of anabolic steroids in weight-trained men. *Physician Sports Med* 11:87–96, 1983.
Bierly J: Use of anabolic steroids by athletes. *Postgrad Med* 82:67–79, 1987.
Wilson JD: Androgen abuse by athletes. *Endocrin Rev* 9:181–199, 1988.

8

Anti-inflammatory Agents

Edward T. Knych

1. THE INFLAMMATORY RESPONSE

Descriptions of inflammation are found in the earliest medical records of civilization. The Greeks referred to it as *phlogsis* and the Romans as *inflammatio*. Cornelius Celsus (c. 30 B.C.E. to 38 C.E.) is generally given credit for describing the four cardinal signs of inflammation as *rubor et tumor cum calore et dolore:* redness and swelling with heat and pain. This nonspecific response of tissues is induced by diverse insults or stimuli. Most observations suggest that the inflammatory response is a beneficial reaction of tissues to injury, leading to removal of the inducing agent and repair of the injured tissue. However, if the stimulus persists, the process may become chronic and produce permanent tissue damage or inappropriate healing.

The inflammatory response is a result of interactions between a number of physiological mechanisms, chemical mediators, and cell types. The complex nature of these interactions permits amplification and preservation of the response. However, the complexity also contributes to variability. After a given inflammatory stimulus, a different time course and outcome is not unexpected because of the variable nature of the elements recruited by the stimulus. Despite its complexity and variablity, the inflammatory response may be divided into the following common events: (1) vasodilatation and hyperemia, (2) increased vascular permeability, and (3) leukocyte infiltration.

The discussion that follows will attempt to provide a broad overview of the anatomical changes occurring in the inflammatory response, the chemical mediators thought to be involved, and the pharmacology of the nonsteroidal anti-inflammatory agents currently available for relieving some of the symptoms of inflammation. It should be emphasized that a discussion of topics as broad and complex as these necessarily will be incomplete and biased by the author's views.

Edward T. Knych • Department of Pharmacology, University of Minnesota School of Medicine, Duluth, Minnesota 55812.

1.1. Vasodilatation and Hyperemia

The changes in the microvasculature which occur at the inflammatory site are often the first to be observed and are critical. The first description of the vascular changes accompanying inflammation, and still referred to as the best, was made by Julius Cohnheim (1839–1884). Vasodilatation and increased blood flow characterize these changes and are critical elements in the response. Increased numbers of leukocytyes and plasma proteins enter the site, continuing the response and leading to eventual resolution. These events account for two of the cardinal signs of inflammation, redness and warmth. How these events are precipitated is not entirely clear, although a number of mediators have been implicated and will be discussed subsequently.

1.2. Increased Permeability

The third cardinal sign of inflammation, swelling, is the result of the accumulation of fluid, called exudate, in the tissues at the site of inflammation. If the process continues, the production of new connective tissue may also add to the swelling. Swelling is not always obvious but may only become apparent with careful observation. Inflammatory swelling is almost always accompanied by pain, either induced by palpation or spontaneous.

The formation of exudate occurs by two mechanisms. The agent inducing the inflammation may be traumatic, directly and mechanically injuring the microvessels, resulting in the leakage of fluids from the injured vessels. In addition, substances released by tissues surrounding the site of inflammation or from the plasma may also induce an increased permeability of the microvessels. The exudate formed by direct traumatic injury to blood vessels will be formed for up to a day or two, or until the injured vessel is repaired or plugged by thrombus. In contrast, the chemically induced exudate formation generally occurs immediately after release of the substances and lasts for a relatively short period of time.

1.3. Leukocyte Infiltration

The most striking histological characteristic of inflamed tissue is the presence of leukocytes. With the initiation of an inflammatory response, leukocytes move from the center of blood vessels (margination) and adhere to the walls of blood vessels near the site of inflammation (adherence). They migrate through the blood vessel wall (diapedesis) and move toward the inflammatory site (chemotaxis). During the initial phase of the response, the predominant leukocytes are neutrophils. After a day or two, the neutrophils are replaced by mononuclear phagocytes (macrophages). These events are only poorly understood although they are undoubtedly initiated and controlled by the release of chemical signals from the tissue or cells near the site of inflammation.

The function of the neutrophils and macrophages is to remove unwanted particulate material, such as bacteria or cellular debris, by the process of phagocytosis. These cells have large numbers of cytoplasmic granules which contain various lysosomal acid hydrolases, neutral proteases, peroxidase, and cationic proteins. With the ingestion of particulate matter, the contents of the cytoplasmic granules are released, accompanied by a burst of metabolic activity and the generation of highly reactive superoxide and hydroxyl radicals. These substances promote the destruction and digestion of the phagocytized material.

1.4. Tissue Damage

Tissue damage resulting from the inflammatory process is produced by several mechanisms. Principal among these are the release of enzymes from the granules of infiltrating leukocytes and the production of reactive oxygen intermediates such as superoxide anions and hydroxyl radicals. However, these enzymes and their products may also initiate and perpetuate the processes of diapedesis and chemotaxis. The inflammatory response, therefore, may require some cellular injury for its initiation. Limiting and removing infiltrating cells, inhibiting the enzymes released by these cells, and scavenging the reactive oxygen products produced are important mechanisms for resolving the inflammatory process. It also follows that incomplete suppression of the inflammatory activity of these cells can contribute to the evolution of a chronic inflammatory condition.

2. MEDIATORS OF THE INFLAMMATORY RESPONSE

The complex process of inflammation is dependent on the interactions between many chemical messages produced by the inflammatory agent or event and perpetuated by events occurring during the inflammatory process. The nature of these chemical mediators and their interactions is the subject of intense investigation. While all the participants in the process have not been identified, a number have been and their role in the process suggested. These mediators are produced either in the plasma or in the cells and tissues participating in the inflammatory process. A brief discussion of several of these substances follows.

2.1. Mediators from Plasma

Mediators of the inflammatory process are produced within the plasma by three interconnected systems: (a) the kinin system, (b) the complement system, and (c) the clotting system. These three systems share the common characteristic of being cascading systems. They consist of a series of proteolytic steps. Each enzymatic step is activated and amplified by the previous step. In this manner, a small signal produces a large response. There is also a complex interaction between each of these systems, each cascade producing factors capable of affecting the other cascades.

2.1.1. The Kinin System

The kinin system produces the peptides bradykinin and kallidin. It begins with the activation of Hageman factor (factor XII of the clotting system). Activation can be produced by a number of agents, including contact with glass surfaces, collagen, basement membrane, or cartilage, and by the action of enzymes such as kallikrein, plasmin, and clotting factor XI. The activated Hageman factor, in turn, activates plasma kallikrein. which converts a high-molecular-weight precursor protein (kininogen) to the nonapeptide bradykinin. Within tissues, kallikrein converts a low-molecular-weight kininogen to the decapeptide kallidin. The kinins produced are rapidly destroyed by kininases and peptidases in plasma or tissue, resulting in a half-life of <1 min. The activation of kallikrein and the cleavage of kininogen to kinin can also be produced by a number of proteases such as plasmin.

Bradykinin produces a number of actions which are characteristic of an acute inflammatory response. At low concentrations, it produces a characteristic slow contraction of smooth muscle, an action which gave bradykinin its name. It also produces a vasodilatation of blood vessels and a fall in systemic blood pressure. The vasodilatation is mediated by the release of a substance, endothelium-derived relaxing factor (EDRF), produced by the endothelial cells which line blood vessels. The chemical nature of EDRF remains to be elucidated. When injected into the skin, bradykinin produces pain and increases vascular permeability, leading to swelling at the site of injection.

2.1.2. The Complement System

The complement cascade is extremely complex, consisting of at least eleven circulating blood proteins that constitute the classic complement pathway, two additional proteins which participate in mediating the alternate complement pathway, and at least six proteins regulating the cascade. The system is activated, primarily, by antigen–antibody reactions. However, activated Hageman factor may also activate the cascade. Details of this complex system are beyond the scope of this discussion.

Most interest in this system has focused on fragments of several of the proteins in the cascade. In particular, the fragments C3a and C5a, formed when the cascade is activated, have been studied intensively. These fragments along with others, may also be produced from their larger parent molecules by the action of various proteases such as trypsin, plasmin, or lysosomal proteases.

C3a and C5a induce the release of histamine, which mediates the increase in vascular permeability. Both fragments stimulate, directly and indirectly, the contraction of smooth muscle. Among the most potent chemotactic substances for neutrophils and monocytes are C5a and related fragments. These substances have also been implicated in the degranulation of neutrophils and in the generation of reactive oxygen intermediates. These actions are indicative of both the significant role played by the complement cascade as well as the potential that inhibitors of this system might have in the control of acute and chronic inflammatory events.

2.1.3. The Clotting System

A cascading system, consisting of more than a dozen plasma proteins, characterizes the series of proteolytic events which results in the formation of fibrin and a stable clot. The intrinsic pathway to fibrin formation is initiated with the activation of factor XII, the Hageman factor. This factor is also capable of activating the kinin and complement systems. In addition, a number of peptides produced during the conversion of fibrinogen to fibrin induce an increase in vascular permeability and are chemotactic. Hageman factor, as well a kallikrein, are capable of initiating the thrombolytic process by activating the enzyme plasmin, which degrades both fibrinogen and fibrin. Plasmin is also capable of activating the classic complement system and the kinin system.

2.2. Mediators from Cells

A large number of chemical mediators are produced during the inflammatory response by involved tissues or blood cells. We will limit our discussion to several of the more important agents: (a) histamine, (b) eicosanoids, (c) reactive oxygen intermediates, (d) lysosomal components, and (e) platelet activating factor.

2.2.1. Histamine

Histamine can be found in most tissues of the body. In tissues, it is found chiefly within granules of mast cells while in blood, it is located in basophils and platelets. It is released from mast cells in response to physical trauma, by certain chemicals, during antigen–antibody reactions, or by C3a and C5a of the complement system. The release of histamine is also initiated by other substances stored with the granules. These include heparin, an eosinophil chemotactic factor, a neutrophil chemotactic factor, and enzymes such as neutral proteases, superoxide dismutase, and peroxidase.

Histamine initiates a characteristic vasodilatation of small-caliber arterioles and venules that results in flushing. The vasodilatation may, in part, be due to the release of EDRF from endothelial cells. Other smooth muscles, including those of large blood vessels, are constricted by histamine. In addition, histamine produces an increase in vascular permeability.

2.2.2. Eicosanoids

The eicosanoids are a diverse group of compounds derived from 20-carbon essential fatty acids. In man, arachidonic acid (5,8,11,14-eicosatetraenoic acid) is the primary precursor. It is found in an esterified form as a component of the phospholipids of cell membranes or other complex lipids. Arachidonic acid is released from these stores in response to a wide variety of mechanical, chemical, and humoral stimuli. With the release of arachidonic acid, there is an increased formation of oxygenated products by one of three pathways: (a) the cyclooxygenase pathway, (b) the lipoxygenase pathway, and (c) the epoxygenase pathway. The cyclooxygenase pathway gives rise to the primary prostaglandins (PGs), PGD_2, PGE_2, and $PGF_{2\alpha}$; to the thromboxanes (TXs), TXA_2 and TXB_2; and to prostacyclin, PGI_2. These are formed through the common precursor endoperoxides PGG_2 and PGH_2. A group of lipoxygenases transform arachidonic acid to either hydroxy (HETE) or hydroperoxy (HPETE) derivatives. In particular, 5-lipoxygenase produces 5-HPETE, the precursor of the leukotriene A_4 (LTA_4). LTA_4, in turn, is converted to either LTB_4 or to the peptide-containing leukotrienes

LTC_4, LTD_4, and LTE_4. The peptide-containing leukotrienes are responsible for the activity characterizing the action of slow-reacting substance of anaphylaxis (SRS-A). More recently, it has been recognized that arachidonic acid can also be metabolized by a series of cytochrome P450 monoxygenases found in the endoplasmic reticulum of cells. This pathway gives rise to a series of epoxides that can be converted to their corresponding diols. In addition, the epoxide pathway is capable of producing HETE derivatives.

The eicosanoids are of extreme importance and interest because of their varied biologic activity and their ubiquitous nature. They are capable of directly mediating responses associated with the inflammatory response and of modulating the response of other agents. The eicosanoids are known to affect many biologic functions. Those important to the inflammatory response include smooth muscle contractility, vascular permeability, chemotaxis, and platelet aggregation. In many areas where eicosanoids have identified functional roles, it is not uncommon for different eicosanoids to possess antagonistic activity. For example, TBX_2 promotes the aggregation of platelets while PGI_2 is antiaggregatory. PGI_2, PGE_2, and PGD_2 are vasodilators while TXA_2, $PGF_{2\alpha}$, and the leukotrienes are vasoconstrictors. LTB_4 is a potent chemotactic agent while LTC_4, LTD_4, and LTE_4 affect permeability. The response generated by eicosanoids, therefore, is unpredictable. It is a function of the mix of eicosanoids and is variable, depending on the tissue, species, and stimulus involved.

The eicosanoids play an important role in modulating the function of other mediators of inflammation. In fact, this may be their most important role. For example, eicosanoids are capable of altering the increases in vascular permeability produced by histamine, bradykinin, LTB_4, or C5a. Low concentrations of $PGF_{2\alpha}$ and PGE_1 enhance histamine release while high concentrations have the opposite effect. This exemplifies the complex interactions which may occur between various proposed mediators of the inflammatory reaction. It also underscores the fact that the particular response produced by a stimulus is dependent upon the mix and quantities of mediators released from the tissues and leukocytes affected.

2.2.3. Reactive Oxygen Intermediates

Reactive oxygen intermediates include superoxide and the hydroxyl radical. These intermediates contain an unpaired electron and are therefore inherently unstable and highly reactive. They can be generated (a) by enzymes such as xanthine oxidase, (b) by small molecules such as flavoproteins, (c) by cellular organelles such as the plasma membrane, (d) in the presence of transition metals such as iron and copper, or (e) by environmental factors such as ultraviolet light.

During the inflammatory process, neutrophils migrating to the site of inflammation are stimulated either by surface contact with particular material, by superoxide, or by complement to increase their oxygen consumption. This respiratory burst also generates superoxide. It is superoxide that is thought responsible for the removal and destruction of cellular debris or the microorganisms present. Hydroxyl radicals are formed from hydrogen peroxide in the presence of catalytic quantities of transition metals in a Fenton reaction or by an iron-catalyzed Haber–Weiss reaction. The hydroxyl radical is particularly reactive and lethal to cells.

Free radical scavengers normally provide protection from these nonselective reactive oxygen intermediates. Superoxide dismutase is an intracellular enzyme capable of catalyzing the conversion of superoxide to hydrogen peroxide. Hydrogen peroxide is enzymatically removed by catalase. Glutathione contains cysteine residues which are preferentially oxidized by the reactive oxygen intermediates and thereby effectively acts as a free radical scavenger. Vitamins E and C also are thought to function as free radical scavengers.

The production of reactive oxygen intermediates by the neutrophils is beneficial since it aids in the destruction and removal of cellular debris or offending organisms during the inflammatory process. The reactive oxygen intermediates also promote the activation of other neutrophils, thereby amplifying the response. However, these intermediates may also spill out into surrounding tissue, causing local tissue destruction and aggravating the inflammatory response. Therefore, serious consequences may result if the production of superoxide or hydroxyl radical is increased or the availability of intracellular free radical scavengers is limited.

2.2.4. Lysosomal Components

A second important group of agents involved in the removal of cellular debris or microorganisms during the inflammatory response is the enzymes of the lysosomes of infiltrating leukocytes. During the process of phagocytosis or cell death, various hydrolytic enzymes are released by these cells. Many of these enzymes operate maximally at acid pH and are thought to function primarily within the vacuoles of phagocytizing cells. Another group of enzymes, operating at neutral or alkaline pH, is thought to be most important in modulating the inflammatory process and contributing to tissue destruction. These neutral hydrolases include collagenase, elastase, and cathepsin. Their function initially may promote the migration of leukocytes through the basement membrane which separates the blood and the interstitial space. The ability of neutral proteases to digest protein and cartilage may result in further tissue damage if their action is not controlled by normally present inhibitors.

2.2.5. Platelet Activating Factor

Platelet activating factor (PAF), identified as acetyl glyceryl ether phosphorylcholine (AGEPC), has recently been implicated as a mediator in the inflammatory response. PAF is produced by neutrophils and monocytes. This lipid mediator has been reported to initiate a number of the reactions characteristic of the inflammatory response. It was first identified by its ability to stimulate platelets to aggregate and release histamine. With regard to neutrophils, PAF is chemotactic, initiates the release of lysosomal enzymes, and stimulates oxygen radical formation. The number and variety of actions attributable to PAF suggest its importance as a mediator of the inflammatory response.

3. PHARMACOLOGY OF ANTI-INFLAMMATORY DRUGS

The use of anti-inflammatory drugs, in particular, the nonsteroidal anti-inflammatory drugs (NSAIDs), in the treatment of sports-related injuries has increased with the growing popularity of sports and exercise. Acute injuries, such as sprains, contusions, and fractures, often are accompanied by bleeding and swelling. The immediate treatment of these injuries with rest, ice, compression, and elevation is intended to limit these symptoms. The addition of NSAIDs to the treatment regimen has been found by most clinical studies to be useful in decreasing the inflammatory symptoms and pain associated with the acute injury. NSAIDs do not appear to differ dramatically among themselves with regard to efficacy. The important considerations in their use are side effects, cost, and compliance. The use of NSAIDs in the treatment of chronic or overuse injuries, such as tendinitis and bursitis, has not been clinically evaluated to the same degree as their use in acute injuries. These injuries are generally treated with reduced activity to allow for healing and with attempts to identify and correct the cause. The few studies that exist suggest that the addition of NSAIDs to the usual treatment is useful in relieving symptoms although they do not differ significantly in efficacy. It should be emphasized that while NSAIDs may provide symptomatic relief of inflammation, they do not arrest the cause or the pathological injury of the inflammatory reaction.

There are many drugs with diverse chemical structures included among NSAIDs. They all share the ability to inhibit the cyclooxygenase enzyme of arachidonic acid metabolism. Thus, they prevent the formation of the prostaglandins, thromboxanes, endoperoxides, and prostacyclin produced by this pathway. The dosage required to inhibit cyclooxygenase closely correlates with their anti-inflammatory potency. Also, all are analgesic and antipyretic as well. The analgesic properties may be useful in relieving the pain associated with inflammation.

NSAIDs also have in common many pharmacokinetic characteristics and adverse side effects. They are acidic drugs and are characterized by a high degree of binding to plasma proteins, in particular, albumin. The high degree of plasma binding gives these drugs the potential to displace other drugs from plasma protiens. Of potential therapeutic importance is the interaction between NSAIDs and anticoagulants. The potential for bleeding is further enhanced by NSAID-induced platelet dysfunction and their potential for inducing gastic bleeding. NSAIDs are rapidly and completely absorbed after oral administration, with peak concentrations occurring within several hours. The onset of clinical action is relatively prompt. The principal pathway for elimination of NSAIDs is hepatic metabolism. The oxidized metabolic products or conjugates are excreted primarily by the kidney with little or no renal clearance of free drug. In addition, many NSAIDs are excreted in feces by the enterohepatic cycle. While hepatic metabolism generally leads to inactivation of NSAIDs, there are several notable exceptions. Both asprin and sulindac are prodrugs. Their anti-inflammatory action is dependent on their hepatic biotransformation to active metabolites.

The most prevalent side effects produced by NSAIDs are gastrointestinal, occurring in up to 20% of patients on full doses of these agents. These range from mild dyspepsia and heartburn to ulceration and gastrointestinal bleeding. Gastrointestinal side effects are most commonly associated with aspirin and less frequently with other NSAIDs. These effects are correlated with the ability of the NSAIDs to inhibit prostaglandin formation. PGE_2 and PGI_2 are the major prostaglandins produced by the gastric mucosa. They normally inhibit the secretion of gastric acids and stimulate the secretion of protective mucus. Inhibition of the formation of these eicosanoids renders the gastrointestinal tract more susceptible to damage. The incidence of these side effects can be reduced by taking these agents with food or antacids. There is continual concern regarding cross-toxicity among these agents. It has been reported that individuals who experience an adverse effect to one NSAID have a 50% chance of developing an adverse effect to a second NSAID. In addition. 25% of those patients who experience a side effect to an NSAID will experience the same side effect to other NSAIDs.

Some individuals are exceedingly sensitive to NSAIDs, displaying reactions ranging from rhinitis and general urticaria to bronchial spasms and respiratory failure. The incidence of mild skin rashes ranges from 1% to 9%. The more severe reactions occur most frequently in individuals with asthma, nasal polyps. or chronic urticaria. Individuals hypersensitive to one NSAID are at high risk of being hypersensitive to other NSAIDs.

Tinnitus occurs commonly (±10%) with aspirin and to a lesser extent with other NSAIDs. NSAIDs can also induce other central nervous system side effects such as dizziness, anxiety, headache, drowsiness, and confusion. More severe central nervous system effects, including depression, disorientation, hallucination, and severe headache, are associated with the use of indomethacin.

Other side effects commonly produced by NSAIDs include platelet dysfunction, which results in an increased bleeding time. This effect is readily reversible when the drug is discontinued, except in the case of aspirin, which is capable of acetylating the cyclo-oxygenase of platelets and irreversibly inactivating it. Since platelets are unable to synthesize new protein, bleeding times may be elevated for 4 to 7 days after discontinuation of aspirin administration, during which time new platelets are being produced. NSAIDs may promote retention of salt and water, leading to edema and hyperkalemia. Hepatic toxicity can occur; this is often asymptomatic but is indicated by elevations in plasma alkaline phosphatase, SGOT (serum glutamic oxalacetic transaminase), and SGPT (serum glutamic pyruvic transaminase) activity. It should be pointed out that much of our knowledge regarding adverse side effects of NSAIDs has been gained during the use of these agents to treat chronic inflammatory diseases such as arthritis.

Three broad categories of NSAIDs exist: (a) the carboxylic acid derivatives, (b) the oxicams, and (c) the pyrazoles. The carboxylic acid derivatives include the salicylates, the acetic acid derivatives, the propionic acid derivatives, and the fenamates. There are more than 60 compounds among these groups that are marketed, somewhere in the world, as anti-inflammatory agents. It is beyond the scope of this discussion to consider all these, and only representative members of each group will be discussed below.

3.1. Carboxylic Acids

3.1.1. Salicylates

Aspirin (acetylsalicylic acid) is the most widely used NSAID and still remains the standard against which all others are judged. It has been estimated that 10 to 20 tons of aspirin are consumed annually. Aspirin is rapidly absorbed, with measurable plasma levels observed within 30 min and peak concentrations at 2 h. Absorption is by passive diffusion and is dependent upon pH, concentration, gastric emptying time, and dissolution rate. Once absorbed, salicylates distribute throughout the body tissues and fluids. Aspirin is a prodrug, being rapidly converted into its active metabolite, salicylic acid, by hydrolysis in the liver. The half-life of aspirin in plasma is about 15 min. Salicylic acid undergoes further hepatic biotransformation, principally to its glycine and glucuronic acid conjugates. These metabolities are excreted by the kidney. The conjugation reactions become saturated at low concentrations. Increasing the dosage produces an increase in the half-life and accumulation may occur.

The use of anti-inflammatory dosages of aspirin is associated with a high incidence of gastrointestinal distress. In addition, gastric ulceration and hemorrhage may occur. Daily aspirin dosages of 1 to 3 g produce a fecal blood loss of 2 to 6 ml. Up to one-half of patients may exhibit mucosal lesions without overt clinical symptoms. In addition, a single dose of aspirin can prolong bleeding time for 4 to 7 days because of irreversible acetylation of platelet cyclo-oxygenase. Other nonacetylated salicylates produce an inhibition of platelet cyclo-oxygenase that is readily reversible upon discontinuation of the drug. Other toxic effects associated with aspirin use are hypersensitivity reactions and tinnitus.

Aspirin may be purchased as plain, buffered, or enterically coated preparations. A low dose (650 mg/day) is analgesic whereas higher doses (3 to 6 g/day) have anti-inflammatory effects. Enteric coatings increase gastrointestinal tolerance but may lead to incomplete absorption. Similarly, buffered preparations may be better tolerated, but alkalinization of the urine may increase excretion in the urine. Other nonacetylated salicylates and their derivatives are also available, both as tablets as well as liquid or topical formulations. Diflunisal (Dolobid) is a salicylic acid derivative which does not require activation by the liver. It has a longer half-life (7.5 to 12 h) than aspirin and therefore requires only twice-daily administration. This may be an important consideration when compliance is a concern. It is also less likely to produce gastrointestinal and auditory side effects.

3.1.2. Acetic Acids

3.1.2a. Indomethacin. Indomethacin (Indocin), introduced in 1963, was among the first nonsalicylate NSAIDs developed. It is one of the most potent inhibitors of cyclo-oxygenase known and is a standard agent in many investigations of the action of eicosanoids. Indomethacin is rapidly absorbed following oral administration. Peak concentrations are observed approximately 2 h after administration. It is bound extensively to plasma proteins. Indomethacin is biotransformed by the liver to inactive metabolites and glucuronic acid conjugates. Metabolites and unchanged drug are eliminated in urine, in part by tubular secretion. There is also an active enterohepatic cycle which leads to elimination in the feces. This latter route contributes to a variable half-life of 2 to 11 h.

While indomethacin is widely used, a high incidence (35% to 50%) of adverse side effects often limits its usefulness. Gastrointestinal complaints consisting of nausea, anorexia, and abdominal pain are most common. Peptic ulcers may occur in 2% to 5% of those administered this agent. Severe headache, dizziness, confusion, depression, and hallucinations are common central nervous system side effects. Hypersensitivity reactions consisting of rashes, itching, urticaria, and asthma have been observed. As many as 20% of those who experience side effects will discontinue usage of the drug.

3.1.2b. Sulindac. Sulindac (Clinoril) is chemically similar to indomethacin. It is a prodrug and owes its anti-inflammatory properties to its sulfide metabolite. The sulfide metabolite is more than 500 times as potent as sulindac as a cyclo-oxygenase inhibitor. Hepatic enzymes first oxidize sulindac to a sulfone and then reduce the sulfone to the sulfide derivative. The half-life of the sulfide is approximately 18 h; therefore, it is administered twice daily. Enterohepatic circulation complicates the pharmacokinetic properties of sulindac and its metabolites. The most common side effects are gastrointestinal disturbances. These are generally mild pain and nausea. Unlike other NSAIDs, sulindac also commonly causes constipation. The incidence of gastrointestinal disturbances is generally lower for sulindac than for indomethacin or aspirin. Central nervous system effects, including drowsiness, dizziness, headache, and nervousness, are frequently reported. Hypersensitivity reactions and prolongation of bleeding time have been observed.

3.1.2c. Tolmetin. Tolmetin (Tolectin) is rapidly and completely absorbed after oral administration. It has a half-life of 1 h. The drug is extensively bound to plasma proteins. Tolmetin is excreted by the kidney either as unchanged drug or as an oxidized or conjugated metabolite. Toxic side effects are experienced by up to 40% of those administered the drug chronically, with gastrointestinal disturbances the most common complaint. Central nervous system effects are similar to those produced by indomethacin but are less common.

3.1.3. Propionic Acids

3.1.3a. Ibuprofen. Ibuprofen (Motrin, Rufen) was the first of the propionic acid NSAIDs to be introduced. It has recently been approved for over-the-counter sale in reduced (200-mg) dosage form. It is equipotent to aspirin as a cyclo-oxygenase inhibitor. It is rapidly absorbed from the gastrointestinal tract with peak concentrations observed at 1 to 2 h. Like all other NSAIDs, it is extensively bound to plasma proteins. Little of this compound is excreted unchanged in the urine. More than 90% is found as oxidized metabolites or glucuronic acid conjugates. Gastrointestinal disturbances are the most commonly experienced adverse effects, although the incidence is generally lower than with either indomethacin or aspirin administration. Nevertheless, 10% to

15% of patients may be required to stop the drug because of adverse side effects. Other side effects reported to occur with ibuprofen include thrombocytopenia, skin rashes, headache, dizziness, blurred vision, fluid retention, and edema.

3.1.3b Naproxen. Naproxen (Naprosyn) has a long half-life (14 h) and is administered twice daily. It has become the most commonly used propionic acid NSAID. Absorption is rapid and complete after oral administration, although it may be reduced by antacids containing aluminum or magnesium. It is excreted in the urine as an inactive metabolite or conjugate. The gastrointestinal and central nervous system side effects common to the other NSAIDs are also observed with naproxen although less often than with indomethacin or aspirin. Less frequently, pruritus or other dermatologic problems have been observed. Jaundice, impairment of renal function, and thrombocytopenia have been reported in a few instances.

3.1.3c. Fenoprofen. Fenoprofen (Nalfon) is rapidly but not completely absorbed after oral administration. In particular, the presence of food may delay and reduce its absorption. Fenoprofen is extensively bound to plasma proteins and metabolized by the liver. Its metabolites are excreted by the kidneys. The half-life is 3 h. Abdominal pain and dyspepsia are the most commonly mentioned side effects of this drug, experienced by one in six patients. Constipation has also been reported with fenoprofen use. Less frequent are central nervous system effects such as dizziness, tinnitus, and confusion. Skin rashes can also occur.

3.1.4 Fenamates

This group of compounds is represented by meclofenamate (Meclomen). This drug is absorbed rapidly, with peak concentrations occurring at 0.5 to 2 h. The half-life in plasma is approximately 3 h. Up to 30% is excreted in the feces by enterohepatic circulation while the remainder is found in the urine as oxidized metabolites or glucuronic acid conjugates. Therapeutically, it is as efficacious as other NSAIDs. The most common side effects are once again observed in the gastrointestinal tract. However, in addition, diarrhea is commonly observed and may be associated with bowel inflammation. A potentially serious side effect, observed in only a few cases, is hemolytic anemia.

3.2. Oxicams

Piroxicam (Feldene) is the only agent in this group available in the United States. It has the distinct advantage of requiring only a single daily dosage because of its long half-life (45 h). Therapeutically, it is equivalent to aspirin and the other NSAIDs, but it is tolerated better. Its absorption is rapid and complete and unaffected by food or antacids. Very little of the drug is excreted unaltered in the urine. Hydroxylation and conjugation are the most prevalent pathways for biotransformation. Excretion is by the kidneys or by an active enterohepatic cycle. Gastrointestinal toxicity may occur in up to 20% of patients. Its effects on the gastrointestinal tract may be reduced somewhat by administration after eating.

3.3. Pyrazoles

Phenylbutazone (Azolid, Butazolidin) is therapeutically the most significant member of this group. Its current use has decreased with the introduction of newer and safer NSAIDs. Its half-life is 50 to 65 h. It is inactivated by hydroxylation and glucuronidation in the liver, and The metabolites are excreted in the urine. Phenylbutazone may be found in synovial fluids for periods up to 3 weeks after cessation of administration. It is capable of inducing hepatic enzymes responsible for the biotransformation of a number of other compounds. It is extensively bound to plasma proteins, and this characteristic has been implicated in therapeutically significant interactions with such agents as the anticoagulant warfarin and the oral hypoglycemic drug tolbutamide.

Adverse side effects are the main reason for the decline in use of phenylbutazone. Gastrointestinal disturbances, including nausea, vomiting, and epigastrc pain, and skin rashes are most commonly reported. Diarrhea, blurred vision, and central nervous system effects common to NSAIDs are also reported. More seriously, phenylbutazone may suppress marrow function, producing agranulocytosis and aplastic anemia. A number of deaths have been reported because of this suppression. Renal toxicity characterized by fluid and electrolyte retention may produce edema.

SUGGESTED READINGS

Bonta IL, Bray MA, Parnham MJ (eds): *The Pharmacology of Inflammation*. New York, Elsevier, 1985.

Calabrese LH, Rooney TW: The use of nonsteroidal anti-inflammatory drugs in sports. *Physician Sportsmed* 14:89–97, 1986.

Flower RJ, Moncada S, Vane JR: Analgesic-antipyretics and anti-inflammatory agents; drugs employed in the treatment of gout, in Gilman AG, Goodman LS, Rall TW, Murad F (eds): *The Pharmacological Basis of Therapeutics*, ed 7. New York, Macmillan, 1985, p 674.

Ford-Hutchinson AW: Leukotrienes as mediators of inflammation. *ISI Atlas of Science: Pharmacology* 1:25–28. 1987.

Hart FD, Huskisson EC: Non-steroidal anti-inflammatory drugs. *Drugs* 27:232–255, 1984.

Larson GL, Henson PM: Mediators of inflammation. *Annu Rev Immunol* 1:335–359, 1983.

Lombardino JG (ed): *Nonsteroidal Anti-inflammatory Drugs*. New York, John Wiley and Sons, 1985.

Lunec J, Griffiths HR, Blake DR: Oxygen radicals in inflammation. *ISI Atlas of Science: Pharmacology* 1:45–48, 1987.

Movat HZ: *The Inflammatory Reaction*. New York, Elsevier, 1985.

9

Effect of Exercise on Fuel Utilization and Insulin Requirements

Michael P. McLane and David L. Horwitz

The hormonal changes that occur during exercise are very important in control of fuel regulation. The observed changes in hormone concentrations, especially insulin, during exercise and the control of fuel regulation that is associated with these changes will be discussed in this chapter. A decrease in insulin concentration and an increase in glucagon concentration from concentrations during pre-exercise rest have been found in many studies.[1–9] Other hormonal changes during exercise include elevations in growth hormone, cortisol, and catecholamines.[5,6] More recent works have clarified the action of these regulatory hormones and have suggested that the decrease in insulin concentration [10–12] and the presence of glucagon [10,13,14] are essential for appropriate regulation of glucose production during exercise.

1. FUEL UTILIZATION

In the resting state, free fatty acids (FFA) are the major fuels of muscle[15] but this changes during exercise. At rest, the brain is the prime site of glucose uptake.[16]

During the first 5 to 10 minutes of exercise, muscle glycogen is the predominant fuel consumed.[17] As exercise continues beyond 10 minutes, the rate of blood glucose uptake by muscle increases 7- to 20-fold compared to pre-exercise rest,[18] depending on the intensity of the work performed. Total blood glucose turnover is increased up to 5 times during severe exercise.[18] Glucose uptake rate peaks at 90 to 180 minutes and then declines slightly.[19] Free fatty acid uptake continues to increase even beyond 180 minutes and FFA becomes the predominant fuel.[19,20] The increase in FFA utilization is directly related to an increase in concentration,[19,20] which indicates that uptake of FFA by exercising muscle is regulated by the rate at which FFA are mobilized from adipose tissue. A recent study indicates that increased lipolysis of muscle triglyceride

Michael P. McLane • Department of Surgery and Department of Physiology, Loyola University Medical Center, Maywood, Illinois 60153. *David L. Horwitz* • Department of Medicine and Department of Nutrition and Dietetics, University of Illinois at Chicago, Chicago, Illinois 60612.

may account for the paradoxical findings of increased FFA oxidation with concomitant decreased plasma FFA concentration in a trained state.[21] In summary, the normal pattern of fuel utilization is triphasic, with muscle glycogen, blood glucose, and free fatty acids successively predominating as the major energy-yielding substrate. Muscle triglyceride stores may play an important role as fuel between the muscle glycogen and blood glucose phases. This triphasic fuel pattern integrates well with the available fuel supplies. At rest, man expends approximately 5 kJ/min; during exercise, this value may increase 20-fold. Carbohydrate stored as muscle glycogen amounts to about 300 to 400 g; as liver glycogen. 80 to 90 g; and in the blood glucose pool, about 20 g.[22] Thus, the total carbohydrate stores represent approximately 8000 kJ, which could alone supply the increased energy need of exercise for about 100 min. The carbohydrate supply is small compared to the potential energy stores as triglyceride in adipose tissue (15 kg = 600,000 kJ).[22] Along with the liver, the kidney can also produce blood glucose, especially in the prolonged fasted state.[23] However, no renal glucose production occurs during normal exercise in postabsorptive man.[18] The lack of change in nitrogen excretion rates during prolonged physical activity[24–27] indicates that protein breakdown does not occur to any significant degree during mild or moderate exercise. However, during prolonged and/or severe exercise, protein catabolism may occur.[28,29] In view of the minor involvement of protein catabolism, the important circulating fuels for muscles during exercise are glucose and FFA. In order to meet the energy demands, rapid regulation of production of these fuels becomes essential. The only known mechanisms that promote increased supplies of these fuels via increasing hepatic glucose output and FFA mobilization from adipose tissue are the glucoregulatory and lipid-mobilizing hormonal and adrenergic regulatory processes,[30] which will be discussed below.

2. SUBSTRATE TURNOVER RATES

To study the rates of production and utilization of the fuels needed by the exercising muscles, two methods were developed. One involves measurement of arterial–venous (A–V) concentration differences across the body region that is either producing or utilizing the fuel along with measurement of the blood flow to that region. The A–V difference multiplied by the flow rate will equal the net uptake or release. The limitations of this method included assay sensitivities too poor to measure the A–V difference[15] and error in determination of blood flow through a particular region. Another limitation is that the calculated product is the *net* balance across an area, rather than the rate of production or utilization. This is particularly important in the splanchnic area[31] where the liver receives some arterial blood from the hepatic artery, but the majority of its blood flow is portal venous blood from the gut. The net splanchnic balance reflects a change in hepatic release (production) or uptake (utilization), a change in uptake or release by the gut, or a combination of these possibilities. Because of these limitations, another method was developed that used tracers (stable or radioactive isotopes of the substrate being studied) to enable calculation of rates of production and utilization of substrates.

Tracer methodology involves analysis of isotope dilution data. Equations were developed that could be used to calculate the rate of turnover using a single-compartment approach with the single-injection technique[32] or using a constant tracer infusion technique.[33] The rates of production and utilization can be determined by using a primed constant infusion and applying equations of DeBodo *et al.*[34] which are based on equations developed by Wall *et al.*[35] and Steele *et al.*[36,37] The DeBodo *et al.* method has been validated in steady state[38] and nonsteady state.[39,40] It is based on stochastic single-compartment analysis of glucose kinetics, in which changes in glucose specific activity and/or concentration do not occur throughout the entire glucose pool but only in a fraction of the entire pool. Cowan and Hetenyi[41] empirically determined that the pool fraction was 0.65.

3. HORMONAL CONTROL OF FUEL REGULATION DURING EXERCISE

Increased energy requirements of exercising muscles are fulfilled by an increased rate of mobilization of fuel substrates. Hormonal milieu and adrenergic nervous system have been studied as two regulatory systems of fuel mobilization and utilization. Although catecholamines are regarded as hormones in some discussions, catecholamines as fuel regulators will be included in the section discussing adrenergic regulation of fuel mobilization.

3.1. Hormonal Control of Glucose Regulation

Glucose utilization by muscles increases during exercise to meet the energy needs. Insulin stimulates glucose uptake and transport in insulin-sensitive tissues (i.e., adipose, muscle, etc.) and therefore is a potential regulator of glucose utilization in exercising muscles. The proposed mechanism would be that exercise causes an increase in insulin concentration which would increase glucose utilization by muscles. The disparate findings of increased glucose utilization and decreased insulin concentration during exercise as compared to pre-exercise rest in many studies[8–10,18] did not appear to support the proposed mechanism. A possible explanation of the disparity is that although there is a decrease in circulating insulin concentration, there is an increased presentation of insulin to the muscle due to an increase in blood flow and increase of capillary surface area.[8] Studies have shown an increase in insulin uptake by muscles during exercise,[42] supporting the idea of increased availability of insulin to exercising muscles.[8] In contrast, *in vitro* studies suggest that muscular contraction and insulin stimulate sugar transport by two different mechanisms.[43,44] Some studies have found or implied that insulin[45,46] or insulin-like, i.e., nonsuppressible insulin-like activity (NSILA),[47] material is released from exercising muscles as a local hormone that increases glucose uptake of muscles. Goldstein[48,49] proposed that a muscular activity factor (MAF) was released by exercising muscles and activated the glucose transport system. These local factors may either directly stimulate glucose uptake or potentiate the effect of insulin. The essential role of insulin in relation to the exercise-induced glucose uptake was shown in several studies. In one study,[50] depancreatized, i.e., insulin-deficient, dogs were exercised and no resulting increase in rate of glucose utilization was seen. Exercise did not increase the rate of glucose utilization in perfused, isolated, skeletal muscle of diabetic rats (i.e., insulin-deficient), but when insulin was added to the perfusate, glucose utilization did increase.[51] Another study,[8] using depancreatized dogs which had insulin therapy discontinued immediately prior to experimentation, showed that exercise caused a rise in the rate of glucose utilization compared to pre-exercise rest rates, but no rise in the metabolic clearance rate of glucose (which is the ratio of glucose utilization rate to the prevailing glucose concentration) occurred, which indicates that the increase in glucose utilization was due to the mass effect of glucose and not directly to exercise. The necessity of insulin for an exercise-induced increase in glucose metabolic clearance rate was also seen in a study comparing depancreatized dogs, chemically induced diabetic dogs, and normal dogs.[52] From the combined data of these and other studies, it can be concluded that insulin is essential for stimulation of glucose utilization.

The increased glucose utilization by muscles during exercise is closely matched by increased hepatic glucose production,[8,50,53] which maintains euglycemia, without which brain cells would starve and cease functioning. In contrast to glucose utilization being primarily regulated by insulin, glucose production is regulated by many factors. Gollnick *et al.*[54] found that glycogenolysis during exercise continues even when many regulatory systems are inactivated, indicating that one or more ineffective glucose production regulatory systems can be compensated for by other systems. The increased glucose output during exercise of brief duration comes predominantly from an acceleration of glycogenolysis.[18] During mild exercise of 3 to 4 hours duration, the relative contribution of gluconeogenesis to total glucose output increases from 25% at rest to 45%.[19,55] During 4 hours of mild exercise, 50 to 60 g of liver glycogen is mobilized, which is about 75% of the hepatic glycogen reserve.[19] Exercise causes a decrease in circulating insulin concentration[3–9,56,57] due to inhibition of insulin secretion rather than an increase in insulin clearance.[8] It has been suggested that the suppression of insulin is mediated by the adrenergic system.[56,58] The decrease in insulin during exercise removes the inhibitory effect of insulin on glycogenolysis and gluconeogenesis effects of hormones such as glucagon, thereby promoting an increase in hepatic glucose production.[8,12,30,59] Hepatic glycogenolysis is very sensitive to the inhibitory effect of small increments in insulin.[60] Richter *et al.*[61] suggest that the decrease in insulin may also act as a restraint on glucose utilization by nonexercising tissue.

Glucagon, another important glucoregulatory hormone, increases 3- to 5-fold during moderate to strenuous exercise.[1–4,7–9] Glucagon is an important stimulator of hepatic gluconeogenesis and glycogenolysis.[62] The adrenergic system has been implicated as the mediator of the exercise-induced increase in glucagon, but whether it is beta-[63,64] or alpha-adrenergic[65] receptor mediated is still unsettled. The essentiality of the presence and/or increment of glucagon during exercise has been studied. Normal dogs were compared to depancreatized, insulin-infused dogs that had resting glucagon levels similar to normal dogs due to extrapancreatic glucagon[66–69] originating from the gastrointestinal tract.[67–69] During exercise, glucose production increased in both groups, but in the normal dogs glucagon increased 3-fold, while in the depancreatized dogs, glucagon remained unchanged[8] (extrapancreatic glucagon has been shown to be unresponsive to exercise and secretagogues[67]). From this study,[8] it was concluded that the increment in glucagon seen during strenuous exercise may not be essential for appropriate glucose production changes. The essentiality of the presence of basal glucagon was studied by suppressing glucagon via somatostatin during exercise in dogs.[7] Glucagon suppression caused attenuation of the increase in glucose production compared to pre-suppression rates. It was concluded that during exercise, glucagon plays an essential role in direct stimulation of hepatic glucose production.

Glucagon may play an indirect role in glucose utilization because glucagon suppression causes a decrease in glucose production. which can cause a decrease in glucose, which can cause the release of catecholamines. The catecholamines can increase lipolysis, which can decrease glucose utilization by muscle,[7] but no direct role for glucagon has been implicated. Concurrent plasma insulin and glucagon elevations by infusions increased glucose turnover while maintaining normoglycemia.[70] Glucagon stimulated glucose production and was not inhibited by insulin infusion rates up to 3000μU/kg·min, while insulin stimulated glucose utilization and was not affected by the concurrent glucagon infusion.

Exercise induces an increase in growth hormone concentration[5,6,58,71] and, in prolonged or strenuous exercise, an increase in cortisol.[5,6,58] The effect and importance of these increases are not yet known, although glucocorticoids may potentiate the effects of epinephrine.[72] Exercise increases epinephrine, which in turn increases glucose production transiently but causes a small (15%) increase in glucose utilization and a 20% decrease in the metabolic clearance rate of glucose even in the presence of a twofold increase in insulin.[72]

An elevated free fatty acid concentration represents one factor that limits glucose utilization in exercising dog,[73,74] the same way as added palmitate decreases glucose utilization by the rat heart had hemidiaphragm.[75] Randle *et al.*[76] noted that the glucose–fatty acid cycle provides a primitive hormone-independent mechanism to maintain glucose, and Paul *et al.*[77] studied the cycle in dogs. Newsholme[78] suggested that increased FFA availability inhibits glucose utilization. In some recent studies, elevated FFA concentration has been found to have a direct inhibitory effect on glucose production *in vivo,*[79,80] and conversely, lowering FFA caused an increase in glucose production *in vitro.*[81]

The type of exercise as well as training and diet have been shown to influence the pattern of hormonal responses.[5,6,58,82] Graded exercise of short duration (5 to 8 min) induced a decrease in insulin; only heavy exercise induced an increase in cortisol, epinephrine. and norepinephrine; and growth hormone was released to the greatest degree with moderate exercise. Training decreased insulin and norepinephrine response to exercise.

Again, it should be suggested that many of these hormonal alterations may be backups to compensate for each other in case one hormone becomes inoperative.

3.2. Hormonal Control of Free Fatty Acid Regulation

Insulin is known to be a lipogenic hormone or antilipolytic hormone.[78] The exercise-induced decrease in insulin has a lipolytic effect and raises FFA concentration[61] and may potentiate lipolytic hormones such as norepinephrine and growth hormone.[74] Conversely, Murray *et al.*[83] showed that exercise during infusion of insulin in diabetic man inhibits FFA mobilization.

Glucagon may indirectly affect FFA regulation. As noted above, in a glucagon-suppressed state, glucose declines. With the decline in glucose, there is a concomitant increase in FFA while glucose utilization is suppressed. However, it is unlikely that glucagon acts directly as a lipolytic hormone because even pharmacological doses of glucagon fail to increase FFA when infused into resting normal dogs[84] or depancreatized dogs.[60]

4. ADRENERGIC CONTROL OF FUEL REGULATION DURING EXERCISE

The adrenergic system is another regulatory system of fuel regulation; hormonal milieu was discussed previously. In many studies concerning exercise, adrenergic receptor blocking agents are used to define the adrenergic control of fuel mobilization during exercise. Therefore, references to the adrenergic nervous system or adrenergic system include all systems or agonists that mediate their actions via the adrenergic receptors, i.e., the adrenomedullary system and the adrenergic nervous system. Thus epinephrine and norepinephrine may be classified as hormones and be functionally included within the adrenergic nervous system.

4.1. Brief History

In 1895, Oliver and Schafer[85] studied the pressor effects of suprarenal (later known as adrenal) extracts. The catecholamines synthesized and secreted by the adrenal medulla (primarily epinephrine in man[86,87] but epinephrine and norepinephrine in rat[87]) are secreted into the circulation and affect many target tissues and metabolic functions. The catecholamines synthesized, stored, and released by postganglionic sympathetic nerve terminals (predominantly norepinephrine in the peripheral nervous system) function as adrenergic neurotransmitters and influence the metabolism of localized sites of innervation.[88] The responses to catecholamines are divided into two major classes.[89] alpha and beta, which are subdivided[90–92] based on potencies of natural and synthetic catecholamines for the receptors mediating the responses. The mechanism of α- and/or β-receptor activation is not yet fully known, but it is generally thought that β-receptor activation causes an increase in cyclic AMP (adenosine-3′,5′-monophosphate) and α-receptor activation is cAMP independent or causes a decrease in cAMP.[88,93] The changes in cAMP might, in fact, mediate both the α and β responses while α- and β-receptors modulate adenylate cyclase in opposing manners.[94] The mechanisms will be discussed further below.

4.2. Adrenergic Control of Glucose Regulation

Soon after the hormonal and metabolic changes that occur during exercise and in response to hypoglycemia were elucidated, the importance of the adrenergic nervous system's involvement in fuel regulation began to emerge. Circulating levels of epinephrine and norepinephrine are increased during exercise.[3,5,6] Norepinephrine increases before changes in glucagon and insulin concentrations occur in response to exercise.[61] In contrast, epinephrine is dependent on both the level of sympathetic activity and on glucose levels,[95] and thus epinephrine increases later than norepinephrine, when glucose begins to decrease.[3] Increased levels of epinephrine is evidence of adrenal medulla stimulation, but norepinephrine may come from either nerves or the adrenal medulla.[96]

Studies,[8,50] of exercising depancreatized dogs have suggested adrenergic control of glucoregulation. Several studies[97–101] have shown the importance of glucagon and epinephrine in counterregulating insulin-induced hypoglycemia. They have shown that an increase in glucagon is the primary counterregulatory process during hypoglycemia in man, with epinephrine being nonessential or secondary. Recent studies[102,103] have shown that in human counterregulation during exercise, adrenergic control, and specifically norepinephrine, is the primary regulator with insulin and glucagon becoming critical only in adrenergic-deficient states. The import of epinephrine for liver glycogenolysis during exercise in rats is controversial.[87,104] Studies[105–107] suggest that catecholamines counterregulate glucose homeostasis via β_2-adrenergic receptors.

Rizza *et al.*[108] showed that in man, physiological concentrations of epinephrine (4 nM) caused a direct transient increase of hepatic glucose production and a sustained suppression of glucose metabolic clearance. The suppression of glucose clearance by epinephrine was also seen in dogs.[109,110] In a subsequent study, *Rizza et al.*[111] showed that glucose production was increased via both α- and β-adrenergic receptors, and the suppression of glucose clearance appeared to be α-adrenergic mediated. However, this study did not control for changes in insulin, and hence the suppression of glucose clearance could have been both α- and β-adrenergic mediated with the β-adrenergic effect being masked by an α-mediated decrease in insulin. Epinephrine (an α and β-adrenergic agonist) produces a transient increase in glucose production and a decrease in glucose utilization, norepinephrine (predominantly an α-adrenergic agonist) produces a smaller transient increase in glucose production and a decrease in glucose utilization, and isoproterenol (a β-adrenergic agonist) produces a lasting maintained increase in glucose production and an increase in glucose utilization.[112] The increase in glucose utilization during isoproterenol possibly results from isoproterenol-induced hypoinsulinemia. A well-controlled study[113] using a pancreatic clamp with portal replacement of insulin and glucagon in dogs demonstrated a direct effect of epinephrine of increasing glucose production by increasing both hepatic glycogenolysis and gluconeogenesis, although the increased gluconeogenesis is an indirect effect of epinephrine mediated by increased alanine and lactate supply from extrahepatic tissue, probably muscle. The existence of direct endogenous α-adrenergic stimulation of hepatic glucose production is controversial.[114,115]

There seems to be a species difference in the import of α- and β-adrenergic stimulation of hepatic glucose production. *In vitro* studies in rodents have indicated that α-receptors are of prime importance[116–118]; in rabbits, β-adrenergic receptors mediate catecholamine-stimulated hepatic glucose production[119]; and in *in vivo* studies in cats, both α- and β-receptor mechanisms appeared to be involved in catecholamine-regulated hepatic glucose production.[120]

In addition to increasing hepatic glucose production and decreasing glucose utilization, epinephrine induces hyperglycemia, in part by interfering with the feedback effects of hyperglycemia on pancreatic β-cell and α-cell function.[121,122]

In a study[123] of dogs in a glucagon- and insulin-suppressed state, glucose metabolic clearance rose during exercise as in normal dogs, then dropped due to the counterregulatory effect of epinephrine release, i.e., epinephrine in a hypoinsulinemic milieu could accelerate both hepatic and muscle glycogenolysis. The increased utilization of FFA by muscle and increased muscle glycogenolysis would inhibit glucose uptake by muscle. In glucagon-suppressed hypoglycemic exercise, glycogenolysis in the muscle is accelerated and could lead to depleted glycogen stores. Thus, the main role of glucagon during exercise could be to preserve muscle glycogen via glucagon's stimulatory effect on hepatic glucose production. The isolated importance of glucagon was further elucidated by maintaining a euglycemic clamp during glucagon suppression in exercise, which eliminated the excessive epinephrine release.[13,14,123] There was little change in glucose production as compared to a state of hyperepinephrinemia, and thus by deductive reasoning, glucagon accounted for 80% of the exercise-induced increase in hepatic glucose production.

4.3. Adrenergic Control of Pancreatic Endocrine Secretions

Since adrenergic regulation of insulin and glucagon secretion would indirectly regulate fuel mobilization as already discussed, it is important to recognize the adrenergic control of pancreatic insulin and glucagon.

Gerich *et al.*[124] roughly characterized the adrenergic control of pancreatic α- and β-cell function in man and concluded that epinephrine stimulated glucagon secretion and that this stimulation was inhibited by β-adrenergic blockers and enhanced by α-adrenergic blockers; the same characterization was found in rats.[64] Glucagon secretion during exercise was due to increased sympathetic activity mediated through β_2-adrenergic receptors.[64]

Robertson and Porte[125] studied the adrenergic control of insulin secretion. Their results showed that there was continuous endogenous β-adrenergic activity that stimulated insulin secretion and α-adrenergic activity that inhibited insulin secretion. The conclusion was drawn that insulin secretion is continually modulated by adrenergic activity in both basal and stimulated (i.e., epinephrine infusion) states, and the importance of characterizing the adrenergic effects on insulin secretion in various diseases that displayed abnormal insulin responses, such as diabetes mellitus, was noted. Also, these authors observed no change in glucose levels when either phentolamine or propranolol was infused. Samols and Weir[126] showed in isolated pancreas that β-adrenergic agonism stimulated insulin and glucagon secretion and α-adrenergic agonism inhibited insulin secretion and moderately stimulated glucagon secretion. Raum *et al.*[127] showed that norepinephrine at chronic low-dose infusion (1.4 μg/min for 3 months) increased glucagon and glucose concentration and inhibited insulin concentration compared to saline infusion. Girardier *et al.*[128] showed that sympathetic stimulation of pancreas *in vivo* increased glucagon secretion and decreased insulin secretion, independent of glucose levels.

A recent study[129] has shown, using a purified rat islet cell preparation, that A cells contain β-adrenoreceptors only (no α-receptors) and that catecholamines, via these receptors. increase cAMP concentration and stimulate glucagon release. They found that B cells contain α_2-receptors only and that catecholamines, via these receptors, in the presence of an adenylcyclase activator such as glucagon will decrease cAMP concentration and inhibit insulin release. This supports previous findings[124,125] that epinephrine inhibits insulin secretion while stimulating glucagon secretion. Since inhibition of insulin secretion by epinephrine is via α-adrenergic activity and stimulation of glucagon secretion by epinephrine is via β-adrenergic receptors, epinephrine activates α-receptors on β cells while activating β-receptors on α cells.

4.4. Adrenergic Control of Free Fatty Acid Regulation

In addition to the adrenergic control of α- and β-cells and the possible direct effect of the adrenergic nervous system on hepatic glucogenesis, the sympathoadrenal system can regulate lipolysis. Glucopenic stress causes a catecholamine induced lipolysis.[130] Epinephrine was implicated as the primary hormone necessary for glycogenolytic and lipolytic response to acute hypoglycemia. Catecholamine-induced lipolysis is mediated predominantly via β_1-receptors but also by β_2-receptors, while catecholamine-induced muscle glycogenolysis is mediated via β_2-receptors.[107] Other studies[131,132] have shown that catecholamines play an important role in mobilization of FFA and glucose.

To study the role of catecholamines in cardiovascular, metabolic, and hormonal homeostasis, many studies have used α-adrenergic and/or β-adrenergic receptor blockades during exercise.[4,64,86,133,134] During exercise, propranolol reduced FFA and glycerol levels and the rate of FFA combustion, indicating that β-adrenergic stimulation promotes lipolysis.[4] A study [133] also showed that propranolol reduced the turnover of FFA and muscle glycogenolysis during exercise, resulting in an increase in glucose uptake by muscle. This, along with the observation that propranolol did not suppress glucose production, suggests that the primary role of catecholamines during exercise is not to regulate hepatic glucose production but to regulate lipolysis and muscle glycogenolysis.[30] Propranolol did not affect the exercise-induced decrease in insulin.[86]

Phentolamine, a nonselective α-adrenergic blocker, impeded the exercise-induced decrease in insulin.[56] α-Adrenergic blocking agents block not only postsynaptic α-adrenergic receptors (mostly α_1 receptors) but also presynaptic α-adrenergic receptors (α_2 receptors) that function to inhibit the release of norepinephrine from axon terminals,[86,135] which is a factor that leads to a large increase in circulating norepinephrine concentration during α-adrenergic blockades. It has been noted that studies using α- or combined α- + β-blockades present problems because of the circulatory effects produced by these blockades that leave the subject unable to exercise.[30]

5. MECHANISMS OF HORMONAL AND ADRENERGIC CONTROL OF FUEL REGULATION

In view of recent trends in research to investigate at the molecular level, it is important to mention some of the proposed mechanisms of control of fuel regulation.

It has been suggested that hormonal regulation alone cannot produce sufficiently precise regulation of metabolic fluxes to meet the energy demands of muscle.[136] Lipolytic lipase and hepatic phosphorylase activity is increased by glucagon, norepinephrine, and epinephrine, and decreased by insulin, but again the hormonal regulation is not sufficient to produce precise regulation of FFA release or glucose 1-phosphate release. respectively.[136] Hormones may increase substrate cycling. This increased cycling increases the sensitivity of enzymes to metabolic regulators (AMP, P_i^+, NH_4^+), which allows rapid and precise adjustments of fluxes to provide sufficient energy for contraction.

Free fatty acid oxidation regulates glucose utilization by the inhibitory effect of citrate on phosphofructokinase (PFKase).[136] However, opposing this inhibition are many PFKase deinhibitors (AMP, P_i^+, NH_4^+, and fructose bisphosphate) that reduce citrate inhibition of PFKase and thereby increase the rate of glycolysis and glucose utilization. This provides a nicely counterbalanced regulation.

Regulation of glucose production via gluconeogenesis occurs by (1) increased supply and uptake of gluconeogenic substrates[19] and (2) metabolic regulation of gluconeogenic enzyme activities. Hormonal regulation of both supply of substrates[137] and gluconeogenic enzyme activities[137–139] translates into hormonal regulation of glucose production via gluconeogenesis.

During heavy exercise and early in the course of submaximal exercise, liver produces glucose primarily by glycogenolysis. During prolonged exercise, gluconeogenesis contributes an ever-increasing fraction of the total glucose requirement. Several mechanisms exist for hormonal regulation of hepatic glycogenolysis. The glucagon- or catecholamine-initiated cAMP-dependent system[140] is best known and involves activation of adenylate cyclase with consequent sequential cascading and activation of phosphorylase. A second system involves catecholamines binding with α-adrenergic receptors and triggering release of CA^{2+} from intracellular binding sites. The free Ca^{2+} activates phosphorylase.[141,142] Another system is the direct neural mechanism for activation of liver glycogen phosphorylase,[143–146] which involves norepinephrine stimulation of the α-adrenergic receptor calcium-mediated system.[144] However, as discussed previously, the direct effect of adrenergic stimulation of hepatic glucose production is species specific and, at this time, very controversial.

Despite the identification of these mechanisms, the role they play during exercise is not known. Conflicting data exist with respect to the effects of glucagon[2] and catecholamines[147,148] on hepatic glucose production during exercise. The need for concentrations of epinephrine[142] higher than concentrations observed during exercise[149] suggests that the physiologically important cathecolamines are not the blood-borne catecholamines from the adrenals but rather the catecholamine neurotransmitters from direct hepatic innervation, which displays increased activity during exercise.[148] Additional studies are required to determine the relative roles of α- and β-adrenergic receptor-mediated effects of catecholamines during exercise on glycogenolysis and gluconeogenesis.

6. OTHER FUEL REGULATORY FACTORS

6.1. Cholinergic Control

The effect of parasympathetic stimulation on fuel regulation is not yet fully elucidated, although it has been found that parasympathetic stimulation increases hepatic glycogen and decreases hepatic glucose release in animals.[150] During parasympathetic stimulation, no change in arterial glucose concentration is observed in spite of reduced glucose production, implying that glucose utilization is reduced, possibly due to an anti-insulin factor that is released from the liver. Acetylcholine infusion stimulated insulin secretion and inhibited glucagon secretion *in vivo*.[151]

6.2. Glucose Autoregulation

Data from *in vivo* studies in dogs[152,153] and in humans[59,107,154–157] support the inverse correlation of hepatic glucose production to glucose concentration, independent of hormonal and neural regulatory factors. i.e., glucose autoregulation. This may be the final regulatory process when all other compensatory processes fail. A possible mechanism for glucose autoregulation has been mentioned previously in the section on mechanisms.

6.3. Dopamine

Dopamine inhibits prolactin release and stimulates glucagon and insulin release independent of adrenergic receptor activation.[158] By these hormonal changes, dopamine may indirectly control fuel regulation.

7. CLINICAL CONSIDERATIONS

7.1. Fuel Utilization in Diabetes

The preceding review of normal fuel utilization predicts the patterns seen in diabetes. In diabetic individuals, fuel utilization will be governed primarily by the relative degrees of insulin deficiency and insulin resistance, and on the adequacy of insulin replacement therapy. Diabetes does not appear to alter FFA transport, as control and diabetic subjects have similar FFA turnover rates.[53,59] In both groups of subjects, FFA uptake depends primarily on concentration. An exception occurs in the presence of ketosis, however, where fractional uptake of FFA is decreased. This is presumably related to preferential muscle uptake of ketone bodies.

Nonketotic diabetic subjects show splanchnic FFA uptake similar to controls, but a greater fraction of the FFA are converted to ketone bodies.[160] With exercise, splanchnic uptake of FFA falls, and in ketotic subjects, an even greater fraction is converted to ketones.[159] If metabolic control of diabetes is good, ketone body metabolism is normal. In insulin deficiency, on the other hand, exercise accelerates lipolysis and ketogenesis, which may not be balanced by the extra muscle consumption. In this case, ketosis is aggravated.

As previously noted, exercise is accompanied by a fall in insulin levels. In the diabetic subject treated with injections of insulin, insulin levels may not fall and, as discussed below, may sometimes rise. Thus, the exercise-mediated fall in insulin will not consistently occur in insulin-treated diabetes. While splanchnic glucose output still increases in response to exercise without a fall in insulin levels, the magnitude of the rise is not as great.[161] This may predispose to hypoglycemia during exercise. Increased muscle uptake of glucose will, of course, further contribute to hypoglycemia.

As noted above, the increased muscle uptake of glucose in exercise does not require an increase in insulin secretion. However, some insulin must be present for this effect of exercise to occur. Thus, the diabetic subject treated with adequate insulin can expect a decline in blood glucose concentration during exercise. However, the underinsulinized subject will see a rise in blood glucose, and possibly progressive ketosis.

There is some flexibility in insulin requirements, however. Zander *et al.*[162] studied subjects with type 1 diabetes either 1 hour or 3 hours after an injection of 4 units of regular insulin. Subjects were considered to be hyperinsulinemic 1 hour after injection and hypoinsulinemic 3 hours after injection, although insulin levels were not measured. Subjects exercised on a bicycle ergometer at an intensity up to 75% of VO_2 max. Although glucose and FFA levels tended to rise in the hypoinsulinemic trial, and fall in the hyperinsulinemic trial, the differences were not statistically or clincally significant, suggesting some leeway in planning exercise programs for persons treated with insulin.

7.2. Exercise Effects on Insulin Requirements

The effects of exercise on stimulating glucose uptake by muscle have been thoroughly discussed. In this manner, exercise has an effect similar to insulin and may reduce insulin requirements. However, exercise also has effects opposing those of insulin, such as increasing splanchnic output of glucose and FFA. In general, the insulin-like effects prevail, and exercise reduces insulin requirements. However, the possibility of exercise resulting in hyperglycemia and ketonemia must be kept in mind.

7.2.1. Exercise and Insulin Absorption

Insulin is generally injected subcutaneously, and its absorption may be related to blood flow in surrounding tissue. This has been demonstrated in studies by Zinman *et al.*[163] When insulin was injected at a rate of infusion designed to maintain high or normal blood glucose levels during exercise, exercise did not appreciably affect blood glucose concentration (Fig. 1). This suggests that the increased muscle uptake of glucose can be compensated for by controlling insulin levels, as happens physiologi-

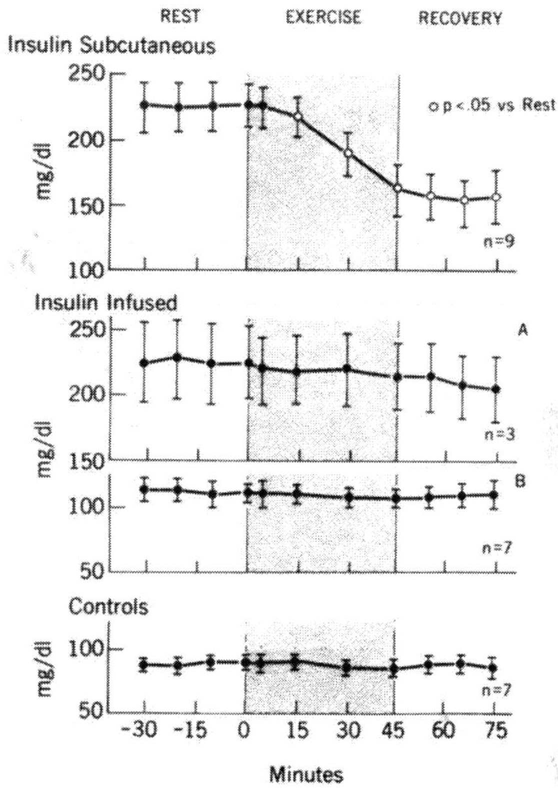

Figure 1. The effect of exercise (shaded area) on plasma glucose (mean ± SEM) in fasting postabsorptive diabetics given one-third their usual insulin dose subcutaneously 1 h prior to exercise (upper panel), or maintained hyperglycemic (middle panel A) or normoglycemic (middle panel B) by constant insulin infusion, and in normal controls (lower panel). From Zinman B, Vranic M, Albisser AM, et al: The role of insulin in the metabolic response to exercise in diabetic man. *Diabetes* 28(suppl 1):76–81, 1979. (Reproduced with permission from the American Diabetes Association, Inc.)

cally in nondiabetic subjects. However, when insulin was given subcutaneously 1 hour before exercise, the plasma glucose dropped markedly. The investigators concluded that this was due to uptake of insulin from the subcutaneous site. To verify this, they studied insulin injection into either the arm or the thigh in the same subject, followed by exercise on a bicycle with the arm immobilized, so only the thigh was exercised. Blood glucose fell after the thigh injection, but not the arm injection.

7.2.2. Exercise and Insulin Sensitivity

In addition to the acute physiological changes seen *during* exercise, there is some evidence that exercise may have lingering effects on intermediary metabolism. Trovati *et al.*[164] have shown that physical training (1 h a day for 6 weeks at 50% to 60% maximum oxygen uptake) results in improved blood glucose control and insulin action (Fig. 2). Following the exercise program, an oral glucose tolerance test yielded lower levels of both glucose and insulin, suggesting increased insulin sensitivity. The mechanism of this change is not known. Over a short term, exhaustive exercise will decrease the affinity of insulin receptors without affecting the receptor number. Interestingly, these effects can be reproduced by incubating pre-exercise cells with post exercise serum, suggesting mediation by a dialyzable serum component.[165]

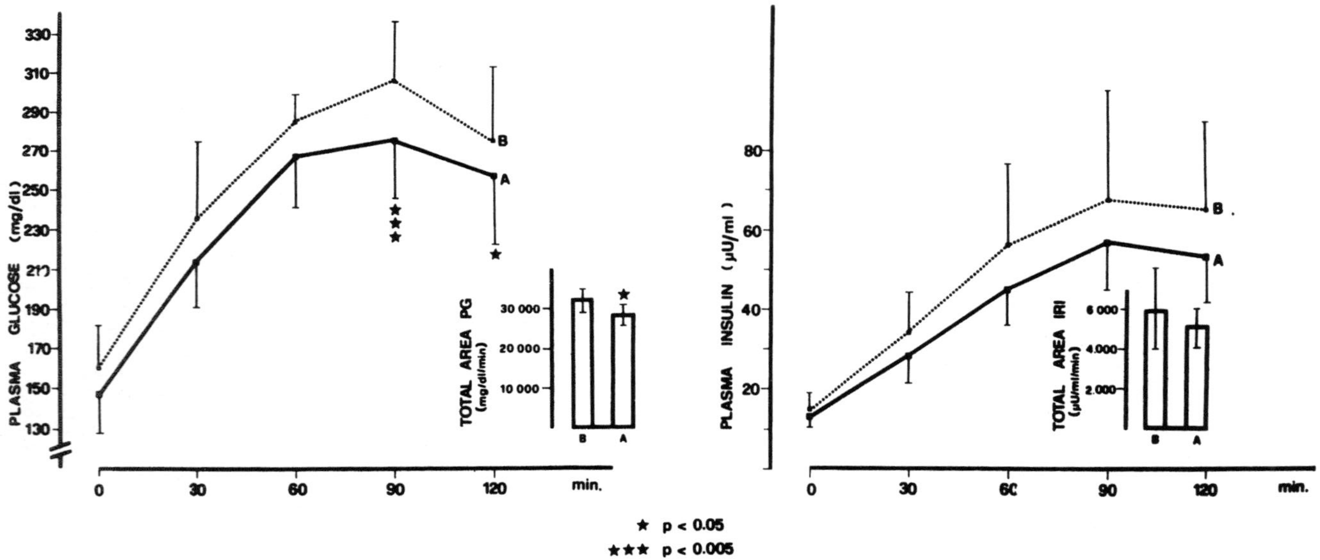

Figure 2. Plasma glucose (left panel) and plasma insulin concentrations (right panel) in five non-insulin-dependent diabetic patients during OGIT before (B) and after (A) a 6-week physical training. Total glucose and total insulin areas under the curves are also pictured. Data are expressed as mean ± SEM. (From Trovati M, Carta Q, Cavalot F, et al: Influence of physical training on blood glucose control, glucose tolerance, insulin secretion, and insulin action in non-insulin-dependent diabetic patients. *Diabetes Care* 7:416–420, 1984. Reproduced with permission from the American Diabetes Association. Inc.)

7.3. Recommendations for Clinical Practice

Exercise has both beneficial and potentially adverse effects in diabetes (Table 1). From a cardiovascular standpoint, exercise can reduce the risk of heart and vascular disease and enhance collateral circulation in diseased areas. On the other hand, diabetic neuropathy may eliminate perception of cardiac pain, thus causing angina of or myocardial infarction during exercise to go unnoticed. Appropriate exercise can help improve glycemic control, while exercise without proper diet or insulin may lead to hypoglycemia. If insulin therapy is insufficient, exercise may elevate glucose levels and lead to ketosis. The psychological benefits of being able to exercise are important to many diabetic patients. However, feet made insensitive by neuropathy, or with impaired circulation due to arteriosclerotic disease, may be more prone to injury.

The beneficial effects of exercise may be optimized, and risks minimized, by using the following guidelines[166,167]:

- Provide an appropriate exercise prescription, based on a careful physical evaluation.
- Patients should be instructed in self blood glucose monitoring, and should test their blood glucose before and after exercise, and during prolonged exercise, until the response to exercise is well characterized.
- Patients should be instructed in the signs and symptoms of hypoglycemia.
- A source of readily available carbohydrate should be available during exercise and afterwards.
- Exercise should be timed for when blood glucose is above fasting, perhaps 1 to 3 hours after a meal.
- If necessary on the basis of blood glucose testing, extra carbohydrate may need to be taken before or during exercise.
- Exercise should be postponed if the blood glucose is above 300 mg/dl.
- If necessary on the basis of blood glucose testing, or because of recurrent hypoglycemia, the insulin dose should be reduced on days exercise is planned.
- Patients should be instructed in proper shoes and other equipment, and should be taught proper foot inspection techniques.
- In a program of graded physical exercise leading to increased fitness, insulin and diet may require periodic evaluation, perhaps every two weeks initially.
- If exercise leads to weight loss, the insulin dose may need to be reduced, because of the relationship of obesity to insulin resistance.

Table 1. Exercise in Diabetes

Benefits	Risks
Cardiovascular	Cardiovascular
Glucose lowering	Hypoglycemia
Psychological	Foot and other injuries

- The site of insulin injection may need to be specified. In particular, rotating injection sites between exercising and nonexercising parts of the body may lead to erratic control. The abdomen tends to be a good injection site to use prior to exercise.

REFERENCES

1. Felig P, Wahren J: Fuel homeostasis in exercise. *N Engl J Med* 293:1078–1084, 1975.
2. Galbo H: *Hormonal and Metabolic Adaptation to Exercise*. New York, Thieme-Stratton Inc, 1983.
3. Galbo H, Holst JJ, Christensen NJ: Glucagon and plasma catecholamine responses to graded and prolonged exercise in man. *J Appl Physiol* 38:70–76, 1975.
4. Galbo H, Holst JJ, Christensen NJ, et al: Glucagon and plasma catecholamines during beta-receptor blockade in exercising man. *J Appl Physiol* 40:855–863, 1976.
5. Hartley LH, Mason JW, Hogan RP, et al: Multiple hormonal responses to graded exercise in relation to physical training. *J Appl Physiol* 33:602–66, 1972.
6. Hartley LH, Mason JW, Hogan RP, et al: Multiple hormonal responses to prolonged exercise in relation to physical training. *J Appl Physiol* 33:607–610, 1972.
7. Issekutz B Jr, Vranic M: Role of glucagon in regulation of glucose production in exercising dogs. *Am J Physiol* 238:E13–E20, 1980.
8. Vranic M, Kawamori R, Pek S, et al: The essentiality of insulin and the role of glucagon in regulating glucose utilization and production during strenuous exercise in dogs. *J Clin Invest* 57:245–255, 1976.
9. Zinman B, Murray FT, Vranic M, et al: Glucoregulation during moderate exercise in insulin treated diabetics. *J Clin Endocrinol Metab* 45:641–652, 1977.
10. Kawamori R, Vranic M: Mechanism of exercise-induced hypolycemia in depancreatized dogs maintained on long-acting insulin. *J Clin Invest* 59:331–337, 1977.
11. Martin MJ, Horwitz DL, Nattrass M, et al: Effects of mild hyperinsulinemia on the metabolic response to exercise. *Metabolism* 30:688–694, 1981.
12. Wolfe RR, Nadel ER, Shaw JHF, et al: Role of changes in insulin and glucagon in glucose homeostasis in exercise. *J Clin Invest* 77:900–907, 1986.
13. Wasserman DH, Lickley HLA, Vranic M: The metabolic role of glucagon during exercise. *Diabetes* 32(suppl 1):24A, 1983.
14. Wasserman DH, Lickley HLA, Vranic M: Interactions between glucagon and other counterregulatory hormones during normoglycemic and hypoglycemic exercise in dogs. *J Clin Invest* 74:1404–1413, 1984.
15. Andres R, Cader G, Zierler KL: The quantitatively minor role of carbohydrate in oxidative metabolism by skeletal muscle in intact man in the basal state: measurements of oxygen and glucose uptake and carbon dioxide and lactate production in the forearm. *J Clin Invest* 35:671–682, 1956.
16. Unger RH: Diabetes and the alpha cell. *Diabetes* 25:136–151, 1976.
17. Reichard GA, Issekutz Jr B, Kimbel P, et al: Blood glucose metabolism in man during muscular work. *J Appl Physiol* 16:1001–1005, 1961.
18. Wahren J, Felig P, Ahlborg G, et al: Glucose metabolism during leg exercise in man. *J Clin Invest* 50:2715–2725, 1971.
19. Ahlborg G, Felig P, Hagenfeldt L, et al: Substrate turnover during prolonged exercise in man: splanchnic and leg metabolism of glucose, free fatty acids, and amino acids. *J Clin Invest* 53:1080–1090, 1974.
20. Issekutz B Jr, Issekutz AC, Nash D: Mobilization of energy sources in exercising dogs. *J Appl Physiol* 29:691–697, 1970.
21. Hurley BF, Nemeth PM, Martin WH III, et al: Muscle triglyceride utilization during exercise: effect of training. *J Appl Physiol* 60:562–567, 1986.
22. Wahren J: Glucose turnover during exercise in healthy man and in patients with diabetes mellitus. *Diabetes* 28(suppl 1):82–88, 1979.

23. Owen OE, Felig P. Morgan AP, et al: Liver and kidney metabolism during prolonged starvation. *J Clin Invest* 48:574–583, 1969.
24. Cathcart EP, Burnett WA: The influence of muscle work on metabolism in varying conditions of diet. *Proc R Soc Biol* 99:405–426, 1926.
25. Hedman R: The available glycogen in man and the connection between rate of oxygen intake and carbohydrate usage. *Acta Physiol Scand* 40:305–321, 1957.
26. Krogh A, Lindhard KG: The relative value of fat and carbohydrate as sources of muscular energy: with appendices on the correlation between standard metabolism and the respiratory quotient during rest and work. *Biochem J* 14:290–363, 1920.
27. Wilson DW, Long WL, Thompson HC, et al: Changes in the composition of the urine after muscular exercise. *J Biol Chem* 65:755–771, 1925.
28. Felig P, Wahren J: Amino acid metabolism in exercising man. *J Clin Invest* 50:2703–2714, 1971.
29. Refsum HE, Stromme SB: Urea and creatinine production and excretion in urine during and after prolonged heavy exercise. *Scand J Clin Lab Invest* 33:247–254, 1974.
30. Vranic M, Berger M: Exercise and diabetes mellitus. *Diabetes* 28:147–167, 1979.
31. Wolfe RR: *Tracers in Metabolic Research: Radioisotope and Stable Isotope/Mass Spectrometry Methods*. New York, Alan R. Liss, 1984.
32. Zilversmit DB, Entenman C, Fishler MC: On the calculation of "turnover time" and "turnover rate" from experiments involving the use of labeling agents. *J Gen Physiol* 26:325–331, 1943.
33. Stetten D Jr, Welt ID, Ingle DJ, et al: Rates of glucose production and oxidation in normal and diabetic rats. *J Biol Chem* 92:817–830, 1951.
34. DeBodo RC, Steele R, Altszuler N, et al: On the hormonal regulation of carbohydrate metabolism; studies with C^{14}glucose. *Recent Prog Horm Res* 19:445–488, 1963.
35. Wall JS, Steele R, DeBodo RC, et al: Effect of insulin on utilization and production of circulating glucose. *Am J Physiol* 189:43–50, 1957.
36. Steele R: Influences of glucose loading and of injected insulin on hepatic glucose output. *Ann NY Acad Sci* 82:420–430, 1959.
37. Steele R, Wall JS, DeBodo RC, et al: Measurement of size and turnover rate of body-glucose pool by the isotope dilution method. *Am J Physiol* 187:15–24, 1956.
38. Hetenyi G Jr, Norwich KH: Validity of the rates of production and utilization of metabolites as determined by tracer methods in intact animals. *Fed Proc* 33:1841–1848, 1974.
39. Radzuik J, Norwich KH, Vranic M: Measurement and validation of nonsteady turnover rates with applications to the inulin and glucose systems. *Fed Proc* 33:1855–1864, 1974.
40. Radziuk J, Norwich KH, Vranic M: Experimental validation of measurements of glucose turnover in nonsteady state. *Am J Physiol* 234:E84–E93, 1978.
41. Cowan JS, Hetenyi G Jr: Glucoregulatorv responses in normal and diabetic dogs recorded by a new tracer method. *Metabolism* 20:360–372, 1971.
42. Berger M, Halban PA, Muller WA, et al: Mobilization of subcutaneously injected tritiated insulin in rats: effects of muscular exercise. *Diabetologia* 15:133–140, 1978.
43. Holloszy JO, Narahara HT: Studies of tissue permeability. X. Changes in permeability to 3-methyl-glucose associated with contraction of isolated frog muscle. *J Biol Chem* 240:3493–3500, 1965.
44. Kolbeck RC, Cavert HM, Wermers GW: Modifiers of sugar transport under the influence of muscular contraction. *Proc Soc Exp Biol Med* 140:1021–1024, 1972.
45. Dieterle P. Birkner B, Gmeiner K-H, et al: Release of peripherally stored insulin during acute muscular work in man. *Horm Metab Res* 5:316–322, 1973.
46. Rennie MJ, Park DM, Sulaiman WR: Uptake and release of hormones and metabolites by tissues of exercising leg in man. *Am J Physiol* 231:967–973, 1976.
47. Couturier E, Rasio E, Conard V: Insulin in plasma and lymph and tissue glucose uptake in the exercising hind limb of the dog. *Horm Metab Res* 3:382–386, 1971.
48. Goldstein MS: Humoral nature of hypoglycemia in muscular exercise. *Am J Physiol* 200:67–70, 1961.
49. Goldstein MS: Humoral nature of the hypoglycemic factor of muscular work. *Diabetes* 10:232–234, 1961.
50. Vranic M, Wrenshall GA: Exercise, insulin, and glucose turnover in dogs, *Endocrinology* 85:165–171, 1969.

51. Berger M, Hagg S, Ruderman NB: Glucose metabolism in perfused skeletal muscle: interaction of insulin and exercise on glucose uptake. *Biochem J* 146:231–238, 1975
52. Issekutz B Jr, Shaw WAS: Glucose turnover in the exercising dog with chemically induced diabetes and the effect of methylprednisolone. *Diabetes* 24:915–921, 1975
53. Wahren J, Hagenfeldt L, Felig P: Splanchnic and leg exchange of glucose, amino acids, and free fatty acids during exercise in diabetes mellitus. *J Clin Invest* 55:1303–1314, 1975
54. Gollnick PD. Soule RG, Taylor AW, et al: Exercise-induced glycogenolysis and lipolysis in the rat: hormonal influence. *Am J Physiol* 219:729–733, 1970.
55. Shaw WAS, Issekutz TB, Issekutz B Jr: Gluconeogenesis from glycerol at rest and during exercise in normal, diabetic, and methylprednisolone-treated dogs. *Metabolism* 25:329–339, 1976.
56. Galbo H, Christensen NJ, Holst JJ: Catecholamines and pancreatic hormones during autonomic blockade in exercising man. *Acta Physiol Scand* 101:428–437, 1977.
57. Hunter WM, Sukkar MY: Changes in plasma insulin levels during muscular exercise. *J Physiol (Lond)* 196:110P–112P, 1968.
58. Galbo H, Richter EA, Hilsted J, et al: Hormonal regulation during prolonged exercise. *Ann NY Acad Sci* 301:72–80, 1977.
59. Jenkins AB, Furler SM, Chisholm DJ, et al: Regulation of hepatic glucose output during exercise by circulating glucose and insulin in humans. *Am J Physiol* 250:R411–R417, 1986.
60. Felig P, Cherif A, Minagawa A, et al: Hypoglycemia during prolonged exercise in normal men. *N Engl J Med* 306:895–900, 1982.
61. Richter EA, Ruderman NB, Scheider SH: Diabetes and exercise. *Am J Med* 70:201–209, 1981.
62. Galbo H, Holst JJ: The influence of glucagon on hepatic glycogen mobilization in exercising rats. *Pflügers Arch* 363:49–53, 1976.
63. Luyckx AS, Dresse A, Cession-Fossion A, et al: Catecholamines and exercise-induced glucagon and fatty acid mobilization in the rat. *Am J Physiol* 229:376–383, 1975.
64. Luyckx AS, Lefebvre PJ: Mechanisms involved in the exercise-induced increase in glucagon secretion in rats. *Diabetes* 23:81–93, 1974
65. Harvey WD, Faloona GR, Unger RH: The effect of adrenergic blockade on exercise-induced hyperglucagonemia. *Endocrinology* 94:1254–1258, 1974
66. Matsuyama T, Foa, PP: Plasma glucose, insulin, pancreatic, and enteroglucagon levels in normal and depancreatized dogs. *Proc Soc Exp Biol Med* 147:97–102. 1974.
67. Muller WA, Girardier L, Seydoux J, et al: Extrapancreatic glucagon and glucagonlike immunoreactivity in depancreatized dogs: a quantitative assessment of secretion rates and anatomical delineation of sources. *J Clin Invest* 62:124–132, 1978.
68. Vranic M, Engerman R, Doi K, et al: Extrapancreatic glucagon and GLI: extrapancreatic glucagon in the dog. *Metabolism* 25(suppl 1):1469–1473, 1976.
69. Vranic M, Pek S, Kawamori R: Increased "glucagon immunoreactivity" in plasma of totally depancreatized dogs. *Diabetes* 23:905–912, 1974.
70. Cherrington AD, Vranic, M: Effect of interaction between insulin and glucagon on glucose turnover and FFA concentration in normal and depancreatized dogs. *Metabolism* 23:729–744, 1974.
71. Schwarz F, Ter Haar DJ, Van Riet HG, et al: Response of growth hormone (GH), FFA, blood sugar, and insulin to exercise in obese patients and normal subjects. *Metabolism* 18:1013–1020, 1969
72. Eigler N, Sacca L, Sherwin, RS: Synergistic interactions of physiologic increments of glucagon, epinephrine, and cortisol in the dog: a model for stress-induced hyperglycemia. *J Clin Invest* 63:114–123, 1979.
73. Colwell JA, Lein A: Quantitative relationship between plasma concentration of fatty acids and glucose in normal and diabetic dogs. *Diabetes* 12:424–428, 1963.
74. Issekutz B Jr, Paul P, Miller HI: Metabolism in normal and pancreatized dogs during steady-state exercise. *Am J Physiol* 213:857–862, 1967.
75. Randle PJ, Newsholme EA, Garland PB: Regulation of glucose uptake by muscle. 8. Effects of fatty acids, ketone bodies, and pyruvate, and of alloxan-diabetes and starvation, on the uptake and metabolic fate of glucose in rat heart and diaphragm muscles. *Biochem J* 93:652–665, 1964.
76. Randle PJ, Garland PB, Hales CN. et al: The glucose fatty-acid cycle: its role in insulin sensitivity and the metabolic disturbances of diabetes mellitus. *Lancet* 1:785–789, 1963.

77. Paul P, Issekutz B Jr, Miller HI: Interrelationship of free fatty acids and glucose metabolism in the dog. *Am J Physiol* 211:1313–1320, 1966.
78. Newsholme EA: Carbohydrate metabolism in vivo: regulation of the blood glucose level. *Clinics Endocrinol Metab* 5:543–578, 1976.
79. Seyffert WA Jr, Madison LL: Physiologic effects of metabolic fuels on carbohydrate metabolism. I. Acute effect of elevation of plasma free fatty acids on hepatic glucose output, peripheral glucose utilization, serum insulin, and plasma glucagon levels. *Diabetes* 16:765–776, 1967.
80. Wolfe RR, Shaw JHF: Inhibitory effect of plasma free fatty acids on glucose production in the conscious dogs. *Am J Physiol* 246:E181–E186, 1984.
81. Shaw JHF, Wolfe RR: Modulation of glucose production by free fatty acids. *Fed Proc* 41:1680, 1982.
82. Galbo H, Holst JJ, Christensen NJ: The effect of different diets and of insulin on the hormonal response to prolonged exercise. *Acta Physiol Scand* 107:19–32, 1979.
83. Murray FT, Zinman B, McClean PA, et al: The metabolic response to moderate exercise in diabetic man receiving intravenous and subcutaneous insulin. *J Clin Endocrinol Metab* 44:708–720, 1977.
84. Issekutz B Jr, Borkow I: Effect of glucagon and glucose load on glucose kinetics, plasma FFA, and insulin in dogs treated with methylprednisolone. *Metabolism* 22:39–49, 1973.
85. Oliver G. Schafer EA: The physiological effects of extracts of the suprarenal capsules. *J Physiol (Lond)* 18:230–276, 1895.
86. Christensen NJ, Galbo H, Hansen JF, et al: Catecholamines and exercise. *Diabetes* 28(suppl 1):58–62, 1979.
87. Richter EA, Galbo H, Sonne B, et al: Adrenal medullary control of muscular and hepatic glycogenolysis and of pancreatic hormonal secretion in exercising rats. *Acta Physiol Scand* 108:235–242, 1980.
88. Malbon CC: Avenues of adrenergic research. *J Lab Clin Med* 94:381–386, 1979.
89. Ahlquist RP: A study of adrenotropic receptors. *Am J Physiol* 153:586–600, 1948.
90. Lands AM, Arnold A, McAuliff JP, et al: Differentiation of receptor systems activated by sympathomimetic amines. *Nature* 214:597–598, 1967.
91. Berthelsen S, Pettinger WA: A functional basis for classifi^ation of α-adrenergic receptors. *Life Sci* 21:595–606, 1977.
92. Langer SZ: Presynaptic regulation of catecholamine release. *Biochem Pharmacol* 23:1793–1800, 1974.
93. Burns TW, Langley PE: Lipolysis by human adipose tissue: the role of cyclic 3′,5′-adenosine monophosphate and adrenergic receptor sites. *J Lab Clin Med* 75:983–997, 1970.
94. Robison GA, Butcher RW, Sutherland EW: Adenyl cyclase as an adrenergic receptor. *Ann NY Acad Sci* 139:703–723, 1967.
95. Galbo H, Christensen NJ, Holst JJ: Glucose-induced decrease in glucagon and epinephrine responses to exercise in man. *J Appl Physiol* 42:525–530, 1977.
96. Landsberg L, Young JB: The role of the sympathetic nervous system and catecholamines in the regulation of energy metabolism. *Am J Clin Nutr* 38:1018–1024, 1983.
97. Abramson EA, Arky RA, Woeber KA: Effects of propranolol on the hormonal and metabolic responses to insulin-induced hypoglycemia. *Lancet* 2:1386–1388, 1966.
98. Clarke WL, Santiago, JV, Thomas L, et al: Adrenergic mechanisms in recovery from hypoglycemia in man: adrenergic blockade. *Am J Physiol* 236:E147–E152, 1979.
99. Cryer PE: Glucose counterregulation in man. *Diabetes* 30:261–264, 1981.
100. Cryer PE, Gerich JE: The relevance of glucose counterregulatory systems to patients with diabetes: critical roles of glucagon and epinephrine. *Diabetes Care* 6:95–99, 1983.
101. Rizza R, Cryer PE, Gerich JE: Role of glucagon, epinephrine, and growth hormone in human glucose counterregulation: effects of somatostatin and adrenergic blockade on plasma glucose recovery and glucose flux rates following insulin-induced hypoglycemia. *J Clin Invest* 64:62–71, 1979.
102. Hoelzer DR, Dalsky GP, Clutter WE, et al: Glucoregulation during exercise: hypoglycemia is prevented by redundant glucoregulatory systems, sympathochromaffin activation, and changes in islet hormone secretion. *J Clin Invest* 77:212–221. 1986.
103. Hoelzer DR, Dalsky GP. Schwartz NS, et al: Epinephrine is not critical to prevention of hypoglycemia during exercise in humans. *Am J Physiol* 251:E104–E110, 1986.

104. Arnall DA, Marker JC, Conlee RK, et al: Effect of infusing epinephrine on liver and muscle glycogenolysis during exercise in rats. *Am J Physiol* 250:E641–E649. 1986.
105. Aigner UA, Muss N, Krempler F, et al: Einfluss einer akuten β_1- und β_1/β_2-rezeptorenblockade auf den kohlenhydrat- und fettstoffwechsel unter belastungsbedingungen. *Dtsch Med Wochenschr* 108:293–298, 1983.
106. Koerker DJ, Halter JB: Glucoregulation during insulin and glucagon deficiency: role of catecholamines. *Am J Physiol* 243:E225–E233, 1982.
107. Lager I: Adrenergic blockade and hypoglycemia. *Acta Med Scand* 672(suppl 1):63–67. 1983.
108. Rizza R, Haymond M, Cryer P, et al: Differential effects of epinephrine on glucose production and disposal in man. *Am J Physiol* 237:E356–E362, 1979.
109. Altszuler N, Steele R, Rathgeb I, et al: Glucose metabolism and plasma insulin level during epinephrine infusion in the dog. *Am J Physiol* 212:677–682, 1967.
110. Sacca L, Sherwin R, Felig P: Effect of sequential infusions of glucagon and epinephrine on glucose turnover in the dog. *Am J Physiol* 235:E287–E290, 1978.
111. Rizza RA, Haymond MW, Miles JM, et al: Effect of α-adrenergic stimulation and its blockade on glucose turnover in man. *Am J Physiol* 238:E467–E472, 1980.
112. Sacca L, Morrone G, Cicala M, et al: Influence of epinephrine, norepinephrine, and isoproterenol on glucose homeostasis in normal man. *J Clin Endocrinol Metab* 50:680–684, 1980.
113. Cherrington AD, Fuchs H, Stevenson RW. et al: Effect of epinephrine on glycogenolysis and gluconeogenesis in conscious overnight-fasted dogs. *Am J Physiol* 247:E137–E144, 1984.
114. Best JD, Ward WK, Pfeifer MA, et al: Lack of a direct α-adrenergic effect of epinephrine on glucose production in human subjects. *Am J Physiol* 246:E271–E276, 1984.
115. Rosen SG, Clutter WE, Shah SD. et al: Direct α-adrenergic stimulation of hepatic glucose production in human subjects. *Am J Physiol* 245:E616–E626, 1983.
116. Exton JH: Minireview: mechanisms involved in alpha-adrenergic effects of catecholamines on liver metabolism. *J Cycl Nuc Res* 5:277–287, 1979.
117. Hutson NJ, Brumley FT, Assimacopoulos FD, et al: Studies on the α-adrenergic activation of hepatic glucose output. *J Biol Chem* 251:5200–5208, 1976.
118. Seydoux J, Brunsmann MJA, Jeanrenaud B. et al: α-Sympathetic control of glucose output of mouse liver perfused in situ. *Am J Physiol* 236:E323–E327, 1979.
119. Muhlbachova E, Chan PS, Ellis S: Quantitative studies of glucose release from rabbit liver slices induced by catecholamines and their antagonism by propranolol and phentolamine. *J Pharmacol Exp Ther* 182:370–377, 1972.
120. Kuo S-H, Kamako JK, Lum BKB: Adrenergic receptor mechanisms involved in the hyperglycemia and hyperlacticacidemia produced by sympathomimetic amines in the cat. *J Pharmacol Exp Ther* 202:301–309, 1977.
121. Beard JC, Weinberg C, Pfeifer MA, et al: Interaction of glucose and epinephrine in the regulation of insulin secretion. *Diabetes* 31:802–807, 1982.
122. Halter JB, Beard JC, Porte D Jr: Islet function and stress hyperglycemia: plasma glucose and epinephrine interaction. *Am J Physiol* 247:E47–E52, 1984.
123. Vranic M, Gauthier C, Bilinski D. et al: Catecholamine responses and their interactions with other glucoregulatory hormones. *Am J Physiol* 247:E145–E156, 1984.
124. Gerich JE, Langlois M, Noacco C, et al: Adrenergic modulation of pancreatic glucagon secretion in man. *J Clin Invest* 53:1441–1446, 1974.
125. Robertson RP, Porte D Jr: Adrenergic modulation of basal insulin secretion in man. *Diabetes* 22:1–8, 1973.
126. Samols E, Weir GC: Adrenergic modulation of pancreatic A, B, and D cells: α-adrenergic suppression and β-adrenergic stimulation of somatostatin secretion, α-adrenergic stimulation of glucagon secretion in the perfused dog pancreas. *J Clin Invest* 63:230–238, 1979.
127. Raum WJ, Swerdloff RS, Garner D, et al: Chronic norepinephrine infusion and insulin and glucagon secretion in the dog. *Am J Physiol* 246:E232–E236, 1984.
128. Girardier L, Seydoux J, Campfield LA: Control of A and B cells in vivo by sympathetic nervous input and selective hyper or hypoglycemia in dog pancreas. *J Physiol (Lond)* 72:801–814, 1976.

129. Schuit FC, Pipeleers DG: Differences in adrenergic recognition by pancreatic A and B cells. *Science* 232:875–877, 1986.
130. Brodows RG, Pi-Sunyer FX, Campbell RG: Neural control of counter-regulatory events during glucopenia in man. *J Clin Invest* 52:1841–1844, 1973.
131. Issekutz B Jr, Allen M: Effect of catecholamines and methylprednisolone on carbohydrate metabolism of dogs. *Metabolism* 21:48–59, 1972.
132. Pequignot JM, Peyrin L, Peres G: Catecholamine–fuel interrelationships during exercise in fasting men. *J Appl Physiol* 48:109–113, 1980.
133. Issekutz B Jr: Role of beta-adrenergic receptors immobilization of energy sources in exercising dogs. *J Appl Physiol* 44:869–876, 1978.
134. Issekutz B Jr: Energy mobilization in exercising dogs. *Diabetes* 28(suppl 1):39–44, 1979.
135. Westfall TC: Local regulation of adrenergic neurotransmission. *Physiol Rev* 57:659–728, 1977.
136. Newsholme EA: The control of fuel utilization by muscle during exercise and starvation. *Diabetes* 28(suppl 1):1–7, 1979.
137. Exton JH: Hormonal control of gluconeogenesis. *Adv Exp Med Biol* 111:125–167, 1976.
138. Hers HG, Hue L: Gluconeogenesis and related aspects of glycolysis. *Annu Rev Biochem* 52:617–653, 1983.
139. Pilkis SJ, Chrisman TD, El-Maghrabi MR, et al: The action of insulin on hepatic fructose 2,6-bisphosphate metabolism. *J Biol Chem* 258:1495–1503, 1983.
140. Exton JH, Blackmore PF, El-Refai MF, et al: Mechanisms of hormonal regulation of liver metabolism. *Adv Cycl Nuc Res* 14:491–505, 1981
141. Exton JH: Mechanisms involved in α-adrenergic phenomena: role of calcium ions in actions of catecholamines in liver and other tissues. *Am J Physiol* 238:E3–E13, 1980.
142. Exton JH, Assimacopoulos-Jeannet FD, Blackmore PF, et al: Mechanisms of catecholamine actions on liver carbohydrate metabolism. *Adv Cycl Nuc Res* 9:441–452, 1978.
143. Edwards AV, Silver M: The glycogenolytic response to stimulation of the splanchnic nerves in adrenalectomized calves. *J Physiol (Lond)* 211:109–124, 1970.
144. Hartmann H, Beckh K, Jungermann, K: Direct control of glycogen metabolism in the perfused rat liver by the sympathetic innervation. *Eur J Biochem* 123:521–526, 1982.
145. Nobin A, Falck B, Ingemansson S, et al: Organization and function of the sympathetic innervation of human liver. *Acta Physiol Scand (Suppl)* 452:103–106, 1977.
146. Shimazu T, Amakawa A: Regulation of glycogen metabolism in liver by the autonomic nervous system. VI. Possible mechanism of phosphorylase activation by the splanchnic nerve. *Biochim Biophys Acta* 385:242–256, 1975.
147. Sonne B, Mikines KJ, Galbo H: Role of autonomic hepatic innervation for glucose turnover during running in rats. *Acta Physiol Scand* 121:13A, 1984.
148. Winder WW, Beattie MA, Piquette C, et al: Decrease in liver norepinephrine in response to exercise and hypoglycemia. *Am J Physiol* 244:R845–R849, 1983.
149. Winder WW, Boullier J, Fell RD: Liver glycogenolysis during exercise without a significant increase in cAMP. *Am J Physiol* 237:R147–R152, 1979.
150. Lautt WW: Hepatic nerves: a review of their functions and effects. *Can J Physiol Pharm* 58:105–123, 1980.
151. Tyler JM, Kajinuma H: Influence of beta-adrenergic and cholinergic agents in vivo on pancreatic glucagon and insulin secretion. *Diabetes* 21:332, 1972.
152. Sacca L, Cryer PE, Sherwin RS: Blood glucose regulates the effects of insulin and counterregulatory hormones on glucose production in vivo. *Diabetes* 28:533–536, 1979.
153. Shulman GI, Liljenquist JE, Williams PE, et al: Glucose disposal during insulinopenia in somatostatin-treated dogs: The roles of glucose and glucagon. *J Clin Invest* 62:487–491, 1978
154. Liljenquist JE, Mueller GL, Cherrington AD, et al: Hyperglycemia per se (insulin and glucagon withdrawn) can inhibit hepatic glucose production in man. *J Clin Endocrinol Metab* 48:171–175, 1979.
155. Sacca L, Hendler R, Sherwin RS: Hyperglycemia inhibits glucose production in man independent of changes in glucoregulatory hormones. *J Clin Endocrinol Metab* 47:1160–1163, 1978.
156. Sacca L, Sherwin R, Hendler R. et al: Influence of continuous physiologic hyperinsulinemia on

glucose kinetics and counterregulatory hormones in normal and diabetic humans. *J Clin Invest* 63:849–857, 1979.

157. Wolfe RR, Shaw JHF, Jahoor F, et al: Response to glucose infusion in humans: role of changes in insulin concentration. *Am J Physiol* 250:E306–E311, 1986.
158. Lorenzi M, Karam JH, Tsalikian E, et al: Dopamine during α- or β-adrenergic blockade in man. *J Clin Invest* 63:310–317, 1979.
159. Hagenfeldt L: Metabolism of free fatty acids and ketone bodies during exercise in normal and diabetic man. *Diabetes* 28(suppl 1):66–70, 1979.
160. Sestoft L. Trap-Jensen J, Lyngsoe J, et al: Regulation of gluconeogenesis and ketogenesis during rest and exercise in diabetic subjects and normal men. *Clin Sci Mol Med* 53:411–418, 1977.
161. Felig P, Wohren J: Role of insulin and glucagon in the regulation of hepatic glucose production during exercise. *Diabetes* 28(suppl 1):71–75, 1979.
162. Zander E, Schulz B, Chlup R, et al: Muscular exercise in type 1 diabetics. II, Hormonal and metabolic responses to moderate exercise. *Exp Clin Endocrinol* 85:95–104, 1985.
163. Zinman B, Vranic M, Albisser AM, et al: The role of insulin in the metabolic response to exercise in diabetic man. *Diabetes* 28(suppl 1):76–81, 1979.
164. Trovati M, Carta Q, Cavalot F, et al: Influence of physical training on blood glucose control. glucose tolerance, insulin secretion, and insulin action in non-insulin-dependent diabetic patients. *Diabetes Care* 7:416–420, 1984.
165. Michel G, Vocke T, Fiehn W, et al: Bidirectional alteration of insulin receptor affinity by different forms of exercise. *Am J Physiol* 247(Endocrinol Metab 9):E153–E159, 1984.
166. Rifkin H, editor-in-chief: *The Physician's Guide to Type II Diabetes (NIDDM).* Alexandria, VA, The American Diabetes Association, 1984, pp 35–36.
167. Vignati L, Cunningham LN: Exercise and diabetes, in Marble A, Krall LP, Bradley RF, et al (eds): *Joslin's Diabetes Mellitus,* ed 12. Philadelphia, Lea & Febiger. 1985. pp 453–464.

10

Drug Abuse in Athletes

Nancy A. Nuzzo and Donald P. Waller

1. INTRODUCTION

> The trainers would bring your medication to your hotel room the night before the game. Empirin compound for men in pain, amphetamine for men expecting pain, specialty drugs for players with chronic injuries, experimental drugs for those who had little body left to sacrifice, including butazolidin for joint pain (a drug also used to treat horses) and of course, sleeping pills.[1]

The above quote certainly was not the first written evidence of man's attempts to modify performance using drugs. An apple for Adam and Eve, mushrooms in the third century B.C., sesame seeds in ancient Greece, bufotein of the legendary Berserkers in Norwegian mythology, coca leaves in South America, pituri of Australian aborigines, and large amounts of coffee for the Army of the Potomac during the Civil War all represent man using current-day knowledge of drugs to increase his ability to perform.[2] Man in general, not just athletes, has always tried to use drugs to elevate the quality of life and the performance of the body.

Major advances in the field of pharmacology, specifically since the late 1940s, have provided modern man with a large number of true miracle drugs. Society has been observing the major changes in health status provided by these drugs. The development of sulfonamides and, shortly thereafter, the penicillins represented a major turning point in the dependence of man upon chemical substances. The success of antibiotics in the fifties resulted in a reverence on the part of the layperson for the doctor who could provide the curative potion. Pharmacologists continued to develop new, more powerful entities capable of altering the function of specific organ systems. The use of drugs to control major disease states gradually developed within man expectations of the ability of drugs to solve all health problems. Many of us have become "chemical junkies" and expect a drug to treat all of our physiological, pathological, and psychological problems and deficiencies.

Modern drugs moved out of the area of health care and into the realm of recreation and self medication during the sixties. Dr. Timothy O'Leary, with the help of the

---

Nancy A. Nuzzo and Donald P. Waller • College of Pharmacy, University of Illinois at Chicago, Chicago, Illinois 60612.

press, publicized the recreational use of drugs. Large numbers of people began to use and accept drugs provided outside of the normal medical channels. At the same time, the media provided a barrage of information on available drugs and their pharmacological effects. A substantial increase in the lay knowledge of drugs occurred. A simple look at the number, types, and potency of over-the-counter remedies available today compared to twenty years ago provides evidence of the lay confidence in self-medication and the increased availability of drugs as a purely consumer commodity.

1.1. Why Do Athletes Abuse Drugs?

The competitive nature of sports is a powerful driving force for athletes to utilize the advances of modern-day science to improve performance and gain a competitive edge. Modern-day athletes have lucrative salaries or scholarships at stake or carry the honor of their school or country when competing. These factors only enhance the competitive nature of man. All types of advances, from batting gloves to fiberglass poles for pole vaulting. have become accepted in order to improve sports performance. The use of pharmacological agents by modern athletes to improve performance is an expected outcome of the availability of powerful new drugs and the social acceptance of self-medication. To the athlete, the benefits of drug abuse outweigh the perceived risks.

Athletes have used a variety of ergogenic aids. Table 1 lists the classes of agents and individual agents both past and present abused by athletes. The ergogenic effects can take many forms. Mechanical, pharmacological, and psychological aids have been developed over many years to maximize performance. Man may be approaching his natural limit of performance.[3] World-class competitors achieve a world record or become world champions with very small changes in performance. There is a great deal of concern among athletic groups that competitors will develop a new manner in which to have a competitive edge. This causes an ever-strengthening circle of events involving the trial use of new and more powerful pharmacological agents.

Intense competition often creates a lack of self-confidence and insecurity in athletes. The chemical boost, whether psychological or ergogenic, becomes an important part of some athletes' ability to continue competing and to deal with competition in spite of self-perceived deficiencies. The use of recreational drugs in athletes may also be a stress-related problem, such as is common for any mental or physical performance-oriented profession.

Athletic competition frequently results in overexertion or injuries. These can have a major impact on performance levels. The availability of drugs that can mask injuries and allow the athlete to continue to perform will provide a short-term solution to the problem of overcoming an injury. Unfortunately, this also frequently leads to increased damage to the tissue and a shortening of a sports career.

1.2. Definition of the Problem

The definition of drug abuse and the decision as to which drugs to ban from competition are difficult and complex. There are medical and ethical considerations.

Table 1. Drugs Banned by the National Collegiate Athletic Association—1986[a]

Psychomotor stimulants		
Amphetamine	Benzphetamine	Chlorphentermine
Cocaine	Diethylpropion	Dimethylamphetamine
Ethylamphetamine	Fencamfamin	Meclofenoxate
Methylamphetamine	Methylphenidate	Norpseudoephedrine
Pemoline	Phendimetrazine	Phenmetrazine
Phentermine	Pipradol	Prolintane
Sympathomimetic amines		
Clorprenaline	Ephedrine	Etafedrine
Isoetharine	Isoprenaline	Methoxyphenamine
Methylephedrine	Phenylpropanolamine	
Miscellaneous central nervous system stimulants		
Amiphenazole	Bemigride	Caffeine[b]
Crolethamide	Cropropamide	Doxapram
Ethamivan	Leptazol	Nikethamide
Picrotoxin	Strychnine	
Anabolic steroids		
Clostebol	Dehydrochlormethyltestosterone	Methandienone
Fluoxymesterone	Mesterolone	Norethandrolone
Methenolone	Nandrolone	Oxymetholone
Oxandrolone	Oxymesterone	
Stanozolol	Testosterone[c]	
Diuretics		
Bendroflumethiazide	Benzthiazide	Clorthalidone
Bumetanide	Chlorothiazide	Flumethiazide
Cyclothiazide	Ethacrynic acid	Hydroflumethiazide
Furosemide	Hydrochlorothiazide	Metolazone
Methyclothiazide	Methyclothiazide	Spironolactone
Polythiazide	Quinethazone	
Triamterene	Trichlormethiazide	
Substances banned for riflery		
Atenolol	Alcohol	Tetoprolol
Nadolol	Pindolol	Propranolol
Timolol		
Street drugs		
Amphetamine	Cocaine	
Marijuana[d]	Methamphetamine	
THC (tetrahydrocannabinol)	Heroin	
	Others	

[a]Modified from Wagner JC: Substance abuse policies and guidelines in amateur and professional athletics. *Am J Hosp Pharm* 44: 305–310, 1987.
[b]If the concentration in urine exceeds 15 μg/m.
[c]If the ratio of the total concentration of testosterone to that of epitestosterone in the urine exceeds 6.
[d]Based on a repeat test.

Stated in simple medical terms, drug abuse occurs when dosages exceed medical standards and/or there is no medical indication for use of the drug. However, ethical considerations make the problem much more complex. Drugs are used by athletes to produce a wide variety of effects leading to improved performance, including increased aggressiveness, increased physical strength, delay of fatigue, increased mental concentration, decreased palpitations, increased body mass, shifts in weight patterns, steady hands, and prevention of anxiety. Some uses of drugs are easy to categorize as being unethical, such as taking drugs to increase muscle strength and endurance or to increase aggressiveness.

Other drugs effects may be beneficial to one type of sport and detrimental to another. Alcohol or propranolol may help the rifle marksman but be inhibitory to the performance of football players. The utilization of antianxiety agents such as Valium to reduce anxiety levels and induce a good night's sleep prior to competion is clearly within the approved medical guidelines for use of such agents. Should such use of a drug be banned due to a potential improvement in the athlete's performance? Propranolol is taken by ski jumpers to prevent palpitations prior to jump runs. Will this directly improve the performance of the athlete? Does it decrease the risk of cardiac problems for the ski jumpers?

Pain alleviation is a primary medical indication for analgesic drugs. When does the administration of an analgesic and/or anti-inflammatory agent become abuse? Pain reduction may permit continued performance of the athlete but may mask warning pain and cause increased or possibly irreversible damage to tissues. Some athletes take analgesics to decrease the pain which will occur during hard training sessions. This can mask pain that is a warning of overexertion or beginning of tissue damage.

It is interesting to note that most drugs are banned because they may positively affect performance. A drug used to decrease pain allows continued participation with the risk of permanent or increased tissue damage. Is this really good medicine or does it constitute drug abuse? It appears that regulations are primarily concerned with the possibility that drugs will affect the outcome of a particular competition and not with what their effects will be on the competitors. Any considerations of drug abuse must be within the context of improper utilization of a drug, whether or not an increase in performance is achieved. A list of drugs banned by the National Collegiate Athletic Association (NCAA) is given in Table 1.

1.3. Breadth of the Problem

Recent autobiographies of professional baseball and football players have detailed the scope of drug abuse in professional sports. Attempts to begin routine drug testing in professional athletics will be most interesting. Since performance is a key to winning, and winning is the basis for large profits, it will be difficult to establish which drugs should be banned and tested for. The illegal recreational drugs, such as heroin and marijuana, can be easily placed on the list.

The current media celebrity status of professional athletes has drawn the attention of young people to this group of people. The use of drugs by professional and college athletes has encouraged drug use by younger athletes. Young athletes model their training and sports lifestyle based upon their perceived impressions of ''model athletes.'' When young athletes experiment with recreational drugs of abuse along with the nonathletes,[4] the drug experimentation may naturally be extended to agents they can use to increase athletic performance. There is little fear of drugs during younger years. The warnings of traditional authority figures including physicians often go unheeded. The young body frequently responds to pharmacological agents in a different or modified way compared to the body of a mature adult. There are major physiological changes occurring during adolescent development with an increased susceptibility to drug alteration and damage. Bone growth, hormones surges, changes in cardiac function are all part of the pubescent adolescent physiology. The abuse of drugs during these important years of physiological development can cause unknown alterations in physiological systems. The adolescent years are also very difficult psychologically. Young athletes may become dependent upon abused drugs to maintain the self-image that was originally built up by and attributed to the use of drugs.

1.4. Drug Research on Agents of Abuse

The development of therapeutic drugs is accompanied by pharmacological testing of efficacy and toxicological testing of safety. The animal models and the patient populations utilized in clinical tests are chosen according to the medical indications of the drug. The use of a drug by an athlete frequently has little relationship to the original pharmacological testing, and the dose may be very different from the amount utilized in clinical trials. For instance, the doses of anabolic steroids currently used by athletes are far in excess of the original doses tested in clinical trials.

The abuse of drugs in athletics presents some special problems related to the risk of side effects. The physiological status of an athlete during heavy exercise creates a special environment for a drug's action. Heat load and physical exercise cause a shift of blood flow, changes in cardiac function, and frequently an increase in core body temperature.[5] Drugs are not tested for side effects under such extreme conditions. British cyclist Simpson collapsed and died after taking amphetamines during the 1967 Tour de France. His death was probably directly related to the tremendous heat production and increased core body temperature during competition.

Several of the classes of drugs routinely abused can cause changes in cardiac function and peripheral resistance. These changes may be deadly in combination with exercise-induced alterations in the physiological status of the body such as heat load, electrolyte balance, fluid balance, and metabolic rate.

Athletes frequently utilize excessive doses to maximize the effects of a drug. In many cases, the liability for side effects make it medically unethical to perform a clinical study using the doses routinely used by athletes. Clinical follow-up of athletes frequently is anecdotal and inaccurate. This makes the scientific data available on drugs of abuse limited and not related to the real life situation. Anabolic steroids have clear pharmacological effects in animal models, and early clinical studies demonstrated minor changes associated with anabolic steroid administration. However, none of the studies utilized the large doses currently used by athletes. Most athletes obtain information from other athletes on which drugs to take and how much drug is needed to achieve the desired effects. The scare tactics of the sixties on the dangers of drugs have created a credibility gap between the medical community and drug users. Several years will pass before the medical community once again becomes the primary source of "reliable" information to the drug abuser.

Placebo effects are extremely powerful. The perceived benefits of drug augmentation of performance are frequently much greater than any actual benefits,[6] particularly when the placebo is identified as a performance enhancer prior to administration. There are few good blind studies which evaluate clinical performance of athletes. Blind clinical studies can be very difficult to perform. A characteristic odor, such as with DMSO, or a psychological effect, such as with amphetamine, can be readily recognized by most subjects so that the drug can often be distinguished from the placebo by the subject. The evaluation of the subject's performance then becomes a study of the perceived effects of the agent and not a truly blind study.

There have been many different classes of drugs abused by athletes. Table 2 lists a wide variety of drug classes or individual agents abused by athletes. Drugs taken by

Table 2. Drugs and Drug Classes Used and Abused by Athletes

Restorative	Nonsteroidal Anti-inflammatory Drugs
	Steroidal anti-inflammatory drugs
	Local anesthetics
	Analgesics
	Analgesic creams and balms
	Oxygen
	Proteolytic enzymes
	Mild sedatives
	Muscle relaxants
	Beta blockers
	Calcium channel blockers
	Erythrocytes
	DMSO
Ergogenic	Antacids
	Laxatives
	Diuretics
	Vasodilators
	Multivitamins
	Iron
	Hormones (HCG, growth hormone)
	Caffeine
	Nicotine
	Stimulants
	Anabolic steroids
	Alcohol
	Cocaine
Recreational	Narcotics
	Depressants
	Marijuana, hashish
	Hallucinogens

athletes fall into three broad categories: (a) restorative agents, (b) ergogenic agents, taken to increase the work potential of the athlete, and (c) recreational agents, taken just to experience a drug effect. No lines are drawn in Table 2 to separate these categories since there is overlap between all of them. Cocaine, for example, is abused for both its ergogenic and recreational effects. The following sections review some of the major drug classes and current established procedures used to enhance performance of athletes.

2. BLOOD DOPING

Blood doping, blood boosting, or blood packing is an attempt to increase the amount of red blood cells (RBCs) available for oxygen transport. Medically, this is defined as induced erythrocythemia or polycythemia. Induced polycythemia usually consists of collecting blood, separating out the RBCs storage of the RBCs, and finally transfusion of the RBCs prior to an athletic event. The athlete usually collects his/her own blood to minimize the possibility of hepatitis and blood-type incompatibility. This must be done 5 to 6 weeks prior to the time of doping to ensure regeneration of lost RBCs. The collection of blood may decrease the ability of the athlete to train, thus negating some of the effects attained at the time of doping.[7]

Refrigeration of whole blood decreases RBC numbers by approximately 60% in 3 weeks; thus, freezing is required to obtain a maximum number of viable red blood cells. Frozen blood only loses approximately 15% of functional RBCs when stored up to two years.[8]

The number and timing of the red blood cell infusions are important. Hemoglobin (Hb) and hematocrit (Hct) remain low for 1 to 2 weeks after blood is removed, followed by a return to normal values over 5 to 6 weeks. The reinfusion of the red blood cells before a return to normal Hb and Hct would decrease the polycythemia achieved. An adequate number of RBCs must also be infused. The minimum amount appears to be about 900 ml or 2 units of blood. The Hb concentration and Hct were found to increase 8% over 24 hours and 11% after 1 week following the reinfusion of 900 ml of blood. The following 15 weeks produced a linear decrease to control values.[7]

Physiologically, an elevated hemoglobin (Hb) concentration increases arterial oxygen content, thereby increasing maximal aerobic power and performance. This is true only if the amount of oxygen delivered to the tissues is the limiting factor for exercising muscle. An increase in maximal aerobic power and/or endurance capacity post-reinfusion has been observed when at least 900 ml of RBCs in saline were infused. However, the oxidative capacity for muscles may not be completely dependent on the amount of oxygen delivered, leading to some question as to the real potential for benefits of artificially induced polycythemia.[7]

The safety of blood doping is a major concern. A transient hypervolemia occurs after blood doping with RBCs, followed by an increase in hematocrit. The hypervolemia is probably too transient to modify athletic performance or create problems due to increased cardiac work load. However, the increase in hematocrit could lead to increases in blood viscosity. Blood flow velocity is inversely related to viscosity. There is an exponential increase in blood viscosity when the hematocrit is greater than 50%.[15] The normal amount of RBCs used in doping can raise the hematocrit almost to 50%. Increases in viscosity can decrease venous return and cardiac output with a concomitant decrease in the transport of oxygen to peripheral tissues. The amount of RBCs added to the blood must be rigidly controlled to achieve a maximal performance-enhancing effect without creating undesirable changes in the vasculature due to changes in viscosity. Great caution must be exercised to ensure that the amount of transfused RBCs does not increase the hematocrit beyond 50% and cause not only a decrease in performance but also shifts in blood circulation and alterations in cardiac function leading to tissue damage.[7]

Induced polycythemia is banned by drug regulatory committees, but detection is difficult because of the difficulty in distinguishing autologous transfused red blood cells from naturally occurring blood cells.[9] Training at high altitudes causes a natural polycythemia and could place a low-altitude-trained athlete at a disadvantage. Should blood doping be permitted to make all competitors have equal RBC concentrations?

The side effects of induced polycythemia in normal individuals appear to be minimal. Electrocardiogram testing during exercise gave no evidence of abnormalities or ischemia after reinfusion.[7] However, studies to detect any long-term physiological effects have not been completed.

The use of induced polycythemia to modulate the RBCs of athletes may be of some benefit to correct deficiencies with minimal side effects. However, it is easy to visualize the abuse of induced polycythemia as excessive amounts of blood are transfused to achieve an ever increasing number of RBCs and maximize performance.

3. BICARBONATE INGESTION

Bicarbonate loading or buffer boosting consists of the ingestion of sodium bicarbonate to increase the body's buffer reserve and counteract the buildup of lactic acid. Energy required for muscle contraction is primarily provided by oxidative processes. However, heavy exercise can deplete oxygen stores and cause a shift to anaerobic glycolysis. Anaerobic glycolysis is self-limiting due to the production of lactic acid. Lactic acid buildup after 1 to 4 minutes of anaerobic glycolysis inhibits anaerobic glycolysis and results in fatigue. The increased buffering capacity of the blood following bicarbonate ingestion may increase the rate of lactic acid removal from muscle cells. This would extend the length of time before lactic acid buildup inhibits anaerobic glycolysis.[10]

Bicarbonate loading is probably beneficial in short-term exhaustive exercise such as running, swimming, and/or cycling.[11] Early studies were inconclusive or did not observe an increase in performance because inadequate doses were administered or performance in primarily aerobic types of exercise was observed. More recent studies demonstrated that bicarbonate ingestion enhanced exercise time to exhaustion.[10,12] The dose at which an increase in performance can be observed is about 300 mg/kg body weight (equivalent to 11 tablets of Alka Seltzer for a 70-kg person).

The most common acute side effect of excessive sodium bicarbonate ingestion is diarrhea.[11] This occurs several hours post-ingestion. The amount of bicarbonate required for effects on performance will cause diarrhea in most subjects. An excessive loss of bicarbonate can occur during diarrhea, which may decrease the buffering of bicarbonate and induce an acidosis. The fluid loss due to diarrhea may also result in some fluid imbalance when added to the potential for loss of water due to perspiration during heavy exercise. It is obvious that the timing of the dose of bicarbonate must be considered by the athlete for both practical and pharmacological reasons.

Chronic bicarbonate ingestion can lead to hypercalcemia and alkalosis. Alkalosis can cause a variety of changes in electrolyte balance and respiration. Alkalosis will depress the central respiratory centers and the peripheral chemoreceptors and lead to hypoventilation and hypercapnia.[13] The potential for alkalosis is exacerbated in athletes when heavy exercise leads to water loss through perspiration. Symptoms of alkalosis include neuromuscular irritability (hyperreflexia, twitching, and possible tetany), which is in part related to a decrease in ionized calcium. Arrhythmias may also develop. Alkalosis also shifts the oxyhemoglobin dissociation curve to the left, making oxygen less available to tissues. The increased lactic acid produced may also lead to an increased anion gap. Precipitation of calcium phosphate in the kidney (nephrocalcinosis) can also occur, resulting in renal insufficiency.[13]

Bicarbonate is readily available in over-the-counter products such as antacids used to buffer acid in the stomach and some analgesic preparations such as Alka Seltzer. The presence of bicarbonate in combination products such as Alka Seltzer could lead to problems. Alka Seltzer contains 100 mg of salicylate. The number of tablets needed to produce a significant bicarbonate load would result in a dose of more than 1 g of salicylate. Bicarbonate loading with Alka Seltzer and concurrent abuse of salicylates could lead to an exaggerated electrolyte imbalance.

Sodium bicarbonate loading is not currently banned from athletic competitions. However, since the concept of enhanced performance is the basis for this practice, sodium bicarbonate falls under the definition of a doping agent. Excessive sodium bicarbonate can be detected in the urine. Therefore, in the future, excessive sodium bicarbonate ingestion could be considered an illegal action in athletic competition.

4. GROWTH HORMONE

Growth hormone (GH) (somatotropin) is used by athletes, alone or in combination with steroid hormones, because of its anabolic effects. (See Chapter 13.) A positive nitrogen and phosphorus balance occurs following growth hormone administration. A positive nitrogen balance is essential for muscle growth. A short-lived increase in serum blood levels of GH is observed during exercise and recovery. However, no studies to date demonstrate increased strength or endurance in association with the administration of growth hormone.[14–16]

GH is normally used by athletes during training to increase muscle mass. Doses are usually small and infrequent. GH is produced by the body in bursts with a short half-life (20 to 30 min). Since of growth hormone is administered for increased muscle mass, the use would be during training in the weeks/months prior to competition. The detection of exogenous growth hormone (extracted from cadavers) would be impossible since it could not be distinguished from naturally produced growth hormone and would have to be measured within 1 h of administration. The distribution through approved pharmaceutical suppliers of growth hormone extracted from cadavers was officially stopped during 1985 because of the possible transmission of the Creutzfeldt–Jakob virus, which causes a fatal, degenerative neurological disease.[17] The current method of producing growth hormone utilizes recombinant-DNA technology. Growth hormone produced by this method may be detectable because it is not an exact duplicate of the natural growth hormone. However, it also has a short half-life and thus there is little chance of it being detected just prior to competition when most drug testing is performed.

Growth hormone is an important hormone with effects on almost every tissue and organ. It is required to achieve normal stature prior to puberty. Children without adequate growth hormone (dwarfism) can achieve normal stature by treatment with exogenous growth hormone. Growth hormone administered to a normal child will also accelerate growth. It is the fear of health officials that physicians will be pressured by parents who want larger children. Excessive growth hormone prior to puberty will cause gigantism. Giant children who survive to become adults have died early in adult life of infection, progressive debility, or hypopituitarism.[18]

In adults, after the closure of the epiphyses in bones, prolonged exposure to growth hormone can result in acromegaly. This condition is characterized by bone and soft tissue deformities without growth in stature. Changes in bony and soft tissues are readily recognized, such as spadelike hands, increased length and thickness of the mandible, frequently resulting in overbite, coarse facial features with enlarged frontal, mastoid, and ethmoid sinuses, enlarged feet, vertebral changes (humpback appearance), and visual field changes. Articular symptoms, from mild arthralgias to severe crippling arthritis, can occur. Skin texture becomes coarse and leathery, and body hair increases and becomes coarse. Excessive sweating combined with unusual oiliness can lead to unpleasant body odor. The tongue is frequently enlarged and furrowed. Peripheral nerves can also be affected due to inappropriate growth of bony or soft tissue around nerves leading to acroparesthesias. Enlargement of the heart and chronic myocardiopathy can also occur. Hepatomegaly with enlarged thyroid, parathyroid, spleen, and pancreas are also observed. The kidney increases in size with enlarged glomeruli and tubules. Inulin clearance, tubular reabsoption of glucose and phosphate, and tubular secretion also increase.[18]

Hormone secretion may also be affected. Hyperthyroidism, increased prolactin levels with gynecomastia, inappropriate lactation, decreased corticotropins, and gonadotropins can occur in association with acromegaly. Growth hormone is also considered diabetogenic due to its ability to decrease glucose uptake into some tissues (e.g., muscle).[18]

The frequencies of manifestations associated with acromegaly are given in Table 3. The effects vary with age and amount of hormone present. The levels of growth hormone associated with acromegaly are inconstant. Acromegaly can occur with abrupt rises at short intervals as well as continuous hypersecretion and elevated blood levels of GH.[17] Children are most sensitive to the effects of growth hormone.

Table 3. Clinical Manifestations of Acromegaly

Symptom	Approximate incidence (%)
Acral enlargement and dermal overgrowth	100
Hyperhidrosis	75
Menstrual dysfunction	65
Headache	60
Peripheral neuropathy (paresthesia, sensory and motor)	60
Male sexual dysfunction	45
Impaired glucose tolerance and diabetes	40
Goiter	30
Cardiac abnormalities	25
Hypertension	25
Galactorrhea (women)	20
Visual field defects	15
Hypothyroidism	Rare
Hypoadrenocorticism	Rare

5. ANABOLIC STEROIDS

Anabolic steroids have been severely abused by professional and amateur athletes to increase muscle mass and strength. (See Chapters 2 and 7.) Testosterone is the male sex steroid primarily responsible for male secondary sex characteristics and has both anabolic and androgenic actions. Anabolic steroids mimic the anabolic actions of testosterone with minimal androgenic effects such as excessive hair growth, aggressive behavior, hirsutism, and acne. Competitors in any athletic event requiring great strength and body mass could benefit from anabolic effects. Anabolic steroids may be even more effective when used by female athletes due to the low natural levels of steroids, such as testosterone, with anabolic character.

Anabolic steroids can be taken orally and/or by intramuscular injection (i.m.). Many athletes use a "stacking" regimen to maximize the anabolic effects, minimize side effects, and decrease the risk of detection. This involves alternating oral and i.m. administration of the anabolic steroids over several weeks.[19,20] A typical anabolic regimen is shown in Table 4.

Studies have shown a significant increase in body size, weight, and strength with the use of anabolic steroids in trained weight lifters who continued workouts while on treatment.[21] Studies have shown the increases in weight did not occur from fluid retention. Anabolic steroid treatment did not increase hemoglobin concentration, reduce subcutaneous fat, or stimulate the central nervous system. A benefit of anabolic steroid use from the athlete's point of view is decreased fatigue; however, no scientific data corroborate this apparently psychological effect.

The actions of anabolic steroids are due to anabolic, anticatabolic, and motivational effects.[21] The anabolic effects are mediated primarily through a shift to

Table 4. Anabolic Steroid "Stacking" Regimen

Weeks	Drug	Route and amount
1–3	Testosterone	Injection, 200 mg/week
	Anabolic steroid	Oral, 10 mg/day
4–6	Testosterone	Injection, 400 mg/week
	Anabolic steroid	Oral, 15 mg/day
7–8	Testosterone	Injection, 600 mg/week
	Anabolic steroid	Oral, 20 mg/day
	Anabolic steroid No. 2 may be stacked	
9–10	Testoserone	Injection, 200 mg/week
	Anabolic steroid	Oral, 20 mg/wk
	Anabolic steroid (No. 2)	Oral, 20–150 mg/wk
11	Testoseterone	Discontinued
	Anabolic steroid	Discontinued
	Anabolic steroid (No. 2)	Oral, 20–150 mg/wk
12	Human chorionic gonadotropin (HCG)	Injection, 500 IU only on last day of week
	Anabolic steroid (No. 2)	Oral, reduced gradually over week period
	HCG	Injection, 1000 IU only on last day of week
13		

[a]No drugs used during final week preceding competition. Some athletes may use a diuretic to increase urine flow and "flush" the system of steroids.

positive nitrogen balance as a result of increased nitrogen retention through improved utilization of ingested protein. This effect may be short-lived due to compensatory mechanisms. An induction of protein synthesis in skeletal muscle cells also occurs through the activation of the synthesis of ribosomal and messenger RNA. A strict drug regimen must be followed to produce increased muscle mass. In addition, the subject must be in continous training throughout steroid administration and must increase dietary protein intake. These criteria are imperative for muscle production. Athletes can develop a chronic negative nitrogen balance during training. This negative state must be present for anabolic steroids to produce the positive nitrogen balance needed to increase muscle tissue. An increase in ingested protein may also be required to raise nitrogen retention and achieve a positive nitrogen balance.

The anticatabolic actions occur primarily when an athlete is in heavy training. Glucocorticosteroid hormones are released from the adrenal cortex in response to the stress of heavy training to cause an elevation of blood glucose through gluconeogenesis in the liver and initiation of catabolism of muscle protein. Muscle catabolism and negative nitrogen balance can result in an undesirable decrease in muscle tissue. The anabolic steroids block the effects of the glucocorticosteroids and increase utilization of ingested proteins to minimize the negative nitrogen balance.[21]

The motivational effects of anabolic steroids are related to a state of euphoria and diminished fatique which enhances training. The real value of this effect is somewhat questionable. A similar effect can be observed in athletes given placebos and told that they have been given anabolic steroids.[21]

The side effects of anabolic steroids depend upon the amount and duration of administration. Short-term treatment usually causes reversible side effects whereas chronic treatment may cause permanent changes. For example, anabolic steroids interrupt the male reproductive system. Normally testosterone is secreted from the testes in response to a pituitary hormone, luteinizing hormone (LH). When testosterone is low, LH is secreted and testosterone production in the testes increases. This cycle allows for normal sperm production (spermatogenesis) in the testes. When anabolic steroids are present, mimicking testosterone action, the body does not release LH to produce more testosterone. The testes undergo atrophy and decreased spermatogenesis occurs. This effect can be reversed. Unfortunately, with extensive long-term use, a male could become infertile permanently. Women taking steroids experience repoductive complications also. In addition to increased facial hair, male-pattern baldness, and deepening of the voice, enlargement of the clitoris and menstrual irregularities may occur. Extended use of steroids could also result in infertility in women.[6,22]

There is some evidence that rapid growth in muscle tissues may not allow for appropriate concomitant strengthening of tendons. Tendinitits may occur and make competing more difficult for some athletes.[6]

The typical regimen of anabolic steroids includes several courses of self-injected steroids. Since the use of anabolic steroids is frequently without medical supervision, there is a potential for contamination of needles. Septic shock and the transmission of disease can result. The current spread of AIDS should be an adequate warning of the problems associated with improper injection of drugs.[6]

Recently, human chorionic gonadotropin (hCG) has begun to be used in conjunction with anabolic steroids to decrease side effects.[22] This commercially available hormone is produced naturally by pregnant women. In early pregnancy, estrogen and progesterone are high, thus inhibiting the release of LH from the pituitary. hCG is secreted by the embryo to mimic LH by stimulating more production of estrogen from the ovary. It seems that the LH-like action of hCG can also occur in the testes. When hCG is administered to males in combination with anabolic steroids, the testes appear to function normally. However, to date no conclusive studies have been done on the long-term effects of hCG and anabolic steroid treatment.

Steroid use has also been associated with increased coronary heart disease and atherosclerosis. These diseases are characterized by low ratios of high-density lipoprotein (HDL)/cholesterol (Ch) in the plasma. Significant decreases in HDL/CH were found in trained weight lifters following standard treatment (oral administration followed by i.m. injection) with anabolic steroids.[23,24] There is growing concern of a rise in athlete deaths from heart problems associated with chronic steroid use.

Anabolic steroid use is also associated with liver abnormalities.[19,21] These disorders are usually reversed upon cessation of steroid treatment. However, chronic use can cause liver tumors as seen in androgen treatment of anemia, kidney disorders, impotence, and hypopitutarism. Blood-filled sacs in the liver (peliosis hepatis) can develop with oral anabolic steroid treatment. These sacs can cause severe hemorrhage and ultimately liver failure upon rupture.

The use of steroids in adolescents is far more serious than in adults. In addition to the side effects listed above, there is premature closure of the epiphyses, causing short stature. Epiphyseal closure normally occurs at puberty with natural increases in endogenous testosterone or estrogen. Additionally, these abnormal increases in steroids can also irreversibly affect the reproductive system of prepubertal males and females, causing permanent infertility.[6,25]

6. ANTI-INFLAMMATORY AGENTS

Anti-inflammatory agents are used by athletes to alleviate pain and swelling due to injury. (See Chapter 8.) Athletic competition and the long hours of preparation for competition frequently lead to overexertion, overt injury of tissues, or tissue damage due to chronic use. Joints, in particular, are damaged or become sore and swollen due to physical stress. Anti-inflammatory agents are used to mask an injury and permit the athlete to continue training and competition.

Anti-inflammatory agents do not improve the performance of a healthy, injury-free athlete. They are usually not included in the list of banned drugs for athletes but are surely one of the most abused categories of pharmacological agents used in sports medicine. Anti-inflammatory agents can permit an athlete to compete at his/her normal level of performance despite injuries which would normally reduce performance or even prevent the athlete from competing. A significant amount of risk may be involved in the administration of such a drug. The masking of pain may exacerbate the injury, leading to permanent damage to a joint or muscle. Precautions should be taken to prevent the unwarranted or unmonitored use of anti-inflammatory agents during treatment for sports injuries. Anti-inflammatory agents must only be used under the supervision of a qualified physician or trainer to decrease the risk of permanent damage to an injury site.

The use of anti-inflammatory agents in professional sports is primarily to make the best use of an investment. However, it is quickly becoming obvious that the improper use of drugs to cover up injuries may result in a shortened lifetime of this investment. The high price of major sports figures dictates the appropriate care of such athletes by highly skilled sports practitioners. However, less prominent athletes may be considered more expendable. The improper use of anti-inflammatory agents in these individuals may be intentional and can lead to shortened sports careers.

College sports programs are also involved. Major sports at big universities have become big business. The glamour and reputation of a school frequently can be enhanced with a successful sports program. The loss of a key athlete during the season could have a major impact on a sports program in future years. The simple use of anti-inflammatory agents may enable a key athlete to continue to participate throughout the season. This carries the risk of shortening a career as with professional athletes.

Young athletes often do not want to project the image of being ''soft'' or being unable to ''take it.'' Pressure from peer groups and coaches in junior sports programs to continue competition in spite of injuries frequently can result in the improper masking of injuries with the self-administration of anti-inflammatory/analgesic agents. The use of injectable anti-inflammatory agents is normally limited because of reduced access and judicious use by physicians in treating sports injuries of younger athletes. However, aspirin and ibuprofen are readily available as over-the-counter products.

There are no good studies that have investigated the use of readily available anti-inflammatory agents such as aspirin in the young athlete population. The abuse may be great since most people consider the over-the-counter drugs, such as aspirin and ibuprofen, harmless. The effectiveness of aspirin has been supported by closely monitored use in some professional sports teams.[26] The use of aspirin prior to training sessions is already prevalent among weekend athletes to prevent or modulate the soreness that usually accompanies infrequent workouts.

Trauma to tissue initiates the process of inflammation. Inflammation is a series of protective measures the body takes to prevent additional damage and facilitate and begin the process of healing. The process includes the production of inflammatory mediators such as leukocytes, fibroblasts, and prostaglandins which destroy the injured tissue and promote healing. Pain and edema at the site of trauma are part of the healing process. Anti-inflammatory drugs interfere with the body's natural defense against injury. These drugs do not speed up the process of healing but impede it. They must be used with great caution in athletes.

6.1. Steroid Anti-inflammatory Agents

The steroid anti-inflammatory drugs, such as prednisolone acetate, triamcinolone acetonide, and methylprednisolone acetate, act to reduce inflammation by inhibiting the recruitment of neutrophils and monocytes into the affected area. Sports-related injury is not a rational indication for the use of steroid anti-inflammatory agents. In some circumstances, such as muscle damage, they may inhibit healing. Steroid anti-inflammatory drugs used to treat sports-related injuries are usually injected in a single dose directly at the injury site such as the interior of bursae and around the area of tendons and ligaments.[26] These agents remain active at the site of action for 5 to 7 days and have potent analgesic as well as anti-inflammatory activity. Extreme care must be taken when continuing activity following drug administration. The strong analgesic effect may give the athlete a lack of pain during exertion, allowing continued activities but possibly promoting further injury.

Steroid anti-inflammatory agents have few pharmacological side effects when used as single injections. However, they should never be used for chronic treatment of sports injuries because of serious and frequently occurring side effects which can decrease performance and endanger the athlete. Pituitary–adrenal function can be suppressed and require months to recover. This decreases the body's ability to respond to stressful situations occurring frequently during competition. Susceptibility to infection is also increased. Fluid and electrolyte disturbances may reduce the athlete's ability to respond to the effects of fluid losses accompanying long workouts in hot environments. Peptic ulcers may occur or preexisting peptic ulcers can be exacerbated.[27]

An interaction between nonsteroidal anti-inflammatory agents, such as aspirin and phenylbutazone, and steroidal anti-inflammatory drugs may increase the risk of ulcers. The pain associated with gastric bleeding can be masked, leading to serious consequences. Behavioral changes may cause the athlete to respond in an abnormal manner to situations occurring during athletic competition. Suicidal tendencies are not uncommon after steroid treatment.[27]

Long-term use of high doses of steroidal anti-inflammatory agents can also cause a myopathy characterized by weakness of the extremity musculature. Steroidal anti-inflammatory agents inhibit DNA synthesis and cell division. This can lead to inhibition of growth in young bodies, especially children.[27]

6.2. Nonsteroidal Anti-inflammatory and Analgesic Agents

Nonsteroidal anti-inflammatory agents act by inhibiting the synthesis of prostaglandins in response to trauma. Prostaglandins are produced during injury to cause vasodilatation and increased vascular permeability. Nonsteroidal anti-inflammatory agents include acetylsalicylic acid (aspirin), pyrazolon derivatives (phenylbutazone, oxyphenbutazone), indomethacin, propionic acid derivatives (ibuprofen, naproxen, fenoprofen), and others. (See Chapter 4.)

The most commonly used agent is aspirin (acetylsalicylic acid). The potential for aspirin abuse is large because it acts as an anti-inflammatory agent and analgesic and is widely available for a reasonable cost. Most laypersons believe aspirin to be safe and without severe liability for side effects. The recent advertisements for the daily use of aspirin to decrease the potential for heart attacks only reinforce the public attitude on the safety of aspirin. Only the potential for aspirin to cause gastrointestinal ulcers and bleeding has caused some concern among users.

The administration of aspirin chronically in large amounts should be accompanied by close clinical monitoring. Gastrointestinal ulcers can form to the extent of perforation of the intestine or stomach and subsequent hemorrhage. Central nervous system disorders can include confusion, lethargy, and headache.[28] The electrolyte imbalances that can occur are relatively unimportant to a normal individual but may be of some concern during heavy exertion during athletic competition.

The use of each of the other nonsteroidal anti-inflammatory agents carries some risk. Propionic acid derivatives, such as ibuprofen, are now available in over-the-counter preparations. Propionic acid derivatives have liabilities for the production of gastrointestinal complications similar to aspirin. In addition, they have some central nervous system effects very undesirable to the athlete, including drowsiness, headache, dizziness, fatigue, and depression.[28] The significantly higher cost and the central nervous system side effects will probably limit the abuse of these agents.

Pyrazolon derivatives such as phenylbutazone were widely used in professional sports during the sixties. There is a risk of bone marrow suppression, including aplastic anemia, following chronic phenylbutazone administration.[28] Phenylbutazone should not be used for longer than five days without close clinical monitoring.

7. PSYCHOMOTOR STIMULANTS

The use of the psychomotor stimulants, e.g., amphetamines and caffeine, is for the simple purpose of improving performance by reducing fatigue and increasing work output. Amphetamines were widely abused during the sixties but their abuse has been decreasing rapidly during recent years. The knowledge of the minimal increases in performance obtained with amphetamine use, the use of substitutes such as caffeine, and the beginning of drug testing programs have probably all played a role in their decreased popularity.

Decreases in amphetamine abuse were followed by increasing consumption of caffeine by athletes. Caffeine or its derivatives are found in foods (chocolate), soft drinks, coffee, some teas, and over-the-counter preparations. Athletes realized that caffeine had less potent but similar stimulant properties to amphetamines. Drinking or ingesting large amounts of caffeine could provide the same effects as taking amphetamines. Current drug testing guidelines now have set limits for caffeine to discourage its abuse.[29]

7.1. Amphetamines

Amphetamines (e.g., amphetamine sulfate, dextroamphetamine phosphate, and phenmetrazine hydrochloride) are taken by athletes as an oral dose within 1 to 2 hours prior to competition. The effects athletes perceive after taking amphetamines are delayed fatigue, increased alertness, uplift of mood, and increased self-confidence.

The influence of amphetamines on athletic performance has been well studied. Amphetamines administered 2 to 3 hours before a swimming competition produced a small but consistent decrease in swim times and an increase in time to exhaustion.[30] Other studies have shown that speed of a task (i.e., sprinting speed) and muscular strength are not affected by amphetamines.[2,31]

Laboratory studies with animals support the positive effects on physical performance demonstrated in man. High doses (10 to 20 mg/kg) of amphetamine were effective in increasing swimming time in rats. However, reduced doses (1.25 to 5 mg/kg) were ineffective.[32] Similar results occurred in treadmill endurance tests.[33]

Amphetamines stimulate the central nervous system by altering neurotransmitter activity at catecholaminergic receptors. The primary effect of amphetamines is to prevent the reuptake of noradrenaline at nerve synapses in the central nervous system. The increase of norepinephrine in the central nervous system mediates the observed effects of amphetamines. Characteristic effects are increased systolic and diastolic blood pressure. Large doses produce tachycardia. Smooth muscle responses are also affected as evidenced by decreased motility in the intestines (constipation), slow gastric emptying (interference with absorption of foods), and stimulation of the urinary sphincter (pain and difficulty in urination). There are also increases in metabolic rate and oxygen consumption.[34]

The mental attitude of athletes is of great importance. Amphetamines have profound effects on the user's mental state. Subjects appear nervous and experience agitation, tremor, anorexia, insomnia, fever, and confusion.[35] Some athletes feel hyped up prior to an event when under the influence of amphetamines and feel they can perform better. Also, some become more aggressive in nature, which can lead to behavior considered overaggressive. Such behavior causes fights and unnecessary sports injuries. The anorectic properties have also led to the abuse of amphetamines in sports with weight classes such as wrestling.[25]

The most serious effects of amphetamine in athletes are alterations in the cardiovascular system including tachycardia, headache, palpitations, and cardiac arythmias. Disruption of thermoregulatory systems can lead to hyperthermia induced hyperpyrexia, cardiovascular shock, and convulsions. Several athletes abusing amphetamines have died while competing on hot sunny days.[35] Chronic use can lead to addiction and withdrawal symptoms

7.2. Caffeine

There has been a recent increase in caffeine abuse by athletes. Since amphetamines and related compounds can be easily detected in the urine and blood, caffeine is used to mimic the central nervous system effects of amphetamines. However, there are conflicting data in the literature as to the affect of caffeine on the central nervous system. Caffeine has direct effects on muscle contraction.[37] It acts on the skeletal muscle by increasing calcium permeability essential for muscle contraction.[36]

Lopes and coworkers[37] observed effects of caffeine on the muscle during exercise *in vivo*. Caffeine (50 mg, orally) given 1 hour before the experiment produced higher muscle tension at low frequencies of muscle stimulation, suggesting a direct effect on muscle contraction. After fatigue, the same effect was seen at low frequencies of stimulation but not with high frequencies. There did not seem to be a difference in endurance times. These studies showed that caffeine may be acting directly on the muscle in addition to the central nervous system in masking fatigue.

Excessive amounts of caffeine are not required for the effects of caffeine. The amount of caffeine in brewed coffee is 100 to 150 mg/8 oz. Tea contains 60 to 75 mg caffeine/8 oz and cola drinks 40 to 60 mg/12 oz. Caffeine tablets available as over-the-counter drug preparations contain 100 mg (NoDoz), 200 mg (Vivarin), and 150 mg with 300 mg dextrose (Quick Pep), to name a few.[38]

Fatalities from caffeine overdose are very low. The lethal dosage is 5 to 10 grams. Symptoms of intoxication include insomnia, restlessness, mild delirium, and sensory disturbances such as tinnitus and flashing of light. Large overdoses of caffeine can produce seizures.[39]

7.3 Summary

Psychomotor stimulants have been abused in sports for many years. Since they must be present in the bloodstream during the sports activity in order to have their stimulatory effects, testing procedures can readily identify these stimulants and their substitutes. Amphetamines probably continue to be abused in sports with no drug testing such as most professional sports. The recent attempts by athletes in events with drug screening to substitute caffeine-containing preparations were an attempt to recover the advantage gained for many years by the administration of amphetamines.

8. SYMPATHOMIMETIC AMINES AND DRUGS USED TO TREAT ASTHMA

Sympathomimetic amines are agents which interact with the sympathetic nervous system. They affect almost all major organ systems in the body. Part of their effects involve stimulatory actions on the heart, the vasculature, and the lungs which could improve performance. The death of a Danish cyclist in the 1960 Olympic Games in Rome from both heat stroke and an overdose of sympathomimetic amines and vasodilator agents pointed out the potential of these agents for abuse and endangering the life of athletes.[40]

Sympathomimetic amines are used primarily by athletes to control asthma and exercise-induced asthma. Most asthmatics develop bronchoconstriction after heavy exercise, sport, or physical activity. A typical asthma response is after 6 to 8 minutes of submaximal exercise with bronchoconstriction peaking 5 to 10 minutes post-exercise. Extreme bronchoconstriction can severely compromise breathing and be fatal. Thus, the control of exercise-induced bronchoconstriction is essential for an asthmatic to compete safely and without respiratory disadvantage with nonasthmatic athletes. Asthmatics make up a significant proportion of athletes, including some of the best in the world. For example, 9% of the competitors on the Australian Olympic teams of 1976 and 1980 were afflicted with current or post-asthma and more than 11% of almost 600 athletes who underwent challenge tests at the 1984 Olympics exhibited exercise-induced asthma.[40]

The primary group of compounds used in the treatment of asthmatics are the sympathomimetic amines. Large changes in the types of sympathomimetic agents and their actions have occurred in the past several years. Agents affecting the sympathetic nervous system are broadly based on six types of actions: (1) peripheral excitation of some smooth muscle such as those in blood vessels supplying skin and mucous membranes, (2) peripheral inhibition of smooth muscle such as those in the wall of the gut, the bronchial tree, and the blood vessels supplying skeletal muscle, (3) improved cardiac function including an increase in heart rate and inotropy, (4), metabolic changes such as an increased rate of glycogenolysis in liver and muscle and the liberation of free fatty acids from adipose tissue, (5) endocrine actions on the secretion of insulin, renin, and pituitary hormones and (6) CNS actions such as respiratory stimulation, wakefulness, increased psychomotor activity, and a reduction in appetite.[40]

Early agents such as adrenaline and ephedrine and isoprenaline were relatively nonspecific in their effects and modified the function of a number of the sympathetic-controlled systems. Such drugs are banned because of their obvious actions on systems such as the heart and the potential for changes in performance. However, modern pharmacology has been able to identify receptor subtypes of the sympathetic system and has developed agents which interact with specific receptor subtypes modulating specific organ function. The ability to differentiate between the B_1 actions, primarily on the heart, the intestinal muscle, and lipolysis, and the B_2 actions, primarily on the smooth muscle of the bronchi, the uterus, and the arteries supplying skeletal muscle, has allowed the development of agents with actions specific for the bronchial tree. This permits a pharmacological correction of the respiratory problems associated with asthma without concomitant changes in the cardiovascular system, or at least minimal effects. Several of the more selective sympathomimetic agents used to treat asthmatics are now approved for use in asthmatics by various regulatory agencies. Some of the sympathomimetic substances and their status with the medical committee of the International Olympic Committee are listed in Table 5.

Epinephrine (adrenaline) is a banned drug. Its principle use is in emergency

Table 5. Status of Some Drugs Used in the Management of Asthma[a]

Permitted drugs
H_1 antagonists
Belladonna alkaloids
Methyl xanthines[b]
Glucocorticoids
Sympathomimetic amines–B_2 agonists[c]
Salbutamol(albuterol)
Terbutaline
Rimiterol
Banned drugs
Sympathomimetic amines–B_2 agonists
Fenoterol
Orciprenaline (metaproterenol)
Isoprenaline (isoproterenol)
Ephedrine
Adrenaline (epinephrine)

[a]Adapted from Fitch KD: The use of anti-asthmatic drugs. *Sports Med* 3:136–150, 1986.
[b]Caffeine is banned if urinary concentation exceeds 15 μg/ml.
[c]Written notification of use is required.

treatment of acute bronchospasm. Ephedrine, which was at one time accepted, is banned due to its cardiac stimulation and mood-altering actions. Terbutaline and salbutamol have been effective in preventing exercise-induced asthma. Rimiterol is also accepted although it has not been extensively evaluated. These drugs do not seem to have any cardiovascular side effects or cause any central nervous system stimulation. These side effects seem to be reduced due to specificity for selected receptors.[40]

Side effects of terbutaline can occur with a 5-mg oral dose in some individuals. The symptoms include nervousness, muscle tremors, headache, tachycardia, palpitations, drowsiness, nausea, vomiting, and sweating. Similar effects are seen with salbutamol and ritodrine. These side effects usually diminish with discontinued use of the drugs.[40]

A wide variety of therapeutic agents are used to control asthma including chromolyn sodium, H_1-antagonists, belladonna alkaloids, methyl xanthines, glucocorticoids, and B_2-adrenoreceptor stimulants.

Chromolyn sodium is used prophylactically and is effective against asthma and exercise-induced asthma. This drug acts by membrane stabilization of mast cells and has no effects on the cardiovascular system or the central nervous system. It is not considered to have any ergogenic effects.[40]

The H_1-receptor antagonists are primarily effective against some manifestations of atopic asthmatics. Depression of the central nervous system is a side effect of these drugs, and thus they would normally be avoided by athletes during competition.[39]

The belladonna alkaloids can produce a bronchodilation but their effectiveness in the treatment of asthma is in question. They are not associated with any significant changes in athlete performance and are used infrequently.[40]

The methyl xanthines, primarily theophylline, are very effective in the treatment of asthma. The drug must be closely monitored to establish appropriate blood levels for therapeutic efficacy. Alterations in the cardiovascular system following theophylline treatment and the close structural similarity of theophylline to caffeine increase suspicions of a potential for changes in performance following its administration.[40] Further studies will be needed to determine what effects theophylline has on sports performance.

The primary side effect of theophylline is gastric upset. It is doubtful that an athlete would risk gastric upset prior to competition by taking a drug with little reputation for improving performance. The current abuse potential for theophylline is very low.

Glucocorticoids are usually considered only in the treatment of severe asthma, and they have little effect on exercise-induced asthma. However, some athletes have tried taking large doses just prior to competition. There is one report that intravenous doses of glucocorticoids can increase cardiac output. Some central nervous system responses such as mood elevation, restlessness, and increased motor activity may occur after large doses of glucocorticoids.[40] The abuse of these agents is not widespread.

9. RECREATIONAL DRUGS

9.1. Introduction

Use of recreational drugs by athletes closely follows trends established in society. Hallucinogens in the sixties, marijuana in the seventies, and cocaine in the eighties represent the primary focus of drug abusers in recent years. Drug use and experimentation primarily occurs in late adolescents and young adults. These age groups are also those primarily involved in amateur and professional sports. The recreational use of drugs by athletes, however, is magnified by the close media coverage given to those individuals in sports. It is interesting to note that some estimates of overall drug use in society indicate a decline in the rate of illiicit drug use.

Cocaine use is clearly on the rise. Intense media coverage of the deaths caused by cocaine, particularly of sports figures, have brought the deadly potential of cocaine into the public eye. However, in 1985, there were 100,000 deaths related to alcohol in the USA and only 613 deaths due to cocaine. Alcohol-related deaths account for more than 30 times the number of deaths attributed to all illegal drugs. Alcohol continues to be the primary recreational drug abused by athletes and society in general.[41] Alcohol is readily available, legal in most areas, and socially acceptable. Cocaine, heroin, hallucinogens, stimulants, and depressants are sold primarily on the black market.

The use of tobacco, as cigarettes, cigars, snuff, or chewing tobacco, is a form of recreational drug abuse. Chewing tobacco use among young teenagers has become a major concern of the medical community. Many sports figures chew tobacco and several have recently been highlighted in commercials. Because sports figures serve as role models, there is concern about their use of chewing tobacco in light of the increasing numbers of young adolescents chewing tobacco.

Generally, recreational drugs cause a decrease in performance and are detrimental to training. The high liability for addiction to recreational drugs makes them especially devastating to sports careers. The news is continuously reporting sports figures being sent to rehabilitation programs.

9.2. Alcohol

Alcohol is the recreational drug most frequently used by both amateur and professional athletes. In a survey of one of the major athletic NCAA conferences, more than 60% of college athletes were regular users of alcohol.[42,43] Alcohol is classified as a depressant and acts primarily on the central nervous system. The action of alcohol takes place in four stages as blood alcohol levels rise. In stage one, there is increased freedom of speech and action, a sense of well-being, and greater self-confidence. Stage two allows the subject to become more talkative, with blurred speech. This is followed in stage three by indistinct and incoherent speech. In stage four, there is uncontrollable behavior with emotional disturbances and reduced sensibility, followed by loss of consciousness.[44]

Recently, alcoholic beverages have been used by marathon runners as a carbohydrate and electrolyte replacement fluid.[43] There are no data to support beneficial effects. There are numerous studies which demonstrate fine motor skill retardation and discoordination under the influence of alcohol. The American Medical Association and the National Safety Council consider an individual intoxicated with 150 mg alcohol/100 ml blood (0.15%) or its equivalent in urine, saliva, or breath.[44]

The toxic effects of alcohol abuse are also well documented. Chronic ingestion leads to addiction and serious neurological and mental disorders such as brain damage, memory loss, sleep disturbances, and psychoses. Liver damage and acute chronic pancreatitis also occur.[45] These disorders can be fatal.

9.3. Marijuana

Marijuana is probably the recreational drug second most frequently abused by athletes.[43] It is used to obtain a general sense of well-being and release from the surrounding environment. Its active ingredient is 1-δ-9-tetrahydrocannabinol (THC). Approximately 50% to 75% of the THC in a marijuana cigarette is absorbed through the lungs when it is smoked. Drug action occurs in 5 to 15 minutes after smoking and has a duration of 3 hours. The primary observed effects are produced by alterations in central nervous system function, but the drug is also found in the liver, lung, kidney, and spleen.[46]

There are no studies to date that indicate any benefits to the athlete from marijuana use. Motor coordination, short-term memory, and perception are impaired. Work motivation, critical to the athlete for adequate training, may be decreased. In chronic users, the toxic effects of marijuana abuse have been decreased plasma testosterone levels, oligospermia, and gynecomastia.[43]

9.4. Cocaine

Cocaine is the third most frequently used recreational drug. However, its abuse is increasing in high school, college, and professional athletics. Abusers describe an "incredible feeling of well-being, a feeling of omnipotence." Cocaine is provided through black market channels and is usually of unknown purity. Cutting agents include lactose, procaine, benzocaine, and lidocaine. Cocaine is usually snorted but the current trend is towards free-basing/smoking cocaine. The cocaine used for this route of administration is called crack. Preliminary evidence indicates that this form of cocaine is much more addictive and causes a very intense, quick drug response.[47] It is a much more deadly than the traditional forms of cocaine because of its very intense and quick action. The death of Len Bias, an amateur basketball player at the University of Maryland, and Don Rogers, a professional football player for the Cleveland Browns, within the past year emphasizes the danger of cocaine abuse. The supply of cocaine has become a major political issue in several South American countries which depend upon cocaine as a major source of revenue.

Cocaine acts on catecholaminergic neurons in preventing reuptake of both norepinephrine and dopamine.[48] The physiological effects of cocaine are similar to those of amphetamines. However, the mood effects are more profound. Moderate effects include both euphoria and dysphoria while strong stimulant effects include irritability, withdrawal, hostility, anguish, fear, and extreme paranoia. These effects would appear to discourage use during competition. However, the increased energy level, hyperactivity, and anorexia produced appeal to some athletes.[49]

The toxic effects of cocaine use are dizziness, tremor, extreme irritability, confusion, and hallucinations. There are also effects on the cardiovascular and respiratory systems which produce chest pain, palpitations, hypertension, sweating, and cardiac armythmias. Extreme cases of cocaine abuse are fatal with hyperpyrexia (increased body temperature) and convulsions.[50]

10. CONCLUSIONS

Drugs are used in sports for three primary reasons:

- as ergogenic aids to augment physical performance,
- as restorative agents to permit continued performance despite injuries, and
- as recreational drugs for coping with problems or for mind- and body-altering experiences.

The use of egrogenic drugs or drugs purported to be ergogenic will be a continuing problem among athletes. Attemps to regulate drugs will be thwarted by the development of new drugs and dosing regimes which make detection difficult or impossible. It is an almost impossible assignment for the analytical chemists to develop methods to detect all types of drug usage. The number of drugs with the potential for abuse will increase continuously as modern science develops new, more powerful and more specific agents to treat disease. Science will continue to probe into the functioning of man and try to gain knowledge which will allow him to artificially control bodily functions. It will be increasingly difficult to separate therapeutic use and abuse of drugs. The primary goal of an athlete or the supporting coach/owner is to be the best. Thus, he/she will use whatever is available to gain an advantage over competitors.

The abuse of restorative drugs will be a problem primarily within the medical community. Each physician or trainer responsible for the career of a sports person will be required to determine if the restorative drug is in the best interests of the health of the athlete. There will certainly be pressures from outside—the fans, the owners, the coaches—to treat an injury and have the athlete return to competition as soon as possible. The close monitoring of drugs used even by health personnel should be performed. This will ensure that the health and safety of all athletes will not be compromised by the pressure of winning at all costs, even at the expense of the health of the athlete.

The recreational use of drugs will always be a problem of society. The failure of Prohibition is a good example of the resistance of society to giving up its recreational drugs. Large amounts of money have been spent to stop or slow the influx of heroin, cocaine, and marijuana into the United States. There has been some success in curbing this flow of drugs, but the effort has not been able to bring about a significant decrease in the use of drugs. Recreational drugs will continue to be a part of society in the forseeable future. This will ensure the availability of these drugs to everyone in society, including athletes, willing to take the risks associated with their use.

Sports have become part of the political arena. The honor of a country and bragging rights for who is the best go along with sports victories. Coaches and medical scientists are continuously monitoring scientific advances leading to a better understanding of the functions of the body and the development of drugs which affect its function. It is difficult to determine the lengths to which a country or sports team will go to develop "super athletes." There have been questions asked about the small stature of female gymnasts from some countries. There is a strong suspicion that drugs may be used to "brake" sexual maturation to keep the gymnasts small in stature, supple, and with reduced bone mass for greater lengths of time. Medroxyprogesterone acetate and cyproterone acetate are both candidates for causing such effects. Restriction of food intake will also delay sexual maturation, but this may also be a form of abuse. Will parents permit or even request growth hormone to be given to their children to ensure a basketball team of seven-foot-tall players?

The definition of what constitutes "abuse" will always be a difficult and complex question to answer. Sports regulatory bodies, professional players' unions, sports owners, sports physicians, trainers, and, of course, the athletes will be required to make increasingly complex decisions regarding drug use.

Some people consider drugs an extension of better sports equipment and training conditions. Opponents say that improved equipment does not cause increased injuries and potentially life-threatening situations. Yet, higher vaults in the pole vault and faster starts by a football player also lead to potential increased injuries.

The increase of drugs in sports has caused sports federations to regulate drug use and identify abusing athletes. Drug testing began in the early 1960s at the Olympic Games and has become a major part of most world-class amateur sporting events.

Approximately 80% of professional cyclists were found to use drugs in past events,[51] but the number of positive drug tests during the 1984 Olympics was less than 2%.[52]

The drug control policy of the International Olympic Committee (IOC) is: (1) to prevent the use of drugs in sports when dangerous and when drugs are employed as doping agents; (2) to prevent drug abuse with the minimum of interference with the therapeutic use of drugs; (3) to ban drugs which can be detected by analytical methods; and (4) to ban classes of drugs based on pharmacological actions rather than individual drugs.[51]

Although these stipulations by the IOC were set up to regulate drug use, there are major abuses of drugs which cannot be detected by analytical methods. For instance, a weight lifter will use steroids months before a competition to build up muscle. By the time of the event, minimal, if any, steroid will be detected. Growth hormone use is also difficult to detect. As analytical techniques are developed, new drugs will be added to the lists of banned drugs. Drug testing programs have probably cut down on the abuse of some drugs in some sports. It is interesting to note that no new weight lifting records have been achieved in the two years since rigorous drug testing was instituted.[54]

A recent symposium on recreational drug abuse in athletes found three main reasons why drug use is a threat to university and professional sports. Firstly, the use of drugs decreases the credibility of the sport among the public. Secondly, drug abuse reduces athletic performance. Thirdly, these drugs are illegal and are criminally connected. Not only does the athlete have to deal with criminals, but there is also a possibility of fixing a game because of debts or blackmail.[53]

The prevention of drug abuse by athletes seems to be in education and in the development of a complete sports medicine program to maximize the ability of each athlete to achieve his/her goals. The athletes must be convinced that no other competitor has the advantage of a super drug, a chemical advantage which cannot be overcome by hard training.

REFERENCES

1. Gent P: Between the white lines. *Dallas Times Herald,* 4 Sept 1983, Magazine section, p 13.
2. Willians MH: *Drugs and Athletic Performance.* Springfield, IL, Charles C Thomas, 1974.
3. Prokop L: The problem of doping. Final report on the international doping conference. FIMS congress, Tokyo, October, 1964. *J Sport Med* 5:88–90, 1965.
4. Toohey JV: Nonmedical drug use among intercollegiate athletes at five American Universities. *Bull Narc* 30:61–64, 1978.
5. Vinger PF, Hoerner EF: *Sports Injuries.* Littleton, MA, PSG Publishing Company, Inc., 1986.
6. Goldman B: *Death in the Locker Room.* South Bend, IN, ICARUS Press, 1984.
7. Gledhill N: Blood doping and related issues: A brief review. *Med Sci Sports Exerc* 14:183–189, 1982.
8. Gledhill N, Buick FJ, Froese AB, et al: An optimal method of storing blood for blood boosting. *Med Sci Sports* 10:40, 1978.
9. Berglund B, Hemmingsson P, Birgegard G: Detection of autologous blood transfusions in cross-country skiers. *Int J Sports Med* 8:66–70, 1987.
10. Sutton JR: Drugs in sport. *Physician Sportsmed* 11:63–101, 1983.
11. Gledhill N: Bicarbonate ingestion and anaerobic performance. *Sports Med* 1:177–180, 1984.

12. Wilkes D, Gledhill N, Smyth R: Effect of acute induced metabolic alkalosis on 800m racing time. *Med Sci Sports Med Exerc* 15:277–280. 1983.
13. Mudge GH: Agents affecting volume and composition of body fluids, in Gilman AG, Goodman LS, Rall TW, Murad F (eds): *The Pharmacological Basis of Therapeutics,* ed 7. New York, Macmillan Publishing Co., 1985, p 865.
14. Vanhelder WP, Radomski MW, Goode RC: Growth hormone responses during intermittent weight lifting exercise in men. *Eur J Appl Physiol* 53:31–34, 1984.
15. Vanhelder WP, Casey K, Goode RC, et al: Growth hormone regulation in two types of aerobic exercise of equal oxygen uptake. *Eur J Appl Physiol* 55:236–239, 1986.
16. Murad R, Haynes RC Jr: Adenohypophyseal hormones and related substances, in Gilman AG, Goodman LS, Rall TW, Murad F (eds): *The Pharmacological Basis of Therapeutics,* ed 7. New York, Macmillan Publishing Co., 1985, pp 1366–1372.
17. Macintyre JG: Growth hormone and athletes. *Sports Med* 4:129–142, 1987.
18. Daughaday WH: The anterior pituitary, in Williams RH (ed): *Textbook of Endocrinology,* ed 7. Philadelphia, WB Saunders Co., 1985, pp 568–613.
19. Lamb DR: Anabolic steroids in athletics: how well do they work and how dangerous are they? *Am J Sports Med* 12(1):31–38, 1984.
20. Bergman R, Leach RE: The use and abuse of anabolic steroids in olympic-caliber athletes. *Clin Orthop Rel Res,* No. 198, September 1985.
21. Haupt HA, Rovere GD: Anabolic steroids: a review of the literature. *Am J Sports Med* 1(6):469–484, 1984.
22. Zurer PS: Drugs in sports. *Chem Eng News* 30:69–78, 1984.
23. Alen M, Rahkila P: Reduced high-density lipoprotein-cholesterol in power athletes: use of male sex hormone derivates, an atherogenic factor. *Int J Sports Med* 5:341–342, 1984.
24. Alen M. Rahkila P, Marniemi J: Serum lipids in power athletes self-administering testosterone and anabolic steroids. *Int J Sports Med* 6:139–144, 1985.
25. Dyment PG: Drugs and the adolescent athlete. *Ped Ann* 13(8):602–604, 1984.
26. Gardiner PF: Anti-inflammatory medications. *Physician Sportsmed* 11(9):71–74, 1983.
27. Haynes RC, Murad F: Adrenocorticotropic hormone; adrenocortical steroids and their synthetic analogs: inhibitors of adrenocortical steroid biosynthesis, in Gilman AG, Goodman LS, Rall TW, Murad F (eds): *The Pharmacological Basis of Therapeutics,* ed 7. New York, Macmillan Publishing Co., 1985, pp 1459–1489.
28. Flower RJ, Moncada S, Vane JR: Analgesic-antipyretics and anti-inflammatory agents; drugs employed in the treatment of gout, in Gilman AG, Goodman LS, Rall TW, Murad F (eds): *The Pharmacological Basis of Therapeutics,* ed 7. New York, Macmillan Publishing Co., 1985, pp 674–715.
29. Wagner JC: Substance-abuse policies and guidelines in amateur and professional athletics. *Am J Hosp Pharm* 44:305–310, 1987.
30. Smith GM, Beecher HK: Amphetamine sulfate and athletic performance. I. Objective effects. *JAMA* 170:542–557, 1959
31. Chandler JV, Blair SN: The effects of amphetamines on selected physiological components related to athletic success. *Med Sci Sports Exerc* 12:65–69, 1980.
32. Bhagat B, Wheeler N: Effect of amphetamine on the swimming endurance of rats. *Neuropharmacology* 12:711–713, 1973.
33. Gerald MC: Effects of (+)-amphetamine on the treadmill endurance performance of rats. *Neuropharmacology* 17:703–704, 1978.
34. Morgan JP: The clinical pharmacology of amphetamine, in Smith DE (ed): *Amphetamine Use, Misuse and Abuse.* Boston, GH Hall & Co, 1979, pp 3–10.
35. Weiner N: Norpinephrine, epinephrine, and the sympathomimetic amines, in Gilman AG, Goodman LS, Rall TW, Murad F (eds): *The Pharmacological Basis of Therapeutics,* ed 7. New York, Macmillan Publishing Co., 1985, pp 145–180.
36. Wood DS: Human skeletal muscle: Analysis of Ca^{2+} regulation in skinned fibers using caffeine. *Exp Neurol* 58:218–230, 1978.
37. Lopes JM, Aubier M, Jardim J, Aranda, JV, Macklem, PT: Effect of caffeine on skeletal muscle

function before and after fatigue. *J Appl Physiol Respirat Environ Exercise Physiol* 54(5):1303–1305, 1983.
38. Scherer JC, in *Lippincott's Nurses' Drug Manual*. Philadelphia, JB Lippincott Co., 1985, p 223.
39. Rall TW: Central nervous system stimulants, in Gilman AG, Goodman LS, Rall TW, Murad F (eds): *The Pharmacological Basis of Therapeutics*, ed 7. New York, Macmillan Publishing Co., 1985, pp 589–603.
40. Fitch KD: The use of anti-asthmatic drugs. Do they affect sports performance? *Sports Med* 3:136–150, 1986.
41. Dollars & Sense, Dec 1986, pp 6–8.
42. Clement DB: Drug use survey: results and conclusions. *Physician Sportsmed* 11:64–67, 1983.
43. Puffer JC: The use of drugs in swimming. *Clin Sports Med* 5(1):77–89, 1986.
44. Weimer WW, Russell JA, Kaplan HL: Ethanol toxicology, in *Alcohols Toxicology*. Park Ridge, IL, Noyes Data Corporation, 1983, pp 27–45.
45. Ritchie JM: The aliphatic alcohols, in Gilman AG, Goodman LS, Rall TW, Murad F (eds): *The Pharmacological Basis of Therapeutics*, ed 7. New York, Macmillan Publishing Co., 1985, pp 372–386.
46. Abel EL: Pharmacology of cannabinoids, in *Marihuana, Tobacco, Alcohol and Reproduction*. Boca Raton, FL, CRC Press, Inc, 1983, pp 1–7.
47. Ovack K: Cocaine unpredictability makes using drug a deadly gamble. *St Petersburg Times* (St Petersburg, FL) 13 July 1986, p F1.
48. Kuchenski R: Biochemical actions of amphetamine and other stimulants, in Creese I (ed): *Stimulants: Neurochemical, Behavioral, and Clinical Perspectives*. New York, Raven Press, 1983, pp 31–61.
49. Post RM, Contel NR: Human and animal studies of cocaine: Implications for development of behavioral pathology, in Creese I (ed): *Stimulants: Neurochemical, Behavioral, and Clinical Perspectives*, New York. Raven Press, 1983, pp 169–203.
50. Jaffe JH: Drug addiction and drug abuse, in Gilman AG, Goodman LS, Rall TW, Murad F (eds): *The Pharmacological Basis of Therapeutics*, ed 7. New York, Macmillan Publishing Co., 1985, pp 532–580.
51. Beckett AH: Use and abuse of drugs in sport. *J Biosoc Sci* (suppl 7):163–170, 1981.
52. Catlin DH, Kammerer RC, Hatton CK, et al: Analytical chemistry at the games of the XXIIIrd Olympiad in Los Angeles, 1984. *Clin Chem* 33:319–327, 1987.
53. Sutton JR: Drugs in sport. *Physician Sportsmed* 11:63–101, 1983.
54. Hersh P: Drug tests take weighty toll. *Chicago Tribune*, 27 July 1987, p 8.

11

Exercise and Immunity

Marc Salit

1. INTRODUCTION

"No pain, no gain" is the often heard rallying cry of today's athlete in training. Both the recreational athlete and the serious competitor undergo strenuous exercise in order to gain improved physical fitness or improved competitive results. Anecdotal reports from these individuals may include references to a perceived reduction in the incidence of infectious disease and an improved sense of well-being.[1,2] The scientific community has also demonstrated an interest in the connection between exercise and host defense against infection. This chapter will review the results of several studies relating exercise to changes in various components of the human immune system. Specifically, the effects of acute bouts of exercise and of chronic training programs on the function of the cellular and humoral compartments of the immune system will be covered. Additionally, studies on the immunopathology of the condition known as exercise-induced asthma will be reviewed.

2. THE IMMUNE SYSTEM

The mammalian immune system provides defense against invasion of the host by foreign, nonself substances (antigens), i.e. pathogenic microorganisms, tumors, tissue grafts, etc. Discussions of the immune system often compartmentalize it into the cellular and humoral components.

The products of a protective cellular immune response are cells capable of killing virus-infected targets or tumors. Other immune cells produce antibody molecules that may be protective. The immune cells also play regulatory roles, orchestrating a host's response to infection. Humoral products include the aforementioned antibodies; these are proteins that bind to specific antigens and effect their removal. Interferons and interleukins are humoral substances that amplify immune responses.

Marc Salit • Baxter Healthcare Corporation, Round Lake, Illinois 60073.

More specifically, the cells of the immune system include the lymphocytes, monocytes, and macrophages, the polymorphonuclear neutrophils (neutrophils, PMN), the basophils, and the eosinophils. The major cellular targets of exercise are the lymphocytes and the neutrophils. Thus, this brief review will focus upon their characterization and function.

Bone marrow-derived lymphocytes, or B cells, respond to the presence of specific antigens when these foreign substances are bound by antibody molecules on the B-cell membrane. The B cells divide and differentiate into plasma cells that secrete copious quantities of antibody capable of binding the antigen that prompted their production. Another product of B-cell division and differentiation is memory B cells, able to respond very quickly to a second antigenic challenge.

Thymus-derived lymphocytes, or T cells, provide antigen-specific modulating and effector functions for the host. Two major types exist: the helper T cells and the cytotoxic/suppressor T cells. A major function of the helper T-cell population, detected in the human by the so-called OKT4 monoclonal antibody, is its ability to interact with and amplify B-cell responses. Helper T cells also interact with other T cells to regulate graft rejection and a reaction known as delayed-type hypersensitivity. The second major T-cell subpopulation, the cytotoxic and suppressive group, may be detected by the monoclonal antibody OKT8. It is the balance between antigen-reactive helper and suppressor T cells that regulates immune responses. The OKT8+ cell subpopulation also generates antigen-specific cytotoxic T lymphocytes that destroy cells infected with sensitizing viruses and certain tumors. T-cell activation also produces memory cells.[3]

The natural killer (NK) cells are large, granular lymphocytes that are spontaneously toxic to certain tumor cells. These reactions are not antigen specific. The killer (K) lymphocytes lyse antibody-coated tumor targets in a reaction called antibody-dependent cellular cytotoxicity. The lytic mechanisms underlying these reactions are unknown except that effector–target contact is required.[4]

Polymorphonuclear neutrophils are circulatory phagocytic cells capable of ingesting and killing bacteria, fungi, and other microorganisms. The killing mechanism includes the cells' use of toxic oxygen species such as hydrogen peroxide and superoxide anions.[5]

The major effectors of humoral immune responses are the immunoglobulin (Ig), or antibody, molecules. Comprising 20% of serum proteins and produced by antigen-activated B lymphocytes, these molecules noncovalently bind to specific antigens. The basic antibody molecule is a four-chain polypeptide structure with an apparent molecular weight of about 150,000 daltons. Called immunoglobulin G or IgG, this molecule binds microorganisms and makes them more palatable to neutrophils. IgG bound to its specific antigen can activate the complement cascade which is able to directly destroy foreign cells like bacteria. A second class of antibody is called IgA. This predominantly dimeric immunoglobulin is found in mucous membrane secretions. IgM, a pentameric structure, has a molecular weight of approximately 900,000 daltons. It is the antibody produced early in immune responses, and its distribution is limited to the intravascular space. IgD, a monomeric molecule found in low concentrations in the serum, may be the type of immunoglobulin found on B-cell membranes. Finally, IgE is the immunoglobulin responsible for allergic reactions. If a mast-cell-fixed IgE binds its specific antigen, vasoactive substances such as histamine and serotonin are released, yielding allergic symptomatology.[6]

Produced predominantly by leukocytes, the interleukins (IL) and the interferons act as modulators of the immune response, IL-1 and IL-2 amplify the expansion of T- and B-cell subpopulations[7] while gamma-interferon regulates the function of macrophages. In addition, interferon prevents viral replication in mammalian cell systems and can inhibit the growth of tumor cells *in vitro* and *in vivo*.[8]

Every immune response includes cellular and humoral aspects. While many responses are protective and advantageous to the host, faulty regulation of the immune system may establish deleterious states such as autoimmune disease or immune deficiency syndromes. In the end, the balance between the various controlling aspects of the immune system may go a long way towards determining the health of the host.

3. EXERCISE EFFECTS ON THE IMMUNE SYSTEM

3.1. Acute Exercise-Induced Leukocytosis

An effect of exercise on white blood cell counts was observed as early as 1935.[9] In this section, the impact of short-term strenuous exercise on the various leukocyte subpopulations of untrained individuals will be considered in detail.

3.1.1. Lymphocytosis

It is now generally accepted that short-term, strenuous exercise leads to lymphocytosis, observed immediately after the cessation of work performed by untrained, healthy individuals.

Hedfors and coworkers have been investigating the response of the immune system to exercise for at least a decade. In their early studies,[12] this group collected blood and prepared highly purified lymphocytes, before and after a session of bicycle ergometry. A marked increase in the number of circulating T and B lymphocytes was noted after exercise. The increases in absolute cell numbers observed were not due to hemoconcentration. The proportion of T cells, detected by a rosette assay, fell whereas the proportion of surface immunoglobulin-bearing cells with receptors for C_3 and IgG-Fc, the B-cell population, rose dramatically. The function of these cells was studied also. Response to the mitogens concanavalin A (Con A), phytohemagglutinin (PHA), and pokeweed mitogen was impaired, as was the response to purified protein derivative (PPD). Therefore, since rising cell counts were coupled with an impairment in mitogenesis, these workers concluded that exercise leads to a mobilization of lymphocytes to the circulation but that these cells may bear qualitative differences from those seen before exercise.

Observations concerning the function of exercise-elicited lymphocytes were extended in 1983 when it was determined that pokeweed-mitogen-induced lymphocyte production of immunoglobulins G, A, and M in 7-day culture was significantly impaired when cells were taken immediately following a brief, strenuous period of bicycling. Similarly, DNA synthesis in response to allogeneic cells was reduced when the responding cells in a mixed lymphocyte culture were obtained during work. Taken together, these observations indicate that exercise changes the composition and function of T-cell subpopulations. These changes are reflected in reduced T-cell responses to allogeneic challenge and a reduction in T-cell-dependent immunoglobulin synthesis.[13]

Corroborating earlier studies, Landmann and coworkers[10] have determined that all lymphocyte subpopulations increase in number following exercise. Using monoclonal antibodies specific for cell-surface markers, it was observed that B-cell counts rose more than those of the T-cell subpopulations, and the suppressor T-cell numbers rose more than those of helper T cells. Therefore, the T cell : B cell and T helper : T suppressor ratios fell as a result of exercise.

Similar results have been obtained by Edwards *et al.*,[11] who also used monoclonal antibodies and fluoresence-activated cell sorting to dissect the lymphocyte response to exercise. Total lymphocytes, total T cells, suppressor T cells, and B cells all increased after a 5-minute period of stair running. A small, insignificant rise in helper T cells was observed.

The mechanism accounting for lymphocytosis following exercise in untrained humans may involve the sympathetic nervous system and its response to physical stress. Exercise-increased levels of adrenaline, noradrenaline, and cortisol[14] have been correlated with changes in lymphocyte counts and the changes in the relative proportions of various cell subpopulations observed in the circulation. Propranolol[15] and prednisone[16] prevent exercise-induced leukocytosis. Thus, lymphocyte traffic as affected by exercise may be regulated by an alpha- and/or beta-receptor mechanism.

3.1.2. Neutrophilia

Few studies have examined the effects of short-term exercise as performed by untrained persons on polymorphonuclear neutrophil counts and function. An interesting citation comes from the apheresis literature, where Christensen and coworkers[17] reported on a method to increase the neutrophil content of transfusion units for neonates with bacterial infection and severe neutropenia. They determined that two minutes of strenuous exercise performed by blood donors led to a 30% increase in the numbers of neutrophils (range 18–55%) recovered from the donated units. While these workers reported that metabolic burst activity was not affected by exercise, Strainer *et al.*[18] determined that a 1-hour session of bicycle ergometry at 50% capacity significantly increased hydrogen peroxide generation by neutrophils. Phorbol myristate acetate was used to elicit peroxide from the cells *in vitro*. Exercise was seen to increase the rate of production and the maximum amount of peroxide generated for up to 3 hours post-exercise.

3.1.3. Natural Killer Cells

The effect of acute exercise on human natural killer cell activity has been examined by several workers including Edwards *et al.*[11] Monoclonal-antibody-based assays showed that acute exercise increased the numbers of NK antigen-displaying cells in the peripheral circulation some fivefold in untrained, healthy individuals. Functional tumor cell (K562) lysis assays demonstrated increases in NK activity when blood was taken immediately after exercise. The effect was transitory, however, as by 1 hour post-exercise, NK activity returned to normal levels.

Targan and coworkers[19] examined augmented NK activity following a short period of moderate exercise and the influence of interferon on this phenomenon. By using both a single-cell cytotoxic assay and the standard ^{51}Cr tumor cell lysis assay, several findings were made. First, exercise produced increases in NK activity by recruiting a "new" population of cytotoxic NK cells. These "new" cells were probably derived from pre-NK cells which were capable of binding tumor targets but were not cytotoxic. Second, the application of exogenous interferon boosted the activity of the exercise-recruited cells. The investigators concluded that interferon had an effect on increasing the capacity of individual effector cells to recycle and take part in many serial tumor target lytic events.

Brahmi *et al.*[20] have demonstrated that while the percentage of cells bearing NK markers increases immediately after intense exercise by more than 50%, the absolute numbers of NK cells in the circulation remains unchanged. NK cell lysis of K562 tumor cell targets was highest immediately after exercise. NK activity reached its lowest point 120 minutes after cessation of work, and 20 hours were required for recovery of full pre-exercise activity levels. The pattern of activity after exercise just described is paralleled by NK cell capacity to bind to target cells. The authors concluded that NK cell numbers are resistant to the depletive and modulatory effects of exercise on other lymphocyte populations and that the increase seen in NK activity after exercise is not due to increased cell numbers. This finding seems to be in direct contrast to that of Edwards *et al.*, who saw fivefold increases of NK cells immediately after exercise. In studies such as these, duration and intensity of exercise, as well as the timing of blood drawing and the mechanics of the assays used, greatly influence the results.

To summarize then, the predominant effect of acute exercise on the immune cells of untrained individuals was the appearance of a marked lymphocytosis immediately after exercise. While B- and T-cell population absolute counts all increased, the B-cell numbers were preferentially affected. Thus, the proportion of lymphocytes carrying T-cell markers decreased relative to B cells. Also, suppressor T cells rose more than helper T cells. Accordingly, both T : B and T helper : T suppressor ratios decreased. These exercise-elicited cells did not seem to function as well as cells taken during rest, as both mitogenesis and immunoglobulin synthesis were suppressed post-exercise.

While acute exercise may transiently affect neutrophil counts, the effect of work on NK cell counts is somewhat controversial. Edwards *et al.* saw fivefold increases in NK counts after 5 minutes of exercise while Brahmi *et al.* observed constant absolute numbers of NK cells before and after standard ergometry. These differences in results may be explained by differences in exercise intensity and in the assay methods employed.

3.2. Effects of Chronic Training on Leukocytes

In this section, studies performed on fit individuals taking part in chronic training regimens will be reviewed. Also to be discussed are the effects of extended exercise periods (e.g., marathon running) on leukocyte populations.

In a study of immune parameters tested before and after a strenuous 6-week training period, Soppi *et al.*[21] observed that bicycle ergometry performed to exhaustion increased lymphocyte counts 100% and 50% in untrained and trained individuals, respectively. Lymphocyte responses to the mitogens Con A and PHA were improved by training. It was proposed that after training, the body's response to physical stress led to a weaker mobilization of lymphocytes into the circulation. When coupled with the observation of enhanced cell function, these investigators concluded that when physical fitness was higher, fewer lymphocytes were required by the host to produce a normal immune response.

Watson *et al.*[22] tested human immune responsiveness before and after a 15-week physical training program consisting of walk/jog/run sessions. The training program caused significant decreases in NK activity, disagreeing with the results of Brahmi *et al.*, who did not see an effect of chronic training on NK function. Training did not significantly affect total circulating leukocvte counts. In agreement with Soppi *et al.*, Watson *et al.* saw enhanced lymphocyte mitogenesis after training. The conditioning program also caused significant increases in the percent of mature T lymphocytes seen in the blood. It should be pointed out that blood samples in this study were drawn some 20 hours after training sessions and that the observed effects were due to the overall training program, and not a single bout of exercise.

The immune function of a group of men training for marathon running was determined by Green and coworkers.[2] Test subjects were not studied immediately after exercise; rather, blood was drawn while individuals were at rest. Ten of 20 runners had slightly decreased lymphocyte counts compared to sedentary controls. Leukocyte function, adjudged by bacterial phagocytosis and killing, and mitogenesis fell within normal limits. It was concluded that an endurance training program, consisting of near-daily, long-distance runs, had no effect on immune function.

It should be pointed out that the work of Soppi *et al.* and Watson *et al.* included conditioning programs of 6 and 15 weeks, respectively, and that the marathon runners tested by Green *et al.* ran 5 to 6 days per week, 30 to 140 miles per week for between 2 and 15 years. Any differences between the two former and the latter studies might be ascribed to the effects of brief versus long-term regimens.

A series of publications have dealt with the *immediate* effects of endurance exercise on immune cell function. While daily exercise may not affect immune response indicators if the athlete is at rest, his actual training session may have profound, though, short-term consequences.

Eskola *et al.*[23] studied the number and function of lymphocytes after a marathon run (26.2 mi in 2.5 hours) and after a moderate run of 7 km in 35 minutes. Though marathon running did not alter lymphocyte counts, cell responsiveness to PHA, Con A, and PPD was significantly depressed. This cell-mediated immune-suppressed state was transient, lasting 24 hours. The ability of marathon runners' lymphocytes to respond to antigen and thereafter produce specific antibody (humoral immunity) was not impaired by the race. A pronounced neutrophilia and increases in plasma cortisol were seen in the marathon runners as well as those subjects taking part in the shorter run. Other immune parameters were unaffected in the 7-km runners.

Marked leukocytosis was the result of a 20-mi run performed by 11 male subjects as reported by Moorthy and Zimmerman.[24] Confirming the result of Eskola *et al.* was the observation that the leukocytosis was due to large increases in neutrophil counts. A 375% increase in these cells was seen 10 to 15 minutes after the race's conclusion. Lymphocyte counts, primarily B cells, increased slightly and, in contrast to the result of short-term exercise, retained good mitogen responsiveness. Moorthy and Zimmerman also saw a rise in plasma cortisol levels as a result of racing stress and were able to inversely correlate the degree of cortisol increase to the miles of prior training performed by the runner.

Several laboratories have seen little change in neutrophil numbers after relatively shorter runs of 8 to 12 mi performed by well-conditioned athletes.[25–27] Hanson and Flaherty's[25] subjects also displayed minimal changes in circulating lymphocyte counts except for a modest though significant rise in antibody-dependent killer cells (K cells).

Nyman[26] studied runners taking part in a 750-mi relay race, each athlete performing an 8- to 12-mi run. Of 20 individuals tested, only 2 showed slight rises in leukocyte counts in blood samples taken during the run.

In summary, subjects taking part in relatively short-term training programs may display lymphocytosis and improved lymphocyte responsiveness to mitogens. Long-term conditioning programs, on the other hand, do not seem to significantly alter immune cell populations. Individuals enduring extreme sports stress (long-distance running) display transient reduced mitogenic responses and increases in circulating neutrophils, killer cells, and cortisol.

The major difference between these results and those produced by acute exercise in untrained individuals seems to be the cell population affected by work. Lymphocytes elicited to the circulation by acute exercise are either not affected by endurance exercise or are transiently elicited but remarginate before the exercise period is completed.[14,28] Likewise, the neutrophil population seems somewhat unaffected by short-term exercise but responds well to endurance running. Perhaps these results are attributable to whether catecholamines (resulting from acute exercise) or corticosteroids (resulting from endurance exercise) are produced by the exertional stress and the differential sensitivity of the various cell types to these immunomodulatory substances.

3.3. Effects of Exercise on Humoral Immune Factors

Circulating immunoglobulins are humoral manifestations of an immune response to several types of infectious agents. Green *et al.*[2] found that well-conditioned athletes had normal levels of circulating IgG, IgA, and IgM when blood specimens were obtained at rest. As previously noted, Hedfors *et al.*[13] determined that *in vitro* production of Ig's by cells taken from untrained individuals after acute exercise was substantially reduced.

Tomasi and coworkers[29] determined the levels of secretory IgA in conditioned Nordic skiers before and after a 20-km race. Prior to the race, these individuals had salivary IgA levels significantly lower than the levels found in age-matched controls. Following the race, the concentration of the immunoglobulin in parotid saliva was reduced to extremely low levels. The authors suggested that the reduction may be due to mucous depletion or a malfunction of mucosal plasma cells due to cold temperatures (and therefore not the exercise). It was speculated that the reduced salivary IgA may increase the athletes' susceptibility to viral and bacterial infection following exertion.

Interleukin-1 (IL-1) is a potent amplifier of inflammatory responses produced by macrophages. The molecule elevates body temperature, promotes production of acute phase proteins, and reduces plasma iron and zinc levels.[30] Cannon and Kluger[31] reproduced several of these effects by injecting rats with plasma taken from acutely exercised humans. They determined that the pyrogen, the molecule that elevated body temperature, was heat denaturable and had a molecular weight of 14,000 daltons. They further determined that mononuclear cells taken from exercised subjects released a similar substance *in vitro*. In a later publication,[32] this group determined that this active material was indeed IL-1. It was found that when untrained or fit individuals performed concentric or eccentric exercise, IL-1 was formed proportionally to creatine kinase, an indicator of muscle damage.[33] Resting IL-1 levels were logarithmically related to the fitness indicator VO_2 max and exercise-evoked IL-1 levels were inversely related to fitness. Therefore, chronic training raises resting plasma IL-1 above untrained, baseline levels but acute exercise performed by untrained individuals results in greater tissue damage and higher circulating IL-1 levels than found in fit persons performing a single period of work.

Recently, it has been determined that the immune system may be regulated to some extent by a group of endogenous opioids known as the enkephalins/endorphins.[34] Exercise raises levels of endorphins in trained and untrained humans and may be responsible for the euphoria or denial of pain associated with endurance training.[35,36] One wonders to what extent the effects of exercise on the immune system are modulated by the endorphins, particularly in light of the idea that the endorphins, the catecholamines, and IL-1, all known immune response modulators, may be found in sections of the brain, especially the hypothalamus.

To summarize the few studies performed relating exercise to humoral immune factors, one might say that exercise performed by untrained individuals may reduce T-cell-dependent immunoglobulin synthesis while Ig levels are unaffected by exertion in well-conditioned athletes. Exercise raises levels of the immunomodulatory substances IL-1 and the endorphins. Obviously, more work remains to be done in this area. Studies designed to demonstrate the effects of exercise on neuroimmunologic control circuits might prove especially interesting.

4. EXERCISE-INDUCED ASTHMA

The most common immunologically medicated pathology of the lung is allergic or atopic asthma. The mechanism underlying the syndrome includes anaphylactic-type reactions involving vasoactive mediator release from mast cells sensitized by IgE which binds a specific antigen (allergen).

Recently, several investigators have identified an asthma-like condition in athletes which apparently does not involve allergen binding by IgE. The symptoms reported include cutaneous angioedema, pruritus and urticaria, respiratory tract obstruction, hyperinflation, choking, coughing, and stridor. Generally, the episodes resemble antigen-induced anaphylaxis, and resolve spontaneously within 30 to 60 minutes. The provocative stimulus in these cases seems to be exercise.[37–39] The magnitude of the respiratory response in this condition does not correlate with either serum IgE levels or the weal diameter of positive allergen skin tests.[40]

At least two mechanisms have been suggested to explain exercise-induced asthma (EIA). The first, a nonimmunologic explanation, involves the need to heat and humidity large volumes of air during exercise. It is suggested that airway cooling and drying may stimulate irritant receptors in the oropharynx and bronchi, leading to bronchoconstriction caused by the vagal efferents.[39]

The second explanation involves the release of mast cell mediators during exercise. Histamine levels rise in plasma during EIA, and cutaneous mast cells demonstrate a loss in the electron density, a fusion of granules with the cell membrane, and a decrease in the number of intact granules.[41] Atopic asthmatics also show increases in plasma concentrations of immunologic mediators called eosinophil or neutrophil chemotactic factors. A statistically significant correlation has been shown to exist between serum histamine or neutrophil chemotactic factor levels and the degree of airflow obstruction after exercise.[42–45]

An interesting paper published by Lee *et al.*[46] attempted to combine these two theories. The authors propose that airway cooling in asthmatic individuals leads to mast cell degranulation and immunologic mediator release which leads directly to symptoms.

Sufferers of exercise-induced asthma maybe experience some relief by administration of cromolyn[39,47] and by maintaining exercise intensity below "tolerance levels."[37]

5. CONCLUSION

Anecdotal reports from persons who engage in exercise programs often include the impression that they are sick less often and that their infrequent infections are less severe than they were before they began training. From some of the evidence reviewed here, one might conclude that there is little immunologic basis for these observations. While short-term, strenuous exercise produces leukocytosis, enhanced competence of the additional cells is either not apparent or is transitory. Chronic training programs, lasting up to 15 weeks, may elicit neutrophilia, but longer-term programs do not seem to significantly alter immune parameters. Extreme sport stress like marathon running or long-distance ski racing may, in fact, reduce a host's response to infectious challenge.

Until such time as a large-scale epidemiologic study is conducted in this area, one is forced to question the value of pain endured for immunologic gain.

REFERENCES

1. Simon HB: The immunology of exercise. A brief review. *JAMA* 252:2735–2738, 1984.
2. Green RL, Kaplan SS, Rabin BS, et al: Immune function in marathon runners. *Ann Allergy* 47(2):73–75, 1981.
3. Klein J: *Immunology, The Science of Self-Nonself Discrimination.* New York, John Wiley and Sons, 1982, pp 445–506.
4. Romano PJ: Cytolytic assays for soluble antigens, in Rose N, Friedman H, Fahey J (eds):, *Manual of Clinical Laboratory Immunology.* Washington, DC, American Society for Microbiology, 1986, pp 72–77.
5. Southwick F, Stossel TP: Phagocytosis, in Rose N, Friedman H, Fahey J (eds): *Manual of Clinical Laboratory Immunology.* Washington, DC, American Society for Microbiology, 1986, pp 326–331.
6. Mehl VS, Penn GM: Electrophoretic and immunochemical characterization of immunoglobins, in Rose N, Friedman H, Fahey J (eds): *Manual of Clinical Laboratory Immunology.* Washington, DC, American Society for Microbiology, 1986, pp 126–137.
7. Durum S, Schmidt J, Oppenheim J: Interleukin 1: an immunological perspective. *Annu Rev lmmunol* 3:263–287, 1985.
8. Merigan T: Interferon—the first quarter century. *JAMA* 248:2513–2516, 1982.
9. Garrey WE, Bryan WR: Variations in white blood cell counts. *Physiol Rev* 15:597, 1935.
10. Landmann RM, Muller FB, Perini C, et al: Changes of immunoregulatory cells induced by psychological and physical stress: relationship to plasma catecholamines. *Clin Exp Immunol* 58:127–135, 1984.
11. Edwards AJ, Bacon TH, Elms CA, et al: Changes in the populations of lymphoid cells in human peripheral blood following physical exercise. *Clin Exp Immunol* 58:420–27, 1984.
12. Hedfors E, Holm G, Ohnell B: Variations of blood lymphocytes during work studied by cell surface markers, DNA synthesis and cytotoxicity. *Clin Exp Immunol* 24:328–335, 1976.
13. Hedfors E, Holm G, Ivansen M. et al: Physiological variation of blood lymphocyte reactivity: T-cell subsets, immunoglobulin production, and mixed-lymphocyte reactivity. *Clin Immunol Immunopathol* 27:9–14, 1983.
14. Robertson AJ, Ramesai KC, Potts RC, et al: The effect of strenuous physical exercise on circulating blood lymphocytes and serum cortisol levels. *J Clin Lab Immunol* 5:53–57, 1981.
15. Ahlborg B, Ahlborg G: Exercise leukocytosis with and without beta-adrenergic blockage. *Acta Med Scand* 187:241–246, 1970.
16. Yu DTY, Clements PJ, Pearson CM: Effect of corticosteroids on exercise-induced lymphocytosis. *Clin Exp Immunol* 28:326–331, 1977.
17. Christensen RD, Hill HR, Anstall HB, et al: Exchange transfusion as an alternative to granulocyte concentrate administration in neonates with bacterial sepsis and profound neutropenia. *J Clin Apheresis* 2:177–83, 1984.
18. Strainer JC, McCarthy DO, Shlafer M, et al: Enhanced hydrogen peroxide generation by human neutrophils following exercise. *Fed Proc* 44(5):1546, 1985.
19. Targan S, Britvan L, Dorey F: Activation of human NKCC by moderate exercise: increased frequency of NK cells with enhanced capability of effector-target lytic interactions. *Clin Exp Immunol* 45(2):352–60, 1981.
20. Brahmi Z, Thomas JE, Park M, et al: The effect of acute exercise on natural killer cell activity of trained and sedentary human subjects. *J Clin Immunol* 5:321–328, 1985.

21. Soppi E, Varjo P, Eskola J: Effect of strenuous physical stress on circulating lymphocyte number and function before and after training. *J Clin Lab Immunol* 8:43–46, 1982.
22. Watson RR, Moriguchi S, Jackson JC, et al: Modification of cellular immune functions in humans by endurance exercise training during β-adrenergic blockage with atenolol or propanolol. *Med Sci Sports Exerc* 18:95–100, 1986.
23. Eskola J, Ruuskanen O, Soppi E, et al: Effect of sport stress on lymphocyte transformation and antibody formation. *Clin Exp Immunol* 32(2):339–345, 1978.
24. Moorthy AV, Zimmerman SW: Human leukocyte response to an endurance race. *Eur J Appl Physiol* 38:271–276, 1978.
25. Hanson PG, Flaherty DK: Immunoloical responses to training in conditioned runners. *Clin Sci* 60(2):225–228, 1981.
26. Nyman CR: Hematological and biochemical observations during a 750 mile relay. *Br J Sports Med* 19:156–157, 1985.
27. Busse WW, Anderson CL, Hanson PG, et al: The effect of exercise on the granulocyte response to isoproterenol in the trained athlete and unconditioned individual. *J Allergy Clin Immunol* 65:358–364, 1980.
28. Steel CM, Evans J, Smith MA: Physiological variation in circulating B-cell:T-cell ratio in man. *Nature* 247:387, 1974.
29. Tomasi TB, Trudeau F, Czerwinski D, et al: Immune parameters in athletes before and after strenuous exercise. *J Clin Immunol* 2:173–178, 1982.
30. Dinarello CA, Wolff SM: Molecular basis of fever in humans. *Am J Med* 72:799–819, 1982.
31. Cannon JG, Kluger MJ: Endogenous pyrogen activity in human plasma after exercise. *Science* 220:617–619, 1983.
32. Cannon JG, Kaplan J, Kluger MJ: Exercise induces monokine secretion from human leukocytes. *Fed Proc* 42(3):464, 1983.
33. Cannon JG, Dinarello CA, Meredith CN, et al: Correlation of plasma IL-1 and creatine kinase activities following exercise. *Fed Proc* 44(5):1546, 1985.
34. Plotnikoff NP, Murgo AJ: Enkephalins-endorphins: stress and the immune system. *Fed Proc* 44:91, 1985.
35. Gambert SR, Garthwaite TL, Pontzer CH, et al: Running elevates plasma beta-endorphin immunoreactivity and ACTH in untrained human subjects. *Proc Soc Exp Biol Med* 168(1):1–4, 1981.
36. Kraemer WJ, Noble B, Culver B, et al: Changes in plasma proenkephalin peptide F and catecholamine levels during graded exercise in men. *Proc Natl Acad Sci USA* 82:6349–6351, 1985.
37. Gunby P: No laughing matter: an "allergy" exercise. *JAMA* 241:2474, 1979.
38. Songsiridej V, Busse WW: Exercise-induced anaphylaxis. *Clin Allergy* 13(4):317–321, 1980.
39. Eggleston P: Exercise induced asthma. *Clin Rev Allergy* 1:19–37, 1983.
40. Schofield NM, Green M. Davies RJ: Response of the lung airway to exercise testing in asthma and rhinitis. *Br J Dis Chest* 74(2):155–163, 1980.
41. Sheffer AL, Fong AK, Murphy GF, et al: Exercise-induced anaphylaxis: a serious form of physical allergy associated with mast cell degranulation. *J Allergy Clin Immunol* 75:479–84, 1985.
42. Lee TH, Brown MJ, Nagy L: Exercise-induced release of histamine and neutrophil chemotactic factor in atopic asthmatics. *J Allergy Clin Immunol* 70(2):73–81, 1982.
43. Soter NA, Wasserman SI, Austen KF, et al: Release of mast-cell mediators and alterations in lung function in patients with cholinergic urticaria. *N Engl J Med* 302(11):604–608, 1980.
44. Ferris L, Anderson SD, Temple DM: Histamine release in exercise-induced asthma (letter). *Br Med J* 1:1697, 1978.
45. Nagakura T, Lee TH, Assoufi BK, et al: Neutrophil chemotactic factor in exercise- and hyperventilation-induced asthma. *Am Rev Respir Dis* 128(2):294–296, 1983.
46. Lee TH, Assoufi BK, Kay AB: The link between exercise, respiratory heat exchange, and the mast cell in bronchial asthma. *Lancet* 1:520–522, 1983.
47. Pepys J: Action of cromoglycate in relation to mediators. *Schweiz Med Wochenschr* 110(6):185–186, 1980.

12

Reproductive Consequences of Athletic Training in Women

Carol Grace Smith and Raymond A. Dombroski

1. WOMEN AND EXERCISE—MODERN TRENDS

Physical exercise and athletic training have become an important part of many women's lifestyles. Thirty years ago, young women and girls were discouraged from participating in such activities. Although boys were expected to participate in athletic training, girls were encouraged not to be too physically active or competitive in sports. Underlying this attitude was the basic belief that female reproductive function might somehow be damaged by too much exercise, especially during menstruation. The beneficial effects of physical fitness on the cardiovascular, musculoskeletal, and metabolic systems are now well recognized for both men and women, and regular exercise has become an important component of a healthful lifestyle. However, the increasing participation of women in athletic training programs has again brought attention to the effects of exercise on reproductive function. The most important of the reproductive changes that frequently accompany intense physical training in women is called athletic amenorrhea or oligomenorrhea. Amenorrhea is a clinical term denoting disruption of the reproductive system with probable anovulation (cycles longer than 90 days duration). The term oligomenorrhea (or irregular cycles) refers to menstrual cycles with inconsistent intervals of 39 to 90 days duration. The terms eumenorrheic, regular, and cyclic are used interchangeably to refer to normal menstrual cycles which recur consistently at intervals of 25 to 39 days duration.

The information available on athletic amenorrhea is incomplete. Some investigators claim that the incidence of amenorrhea among athletes is no different than among the general population, i.e., about 2%, whereas others report the incidence among athletes to be as high as 40%.[1] It is not known whether athletic amenorrhea represents a single entity or multiple entities sharing a common syndrome. Several factors appear to contribute to the problem, including the particular athlete's body size and composition,[2] the physical stress of the specific sport or activity,[3] the severity of the training

Carol Grace Smith and Raymond A. Dombroski • Department of Obstetrics and Gynecology, The University of Texas Health Science Center at San Antonio, San Antonio, Texas 78284.

regimen,[4] the age and reproductive maturity of the athlete,[5] the dietary intake,[6] and the degree of psychological stress associated with athletic performance.[7] We will review here the pathophysiology of athletic amenorrhea, what is known about its causes, the possible consequences of this syndrome, and current recommendations for treatment. Following this discussion, we will briefly review the topic of exercise and pregnancy.

2. BACKGROUND

2.1. Physiology of the Menstrual Cycle

A simplified diagram of the normal menstrual cycle is shown in Fig 1. The onset of menstruation is generally designated as day 1. The cycle is approximately 28 days in length, with ovulation occurring at midcycle. Cyclic changes in the gonadotropic hormones, luteinizing hormone (LH) and follicle-stimulating hormone (FSH), are shown in the top panel. FSH causes follicular growth within the ovary and the secretion of estrogen. FSH and LH act together to complete follicular development and to induce

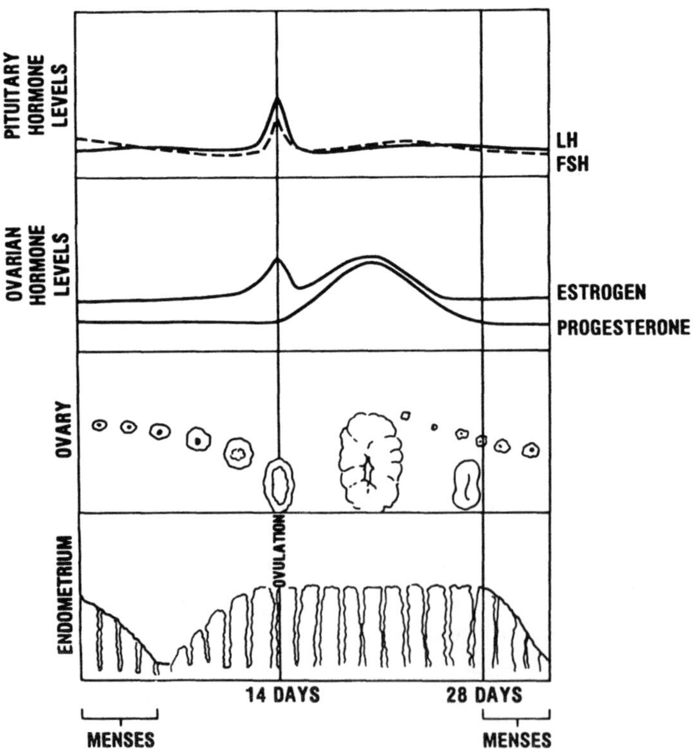

Figure 1. Normal menstral cycle.

ovulation at approximately day 14 of the cycle. The corpus luteum forms on the ovary following ovulation and secretes estrogen and progesterone (second and third panels). If conception and pregnancy do not occur, the corpus luteum ceases functioning and the cycle ends with the occurrence of menstruation. The bottom panel shows growth of the endometrium. In the first half of the cycle (follicular phase), endometrial growth depends on estrogen produced by the maturing follicle. In the second half of the cycle (luteal phase), endometrial growth is dependent on estrogen and progesterone secreted by the corpus luteum. At the end of the cycle, the corpus luteum decreases its secretion of steroids and the endometrium is sloughed off during menstruation.

The menstrual cycle is initiated at the time of puberty by the maturation of the hypothalamic–pituitary–gonadal complex. The hypothalamus secretes, in pulses, a hormone called gonadotropin-releasing hormone (GnRH), which stimulates the pulsatile release of LH and FSH by the pituitary gland. LH and FSH stimulate ovarian functions (as described above), and ovarian steroid hormones, in turn, modulate hypothalamic–pituitary activity. Maintenance of the menstrual cycle depends upon the continued pulsatile secretion of GnRH. This pulsatile secretion is generated by neural activity within the hypothalamus. There are several ways this neural activity can be influenced. The most physiologically important way is the feedback control exerted by ovarian steroid hormones. Excesses or imbalances in steroid hormones can inhibit hypothalamic activity and GnRH secretion. Higher centers within the brain can impinge on the hypothalamic pathways and alter the concentrations of neurotransmitters or endogenous opioid peptides. For example, psychological stress is thought to impair reproductive function through higher brain centers. Diets deficient in certain amino acids can alter neurotransmitter synthesis, and this might affect secretion of GnRH. Lastly, pharmacological amounts of steroid hormones (e.g., oral contraceptives or anabolic steroids) and certain drugs of abuse can inhibit hypothalamic neural activity and GnRH secretion.

2.2. Pathophysiology of the Menstrual Cycle

Amenorrhea has been classified by cause into three types: (1) anatomic, caused by abnormal anatomy of the genital tract that prevents menstrual bleeding; (2) ovarian, caused by failure of the ovaries to develop or respond to gonadotropic stimulation; and (3) chronic anovulation, caused by a defect in the CNS–hypothalamic–pituitary system or by a disturbance in the steroid hormone feedback control.[8] Amenorrhea in athletes has been tentatively placed under the general classification of chronic anovulation. This classification is based on steroid hormone and gonadotropin concentrations and on the absence of both anatomic obstruction and ovarian failure. Developing reproductive dysfunction usually follows a progression of increasingly severe events: (1) luteal phase deficiency with inadequate progesterone concentrations and decreased luteal phase length, (2) anovulation with apparently normal estrogen concentrations, and (3) anovulation with less-than-normal estrogen concentrations.[9] It is likely that women who develop athletic amenorrhea follow this same progression of dysfunction. Thus, infertility due to inadequacy of luteal function may be considerably more extensive than the syndrome of athletic amenorrhea, and we cannot assume that all women who experience vaginal bleeding at regular intervals have normal ovulatory and luteal phase function.[10]

3. HORMONAL MODULATION IN EXERCISE

3.1. Acute Response of Gonadotropins, Prolactin, and Steroids to Exercise

In order to understand the role of endocrine disruption in athletic amenorrhea, many investigators have examined the acute effects of exercise on reproductive hormones. Hormone concentrations have been measured before, during, and after strenuous exercise in trained and untrained athletes to determine if acute changes in hormones might be the cause of the observed changes in the menstrual cycle. Changes that have been observed in gonadotropins, prolactin, and steroid hormone concentrations with acute exercise are summarized below.

3.1.1. LH and FSH

The pulsatile pattern of gonadotropin secretion makes it difficult to separate exercise-related changes from normal pulsatile release of the hormones. Frequent sampling and evaluation of both pulse frequency and pulse amplitude are necessary to document changes in gonadotropin secretion. Changes in feedback control caused by exercise-induced alterations in steroid hormones must also be considered. Perhaps the best information on the effects of exercise on gonadotropin secretion comes from studies in men. Both the frequency and amplitude of gonadotropin pulses were decreased in male marathon runners as was the responsiveness to exogenous GnRH. During short-term intense physical exercise, however, gonadotropin concentrations remained stable in these highly trained athletes, although significant increases in testosterone, cortisol, and prolactin were observed.[11] These investigators hypothesized that the deficiency of hypothalamic GnRH in these athletes might be caused by prolonged, repetitive elevations of gonadal steroids produced by their daily exercise. Exercise in active, but untrained, male volunteers was associated with an acute increase in all of the hormones studied, including gonadotropins.[12] Because the increase in testosterone was simultaneous with the increases in LH and FSH, these observers concluded that the exercise-associated increase in testosterone was not caused by gonadotropin stimulation. Another study showed an increase in both free and total testosterone during exercise in normal men, without any effect on gonadotropin concentrations.[13] The apparent dissociation of gonadotropin and sex steroid concentrations that seems to occur with exercise may be caused by activation of the endogenous opioid peptide (EOP) system, resulting from the stress of strenuous exercise.[14,15] The inhibitory effect of the hypothalamic peptides on GnRH secretion has been demonstrated.[16] Cumming and Rebar have described a reduction in LH pulse frequency in women following 60 minutes of exercise. Normal pulse frequency (90 to 100 minutes between pulses) was virtually abolished for up to 6 hours following exercise.[17] These investigators suggest that the increase in sex steroids that occurs with exercise (see Section 3.1.3) is not mediated by gonadotropin stimulation, but that some other direct gonadal stimulus may be responsible for the effect.

3.1.2. Prolactin

There is general agreement that the acute effect of exercise on prolactin is an increase in circulating concentrations. This increase in prolactin secretion has been observed in trained and untrained athletes during submaximal and maximal exercise.[18,19]

3.1.3. Steroid Hormones

Circulating concentrations of the sex steroids, testosterone, estradiol, and progesterone, rise during exercise in women and return to normal within an hour or two after cessation of exercise.[17] Studies have shown that estradiol concentrations increase in response to maximal exercise, but not necessarily to exercise at a lesser intensity.[20] In one group of untrained subjects, estradiol concentrations were increased by exercise during the luteal phase of the cycle, but not during the follicular phase.[21] In untrained women, several studies have demonstrated exercise-induced increases in progesterone concentrations during the luteal phase of the cycle.[22,23] Some of the increase in plasma concentrations of steroid hormones is probably due to a decreased clearance of sex steroids during exercise, a response that has been shown for estradiol and which is probably due to the decreased hepatic and renal blood flow during exercise.[24] Anticipation of exercise causes an increase in testosterone and cortisol concentrations in male athletes, and a similar effect contributes to the increase in female sex steroids. Lastly, it seems likely that some stimulus other than LH is responsible for the increases in gonadal steroid concentration that are associated with exercise.[17]

3.2. Long-Term Effects of Athletic Training on Hypothalamic–Pituitary–Gonadal Function

Baker *et al.* have reported lower levels of estradiol and sex-hormone-binding globulin (SHBG) among amenorrheic runners than among cycling runners or nonrunners.[25] These investigators hypothesized that the reduction in SHBG was caused by low estradiol concentrations in the amenorrheic runners. Schwartz *et al.* have reported estrone and estradiol concentrations within normal ranges among these groups, but the ratio of estrone to estradiol was significantly higher in runners than in nonrunners.[7] An increased estrone/estradiol ratio is indicative of increased peripheral conversion of androgens to estrone or decreased ovarian secretion of estradiol. These investigators interpreted their findings as indicating the absence of ovarian follicular activity in amenorrheic runners and altered steroid metabolism in all runners. No physiologically significant differences have been found between amenorrheic and cycling runners and nonrunners in other important adrenal and ovarian steroids, including androstenedione, dehydroepiandrosterone, dehydroepiandrosterone sulfate, and testosterone, so there is little evidence that an altered steroid mechanism causes athletic amenorrhea.[7,12,25]

Gonadotropin concentrations in women with athletic amenorrhea appear to be in the low-to-normal range for the early follicular phase, with noncyclic ovulatory discharge of hormones.[25,26] Two studies of four amenorrheic runners indicate that the pituitary can respond to exogenous GnRH with an appropriate release of gonadotropins.[26,27] These observations have led to the tentative conclusion that the hypothalamus might not be properly secreting GnRH in athletic amenorrhea. Such a defect could result directly in depressed gonadotropins and indirectly in reduced ovarian steroids.

Several studies have observed changes in the luteal phase of regularly cycling athletes.[10] Concentrations of FSH, progesterone, estradiol, and 17α-hydroxyprogesterone were all significantly lower in the luteal phase of swimmers than in untrained controls.[28] Shortened luteal phase lengths have been reported in regularly cycling athletes. In one runner, the length of the luteal phase was negatively correlated to the average weekly distance run during the luteal phase.[29] These data may represent early changes in the progression of the syndrome of athletic amenorrhea and may also indicate that athletic infertility, caused by inadequate luteal function, may be an additional consequence of athletic training in women.

3.3. Risks of Athletic Amenorrhea

If left untreated, disruption of reproductive hormones by athletic training has potential consequences other than temporary infertility. Restoration of a normal menstrual cycle is beneficial even if pregnancy is not desired. In the normal menstrual cycle, estrogen and progesterone maintain the health of the reproductive tract and contribute to the health of other tissues, including breasts, skin, hair, and bones. Estrogen stimulates the growth of the endometrium and progesterone protects the endometrium from excessive growth stimulation. Women who have normal estrogen levels but do not ovulate do not produce progesterone to protect the endometrium from overstimulation. These women are at increased risk of endometrial hyperplasia and adenocarcinoma. Women who have very low levels of estrogen do not have this risk, but can experience symptoms similar to menopause, including atrophic vaginitis and urethritis. In addition. estrogen deficiency enhances bone resorption of calcium, decreases calcium reabsorption by the kidneys, and decreases dietary absorption of calcium, all of which contribute to an increased risk of developing osteoporosis. Although exercise promotes bone density, there are no data showing that exercise compensates for a deficiency of estrogen, and recent studies show that women athletes with menstrual irregularity have an increased incidence of musculoskeletal injuries.[30]

Therapeutic options for management of athletic amenorrhea have recently been published.[9] Frequently, a reduction in exercise or an increase in body weight will restore ovulation and regular cycling. If the woman does not want to change her training or weight or if the change fails to reinstitute ovulation, other hormonal therapy is recommended. For example, oral contraceptives can be used since they provide both estrogen and progesterone replacement. Clearly, the dangers of hormone deficiencies are greater than the risks of hormone replacement therapy.

4. EXERCISE AND PREGNANCY

Women in increasing numbers are participating in exercise programs during pregnancy. These programs may be self-styled or organized and supervised by a variety of professionals. The reasons for participation in exercise during pregnancy vary. Some already-fit women wish to maintain fitness during a pregnancy. Some hope to limit the gain in weight which accompanies pregnancy. Some believe that their offspring will be healthier as a result of regular exercise during pregnancy. Others believe that their labors will be shorter or less painful.

Whatever the motivation, these women and the physicians and midwives caring for them often express concern as to the impact of exercise on pregnancy and how pregnancy influences the ability to exercise. They want to know what types and levels of training are "safe" for the pregnant woman and her fetus. They also question whether exercise in certain circumstances might be deleterious to pregnancy.

4.1. Limitation of Available Studies

Inherent difficulties exist in the design and interpretation of studies assessing the effects of exercise on pregnancy.[31] These problems limit the ability to answer the questions posed above.

During normal pregnancy, cardiovascular function is markedly altered. Furthermore, the degree of alteration relative to the nonpregnant state varies with gestational age. Thus, basal levels of many of the parameters which reflect exercise performance during pregnancy vary.[32] Selection of appropriate controls in the background of changing variables is difficult. Individual variations in the degree of alteration of baseline values and in the response to a given work load are additional complications.

The weight gain and change in posture that accompany normal pregnancy affect the ability of the pregnant woman to perform weight-bearing exercise. Many studies have attempted to circumvent this problem by utilizing non-weight-bearing exercises to compare pregnant and nonpregnant exercise performance. However, during bicycle ergometer exercise in a sitting position, the mechanical effects of the gravid uterus coupled with increased vascular capacitance accentuated in the upright posture markedly affect venous return.[33] Evaluation of exercise performance during pregnancy, as a result, requires attention to factors which may directly or indirectly influence commonly measured cardiopulmonary parameters.

Because of the many variables involved, clear-cut conclusions regarding the effect of exercise on pregnancy outcome are difficult to make. Appropriately controlled, prospective studies of sufficient size are lacking.

Finally, due to ethical and legal limitations, most studies of exercise in pregnancy have been limited to the study of moderate exercise. Little is known about maximal exercise performance during pregnancy. Additionally, the parameters evaluated are generally those which may be measured noninvasively or approximated by noninvasive techniques. The bulk of solid physiological data available has been obtained from animal studies. Applicability of these findings to humans may not be valid due to differences in posture, heat elimination, and the levels of stress experienced by the subjects.

4.2. Physiological Alterations of Normal Pregnancy

Striking changes occur in many physiological parameters during pregnancy (Table 1). They reflect adaptations of the maternal organism which are important for normal fetal growth and development. Changes in the cardiovascular and respiratory systems alter the parameters by which exercise performance is assessed. These factors will be briefly reviewed.

4.2.1. Cardiovascular Changes

Blood volume increases early in pregnancy and levels reached by the third trimester are an average of 40% to 50% greater than nonpregnant levels.[34] This increase in blood volume affects both overall cardiac output and regional blood flow.

Resting cardiac output during normal human pregnancy is increased an average of 40% over nonpregnant levels.[32] The magnitude of the increase shows wide individual variability. The majority of the increase in cardiac output is accomplished early in gestation and is primarily due to an increase in stroke volume. Resting heart rate rises progressively during early and mid-pregnancy. At 36 weeks, the heart rate is 10 to 15 beats per minute faster than the nonpregnant rate.[35] Cardiac output declines modestly during the last few weeks of pregnancy. Posture influences both cardiac output and stroke volume, especially during the third trimester. At term, stroke volume in the supine position is lower than in the nonpregnant state due to the mechanical effect of the gravid uterus on venous return.[36]

4.2.2. Respiratory Changes

Oxygen consumption at rest increases with advancing gestational age. At term, oxygen consumption is 20% to 30% greater than that of nonpregnant controls.[37–39] The increase in resting oxygen consumption during pregnancy is primarily attributable to demands of the fetus, placenta, and uterus.[40] When normalized to body weight, resting metabolic rate appears to be unaffected by gestational age.[41]

Table 1. Physiological Alterations of Normal Pregnancy

Parameter	Change in pregnancy
Blood volume	Increased
Heart rate	Increased
Cardiac output	Increased
Oxygen consumption	Increased
Ventilation	Increased

Minute ventilation is elevated during pregnancy, reflecting a progesterone-mediated, heightened sensitivity of chemoreceptors to carbon dioxide.[38,42] The increase in ventilation is accomplished by an increase in tidal volume.[43,44] Respiratory frequency at rest appears to be unchanged during pregnancy.

The composition of blood gases is altered during pregnancy, reflecting the alterations in ventilation outlined above. Arterial pH is higher and pCO_2 is lower than in the nonpregnant individual. The level of arterial oxygen tension and the percent of saturation are essentially unchanged. Because the rise in cardiac output is proportionately greater than the increase in oxygen consumption, arteriovenous oxygen content difference declines.[45]

4.3. Effect of Pregnancy on Exercise Performance

Whether the physiological burden of pregnancy changes the individual's ability to adapt to the stress of aerobic exercise has been the subject of several investigations. Aerobic exercise involves the repetitive use of major muscle groups in such a fashion that a submaximal increase in cardiopulmonary function ensues. Cardiopulmonary and regional vascular circulations are adjusted to ensure an adequate delivery of oxygen and nutrients to, and removal of wastes from, the exercising muscle groups. Below the anaerobic threshold, arterial oxygen and carbon dioxide content remain unchanged due to an efficient matching of supply and demand.[46,47] Thermoregulatory and metabolic alterations to maintain organ homeostasis also occur. Maternal adaptations to pregnancy may alter the ability to respond to the stress of exercise (Table 2).

4.3.1. Exercise Efficiency

Pregnancy results in less efficient performance of weight-bearing exercise. For a given weight-bearing task, the pregnant individual consumes more oxygen than in the nonpregnant state. The increased oxygen consumption has been attributed to the greater weight of the pregnant individual and encumbrance by the fetus.[41,43,44] Several observers have concluded that moderate non-weight-bearing exercise during pregnancy is performed with efficiency comparable to that in the nonpregnant state.[43,48,49] However, others have suggested that exercise efficiency declines progressively by a small amount during pregnancy.[37,39] Those investigators finding decreased non-weight-

Table 2. Effect of Pregnancy on Exercise Performance

Parameter	Change in pregnancy
Efficiency	Unchanged
Maximum increase in cardiac output	Decreased
Maximum increase in ventilation	Decreased

bearing exercise efficiency ascribed the increased oxygen consumption to increases in cardiac work as well as the increased work of ventilation.

Decreased efficiency in the performance of weight-bearing exercise is responsible for the voluntary curtailment of such activities during pregnancy. Several investigators have noted that physically fit women who engaged in regular weight-bearing exercise programs prior to pregnancy voluntarily either ceased or diminished the duration and intensity of such exercise during pregnancy.[50–53] Similarly, in a group of healthy, but untrained. pregnant women, self-paced walking was found to be slower at term than earlier in pregnancy or in the nonpregnant state.[41]

4.3.2. Cardiac Responses to Exercise in Pregnancy

The increased oxygen needs of exercise are met by increases in cardiac output. The degree to which cardiac output may be maximally increased defines cardiac reserve. Cardiac reserve is directly related to ventricular stroke volume and the difference between the resting and maximal heart rate. Because resting heart rate and stroke volume are elevated during pregnancy, cardiac reserve in the pregnant individual is potentially limited.

Bader *et al.* noted that the increase in cardiac output with exercise was similar in nonpregnant and pregnant individuals.[54] In this study, cardiac output during exercise was found to be augmented through increases in both the stroke volume and heart rate. Similarly, Guzman and Caplan reported that the increase in heart rate and cardiac output with increasing work load was the same in the pregnant and the nonpregnant state.[49] These authors concluded that the cardiac response to exercise was not altered by pregnancy. It was suggested, however, that the pregnant individual might reach a maximum work capacity at a lower absolute level of work than when not pregnant. In contrast, Ueland *et al.* found that the increase in cardiac output with moderate exercise became progressively smaller as pregnancy advanced.[32] Women in early and late pregnancy experienced similar increases in heart rate; however, the increment in stroke volume with exercise was diminished in late pregnancy.[32] These investigators concluded that cardiac reserve declined as pregnancy advanced, due to venous pooling and limitation of venous return. Morton *et al.* also found that cardiac response to exercise in late gestation was dominated by factors influencing venous return.[33] Though cardiac output during exercise was similar, heart rate was higher and stroke volume lower in late gestation as compared to postpartum determinations. This group also noted that stroke volume consistently experienced a dramatic decrease immediately following exercise in late gestation.

4.3.3. Ventilatory Response to Exercise in Pregnancy

The rate and depth of ventilation are increased in response to exercise in pregnant women. During pregnancy, oxygen consumption, carbon dioxide production, and expiratory minute volume at rest are increased.[37–39,42–44] The ventilatory equivalent (volume of air expired per volume of oxygen consumed) is also elevated during pregnancy and underscores the fact that ventilation is elevated out of proportion to the amount of oxygen utilized.[43] That is, hyperventilation is characteristic of pregnancy.

The hyperventilation of pregnancy is maintained and accentuated with moderate exercise. Despite similar exercise efficiency, the ventilatory response to a moderate work load is increased.[44] Edwards *et al.* found that oxygen consumption, carbon dioxide production, and ventilation increased more rapidly after exercise onset in pregnant women than in postpartum women.[38] The faster response rate of pregnant women was a short-lived phenomenon. After 75 to 90 seconds of exercise, the difference between the two groups was no longer apparent. This was attributed to the rapid delivery of venous blood to the lungs by muscular compression of the capacitance vessels of the lower extremities. The volume of this blood is greater in the pregnant individual due to hormonal effects on venous capacitance vessels.

During moderate non-weight-bearing exercise, oxygen consumption is higher during pregnancy than in the nonpregnant state. This difference is attributed to the increase in weight and fetal demands during pregnancy. The increment in oxygen consumed and carbon dioxide produced relative to resting levels for a given work load has been found in several studies to be unchanged during pregnancy.[38,39,48,49] In contrast, Pernoll *et al.*, in a longitudinal study of 12 healthy, but untrained, pregnant patients, demonstrated an increase in oxygen consumption and oxygen debt incurred by a standard exercise regimen.[37] In a similar study by the same group, this difference was not apparent in women who had exercised regularly before and during pregnancy.[42] At exercise levels approaching maximal oxygen consumption, pregnant patients lag behind nonpregnant controls in their ability to increase oxygen consumption, minute ventilation, and respiratory frequency.[44]

It thus appears that the cardiopulmonary responses to exercise during pregnancy are similar to those of the nonpregnant individual at low to moderate levels of exercise intensity. Cross-sectional studies fail to demonstrate any difference attributable to pregnancy in oxygen consumption increases over basal levels. Longitudinal studies, however, suggest that untrained pregnant women may utilize more oxygen in performance of a standard work load, whereas trained women do not. At work levels approaching maximum, absolute increases in cardiac and pulmonary function may be limited during pregnancy due to increased demands in the basal state.

4.4. Exercise Effects on the Fetus

Concern has been expressed that exercise during pregnancy may have detrimental effects on the fetus. Potential hazards to the fetus of maternal exercise include hypoxia, limitation of nutrients, hyperthermic effects, and premature uterine activity.[55] On the other hand, improved fetal outcome might occur if the conditioning effects of regular exercise on maternal cardiopulmonary performance resulted in increased placental perfusion (Table 3).

4.4.1. Acute Effects

Animal studies provide most of the data regarding the acute effects of maternal exercise on uterine blood flow and fetal oxygenation. In animals and in man, exercise induces a catecholamine-mediated reduction in visceral blood flow so that the meta-

Table 3. Effects of Maternal Exercise on Fetus

Parameter	Effect of maternal exercise
Acute	
Uterine blood flow	Decreased
Oxygen delivery to fetus	Unchanged
Fetal oxygen consumption	Unchanged
Chronic	
Gestational age at time of delivery	Decreased
Birth weight	Decreased

bolic demands of the exercising muscle groups may be met. Maternal exercise in goats and sheep results in a reduction in uterine blood flow proportional to the level of exercise.[56–59] The reduction in blood flow appears to be the result of alpha-adrenergic stimulation of the uterine vasculature.[56] Hemoconcentration, which accompanies exercise, partially offsets the effect of decreasing blood flow by increasing the amount of oxygen delivered per unit volume of blood. Furthermore, fetal extraction of oxygen from maternal blood increases in response to diminished supply. Thus, short of maternal exhaustion, mechanisms exist that maintain fetal oxygenation at a near-normal level.[57–59]

Several studies in humans have noted that maternal exercise is followed by an elevation of the fetal heart rate.[60–63] It is unclear whether this represents a response to diminished oxygen delivery or to nonspecific stimulation of the fetus, or whether it occurs as a result of transplacental passage of maternal catecholamines. Others have found that fetal biophysical and cardiac response to moderate maternal exercise is minimal.[64–66] In a small sample, Jovanovic *et al.* noted bradycardia on fetal heart rate tracings monitored during the performance of bicycle ergometer exercise.[67] Confirmation of this finding was documented in one instance by ultrasonographic imaging of the fetal heart. Similarly, Artal *et al.* noted fetal bradycardia in 3 or 19 subjects during symptom-limited maximal treadmill exercise.[68] In these observations and those noting tachycardia, fetal heart rate changes associated with maternal exercise were short-lived phenomena, resolving promptly following cessation of exercise. Fetal tachycardia and bradycardia are common responses to decreased oxygenation. These findings thus suggest that the human fetus is transiently stressed during maternal exercise.

During maternal exercise in the human, maternal venous lactate concentrations are significantly elevated. With moderate levels of exercise, hypoglycemia and acidemia do not develop.[64,67] Maternal levels of epinephrine and norepinephrine are consistently elevated during exercise.[64,68] In addition to the above-mentioned effects on uterine blood flow, elevated maternal catecholamines (specifically norepinephrine) could potentially precipitate uterine contractions. Veille *et al.*, however, noted no increase in uterine activity following either weight-bearing or non-weight-bearing exercise in the third trimester.[69]

Maternal thermoregulation during work and exercise is important due to the potentially adverse effect of hxperthermia on fetal growth and development. Jones *et al.* demonstrated that in previously conditioned women, the ability to maintain thermal balance during exercise is unaffected by pregnancy.[70]

4.4.2. Chronic Effects

Chronic physical work during pregnancy is associated with the birth of infants smaller than gestationally age-matched controls.[71,72] Working conditions that result in high levels of maternal fatigue have been found to increase the risk of premature birth.[73] Although other differences exist between women who, out of economic necessity, must perform heavy physical work for long hours during pregnancy and those who pursue physical exercise in their leisure, the effects on pregnancy outcome may be similar.

Pomerance *et al.* determined the fitness level of a group of healthy pregnant women in the third trimester.[74] It is unclear whether any of these women were involved in regular exercise programs. No correlation between maternal fitness level and gestational age at delivery, infant size, Apgar score, or pregnancy complications was found.[74] It is notable that women who delivered prematurely were excluded from this study. Erkkola and Rauramo determined maternal venous and umbilical artery pH levels at the end of labor and compared these with the subject's level of fitness.[75] Fit women and their offspring were found to have higher pH levels. However, the differences between fit and less fit women were not statistically significant.[75]

Jarrett and Spellacy examined pregnancy outcome in 67 women who jogged on a regular basis before and during pregnancy.[53] Subjects were recruited by newspaper advertisement and were subsequently asked to complete a questionnaire. Complications reported in these pregnancies were low. No correlation between the level of maternal exercise and fetal weight or gestational age was found. The limitations of such a study are obvious. Clapp and Dickstein conducted a prospective evaluation of the effect on pregnancy outcome of regular endurance exercise at or above a level necessary to maintain conditioning.[50] When matched sedentary controls and women who stopped exercise prior to 28 weeks were compared, 29 women who continued to exercise gained less weight, had smaller babies, and were more likely to deliver earlier. Mean gestational age was almost 13 days less and infant birth weight almost 900 g less in the exercising women, and 38% of this group gave birth to infants who were small for gestational age. In a subsequent study, a strong inverse relationship was found between exercise intensity and both pregnancy weight gain and infant birth weight.[76] Infant anthropometric data suggested that birth weight was diminished by factors affecting nutritional support. Thus, the decrement was not due to the effect of shorter gestation or constitutional smallness, but to factors which adversely affected fetal growth.

4.5. Conclusions: Exercise and Pregnancy

In summary, pregnancy and exercise both represent stresses to the mother. The healthy woman possesses reserves adequate to respond to these stresses. Pregnancy itself appears not to influence the efficiency with which non-weight-bearing exercise is performed. However, due to fetal encumbrance and weight gain, weight-bearing exercise is performed with less efficiency and generally at a slower rate. The combination of these factors leads the majority of women to curtain exercise performance during pregnancy. Furthermore, the physiological burden of pregnancy most likely limits maximal exercise capacity.

Moderate-level aerobic exercise probably represents a stress to the fetus due to factors that affect uterine blood flow and fetal oxygenation. Protective mechanisms exist to limit these adverse effects. In the short term, the normal fetus tolerates maternal exercise well; however, when exercise is performed chronically during pregnancy, maternal weight gain and fetal growth may be limited. Larger prospective studies are needed to confirm preliminary reports and to elucidate the mechanisms involved.

A direct benefit of exercise on pregnancy is difficult to document. Regular exercise, in addition to its training effects, has psychological and social benefits. Exercise improves one's sense of well-being and is an enjoyable activity. The value of these benefits is difficult to quantify.

If a pregnant woman wishes to participate in an exercise program, it is suggested that she do so under medical guidance. The presence of pregnancy complications that may limit uteroplacental perfusion or increase the risk of premature labor is a prohibitive risk. Exercise during pregnancy should be limited to aerobic activities at moderate levels (less than 70% predicted maximal heart rate) done 3 or 4 times a week. Such a level of performance is sufficient to maintain cardiovascular fitness but is unlikely to pose a major threat to the fetus. Adequate warm-up and cool-down periods may limit blood volume shifts that might adversely affect cardiac output. Nutritional support should be provided to ensure adequate maternal weight gain, and attention should be paid to signs of premature uterine activity or suggestions of inadequate fetal growth.

REFERENCES

1. Loucks AB, Horvath SM: Athletic amenorrhea: a review. *Med Sci Sports Exerc* 17:56–72, 1985.
2. Carlberg KA, Buckman MT, Peake GT, et al: Body composition of olig/amenorrheic athletes. *Med Sci Sports Exerc* 15:215–217, 1983.
3. Sanborn CF, Martin BJ, Wagner WW: Is athletic amenorrhea specific to runners? *Am J Obstet Gynecol* 143:859–861, 1982.
4. Warren MP: The effects of exercise on pubertal progression and reproductive function in girls. *J Clin Endocrinol Metab* 51:1150–1157, 1980.
5. Speroff L, Redwine DB: Exercise and menstrual function. *Phys Sports Med* 8:42–52, 1980.
6. Deuster PA, Kyle SB, Moser PB, et al: Nutritional intake and status of highly-trained amenorrheic and eumenorrheic women runners. *Fertil Steril* 46:636–643, 1986.
7. Schwartz B, Cumming DC, Riordan M, et al: Exercise-associated amenorrhea: a distinct entity? *Am J Obstet Gynecol* 141:662–670, 1981.
8. Yen SSC: Chronic anovulation due to CNS–hypothalamic–pituitary dysfunction, in Yen SSC, Jaffe RB (eds): *Reproductive Endocrinology and Clinical Management*. Philadelphia, W.B. Saunders Co, 1986, p 500.
9. Shanegold M: Causes, evaluation and management of athletic oligo-/amenorrhea. *Med Clin North Am* 69:83–95, 1985.

10. Prior JC, Cameron K, HoYuen B, et al: Menstrual cycle changes with marathon training: anovulation and short luteal phase. *Can J Appl Sport Sci* 7:173–177, 1982.
11. MacConnie SE, Barkan A, Lampman RM, et al: Decreased hypothalamic gonadotropin-releasing hormone secretion in male marathon runners. *N Engl J Med* 315:411–417, 1986.
12. Cumming DC, Brunsting LA, Strich G, et al: Reproductive hormone increases in responses to acute exercise in men. *Med Sci Sports Exerc* 18:369–373, 1986.
13. Vogel RB, Books CA, Ketchum C, et al: Increase of free and total testosterone during submaximal exercise in normal males. *Med Sci Sports Exerc* 17:119–123, 1985.
14. Farrel PA: Exercise and endorphins—male responses. *Med Sci Sports Exerc* 17:89–93, 1985.
15. McArthur JW: Endorphins and exercise in females possible connection with reproductive dysfunction. *Med Sci Sports Exerc* 17:82–88, 1985.
16. Robert JF, Quigley ME, Yen SSC: Endogenous opiates modulate pulsatile luteinizing hormone release in humans. *J Clin Endocrinol Metab* 52:583–585, 1981.
17. Cumming DC, Rebar RW: Hormonal changes with acute exercise and with training in women. *Sem Reprod Endocrinol* 3:55–64, 1985.
18. Shanegold MM, Gatz ML, Thysen B: Acute effects of exercise on plasma concentrations of prolactin and testosterone in recreational women runners. *Fertil Steril* 35:699–702, 1981.
19. Baker ER, Mathur RS, Kirk RF: Plasma gonadotropins, prolactin, and steroid hormone concentrations in female runners immediately after a long distance run. *Fertil Steril* 38:38–41, 1982.
20. Cumming DC, Belcastro AN: The reproductive effects of exertion. *Curr Prob Obstet Gynecol* 5:1–42, 1982.
21. Bonen AW, Ling K, MacIntyre R, et al: Effects of exercise on the serum concentrations of FSH, LH. progesterone and estradiol. *Eur J Appl Physiol* 42:15–23, 1979.
22. Cumming DC, Rebar RW: Exercise and reproductive function in women. *Am J Indust Med* 4:113–125, 1983.
23. Jurkowski JE, Jones WC, Walker EV, et al: Ovarian hormonal responses to exercise. *J Appl Physiol* 44:109–114, 1978.
24. Keizer HA, Poortman J, Bunnik GSJ: Influence of physical exercise on sex-hormone metabolism. *J Appl Physiol* 48:765–769, 1980.
25. Baker ER, Mathur RS, Kirk RF, et al: Female runners and secondary amenorrhea: correlation with age, parity mileage, and plasma hormonal and sex-hormone-binding-globulin concentrations. *Fertil Steril* 36:183–187, 1981.
26. McArthur JW, Bullen BA, Beitins IZ, et al: Hypothalamic amenorrhea in runners of normal body composition. *Endocrinol Res Commun* 7:13–25, 1980.
27. Wakat DK, Sweeney KA, Rogol AD: Reproductive system function in women cross-country runners. *Med Sci Sports Exerc* 14:263–269, 1982.
28. Bonen A, Belcastro AN, Ling WY, et al: Profiles of selected hormones during menstrual cycles of teenage athletes. *J Appl Physiol* 50:545–551, 1981.
29. Shanegold MR, Freeman R, Thysen B, et al: The relationship between long-distance running, plasma progesterone and luteal phase length. *Fertil Steril* 31:130–133, 1979.
30. Lloyd T, Triantafyllou SJ, Baker ER, et al: Women athletes with menstrual irregularity have increased musculoskeletal injuries. *Med Sci Sports Exerc* 18:374–379, 1986.
31. Lotgering FK, Gilbert RD, Longo LD: The interactions of exercise and pregnancy: a review. *Am J Obstet Gynecol* 149:560–568, 1984.
32. Ueland K, Novy MJ, Peterson EN, et al: Maternal cardiovascular dynamics. IV. The influence of gestational age on the maternal cardiovascular response to posture and exercise. *Am J Obstet Gynecol* 104:856–864, 1969.
33. Morton MJ, Paul MS, Campos GR, et al: Exercise dynamics in late gestation: Effects of physical training. *Am J Obstet Gynecol* 152:91–97, 1985.
34. Chesley LC: Plasma and red cell volumes during pregnancy. *Am J Obstet Gynecol* 112:440–450, 1972.
35. Clapp JF: Maternal heart rate in pregnancy. *Am J Obstet Gynecol* 152:659–66, 1985.
36. Metcalfe J, McAnulty JH, Ueland K: Cardiovascular physiology. *Clin Obstet Gynecol* 24:693–710, 1981.

37. Pernoll ML, Metcalfe J, Schlenker TL, et al: Oxygen consumption at rest and during exercise in pregnancy. *Respir Physiol* 25:285–293, 1975.
38. Edwards MJ, Metcalfe T, Dunham MJ, et al: Accelerated respiratory response to moderate exercise in late pregnancy. *Respir Phys* 45:229–241. 1981.
39. Ueland J, Novy MJ, Metcalfe J: Cardiorespiratory responses to pregnancy and exercise in normal women and patients with heart disease. *Am J Obstet Gynecol* 115:4–10, 1973.
40. Clapp JF: Cardiac output and uterine blood flow in the pregnant ewe. *Am J Obstet Gynecol* 130:419–423, 1978.
41. Nagy LE, King JC: Energy expenditure of pregnant women at rest or walking self-paced. *Am J Clin Nutr* 38:369–376, 1983.
42. Pernoll ML, Metcalfe J, Kovach PA, et al: Ventilation during rest and exercise in pregnancy and post partum. *Respir Physiol* 25:295–310, 1975.
43. Knuttgen HG, Emerson K: Physiological response to pregnancy at rest and during exercise. *J Appl Physiol* 36:549–553, 1974.
44. Artal R, Wiswell R, Romem Y, et al: Pulmonary responses to exercise in pregnancy. *Am J Obstet Gynecol* 154:378–383, 1986.
45. Pauerstein CJ: Physiology of the pregnant woman in Pauerstein, CJ (ed): *Clinical Obstetrics*. New York, Wiley Medical, 1987, pp 65–82.
46. Wasserman K, Whipp BJ, Castagna J: Cardiodynamic hyperpnea: hyperpnea secondary to cardiac output increase. *J Appl Physiol* 36:457–464, 1974.
47. Wasserman K: Breathing during exercise. *N Engl J Med* 298:780–785, 1978.
48. Seitchik J: Body composition and energy expenditure during rest and work in pregnancy. *Am J Obstet Gynecol* 97:701–713, 1967.
49. Guzman Ca, Caplan R: Cardiorespiratory response to exercise during pregnancy. *Am J Obstet Gynecol* 108:600–605, 1970.
50. Clapp JF, Dickstein S: Endurance exercise and pregnancy outcome. *Med Sci Sports Exerc* 16:556–562, 1984.
51. Hutchinson PL, Coreton KJ, Sparling PB: Metabolic and circulatory responses to running during pregnancy. *Phys Sports Med* 9(8):55–61, 1981.
52. Zaharieva E: Olympic participation by women. *JAMA* 221:992–995, 1972.
53. Jarrett JC, Spellacy WN: Jogging during pregnancy: an improved outcome? *Obstet Gynecol* 61:705–709, 1983.
54. Bader RA, Bader ME, Rose DJ: Hemodynamics at rest and during exercise in normal pregnancy as studied by cardiac catheterization. *J Clin Invest* 34:1524–1536, 1955.
55. Botti JJ, Jones RL: Aerobic conditioning, nutrition and pregnancy. *Clin Nutr* 4:14–17, 1985.
56. Hohimer AR, Bissonnette JM, Metcalfe J, et al: Effect of exercise on uterine blood flow in the pregnant Pygmy goat. *Am J Physiol* 246:H207–212, 1984.
57. Clapp JF: Acute exercise stress in the pregnant ewe. *Am J Obstet Gynecol* 136:489–494, 1980.
58. Lotgering FK, Gilbert RD, Longo LD: Exercise responses in pregnant sheep: oxygen consumption, uterine blood flow and blood volume. *J Appl Physiol* 55:834–841, 1983.
59. Lotgering FK, Gilbert RD, Lawrence LD: Exercise responses in pregnant sheep: blood gases, temperatures and fetal cardiovascular system. *J Appl Physiol* 55:842–850, 1983.
60. Collings CA, Curet LB, Mullin JP: Maternal and fetal responses to a maternal aerobic exercise program. *Am J Obstet Gynecol* 145:702–707, 1983.
61. Clapp JF: Fetal heart rate response to running in midpregnancy and late pregnancy. *Am J Obstet Gynecol* 153:251–252, 1985.
62. Hauth JC, Gilstrap LC, Widmer K: Fetal heart rate reactivity before and after maternal jogging during the third trimester. *Am J Obstet Gynecol* 142:545–547, 1982.
63. Collings C, Curet LB: Fetal heart rate response to maternal exercise. *Am J Obstet Gynecol* 151:498–501. 1985.
64. Platt LD. Artal R, Semel J, et al: Exercise in pregnancy: II. Fetal responses. *Am J Obstet Gynecol* 147:487–491, 1983.
65. Sorensen KE, Borlum K: Fetal heart function in response to short-term maternal exercise. *Br J Obstet Gynaecol* 93:301–313, 1986.

66. Pijpers L, Wladimiroff JW, McGhie J: Effect of short-term maternal exercise on maternal and fetal cardiovascular dynamics. *Br J Obstet Gynaecol* 91:1081–1086, 1984.
67. Jovanovic L, Kessler A, Peterson CM: Human maternal and fetal response to graded exercise. *J Appl Physiol* 58:1719–1722, 1985.
68. Artal R, Paul RH, Romem Y, et al: Fetal bradycardia induced by maternal exercise. *Lancet* 2:258–260, 1984.
69. Veille J, Hohimer R, Burry K, et al: The effect of exercise on uterine activity in the last weeks of pregnancy. *Am J Obstet Gynecol* 151:727–730, 1985.
70. Jones RL, Botti JJ, Anderson WM, et al: Thermoregulation during aerobic exercise in pregnancy. *Obstet Gynecol* 65:340–345, 1985.
71. Naeye RL, Peters EC: Working during pregnancy: effects in the fetus. *Pediatrics* 69:724–727, 1982.
72. Tafari N, Naeye RL, Gobezie A: Effects of maternal undernutrition and heavy physical work during pregnancy on birth weight. *Br J Obstet Gynaecol* 87:222–226, 1980.
73. Mamelle N, Laumon B, Lazar P: Prematurity and occupational activity during pregnancy. *Am J Epidemiol* 119:309–322, 1984.
74. Pomerance JJ, Gluck L, Lynch VA: Physical fitness in pregnancy: its effect on pregnancy outcome. *Am J Obstet Gynecol* 119:867–875, 1974.
75. Erkkola R, Rauramo L: Correlation of maternal physical fitness during pregnancy with maternal and fetal pH and lactic acid at delivery. *Acta Obstet Gynecol Scand* 55:441–446, 2976.
76. Clapp JF, Wesley M: Selective aspects of pregnancy outcome in recreational runners. Abstract No. 129. Society for Gynecological Investigation, 34th Annual Meeting, Atlanta, Mar 18–21, 1987.

13

Human Growth Hormone

Michael J. Thomas and John A. Thomas

1. INTRODUCTION

Human growth hormone (hGH) was discovered over three decades ago, and evidence of its therapeutic effectiveness was quickly recognized. Until recently, however, the therapeutic use of hGH was limited due to its scarcity and relatively high cost. Prior to recombinant-DNA-dervived (rDNA) hGH, the only source was from the pituitary glands of cadavers. In the human pituitary gland, approximately 10% of the dry weight of pituitary tissue is growth hormone.

In 1963, the National Pituitary Program was established to provide hGH for growth-hormone-deficient children. By the early 1970s, the Program was providing upwards of 200,000 I.U. of this scarce protein hormone.[1] Into the 1980s, the total amount and distribution of cadaveric hGH was approximately 900,000 I.U. Despite improvements in purification and yield of cadaveric hGH, therapeutic needs outstripped the supply of this hormone. It was estimated that only about 2,500 children could be treated annually, or about 1 in 4 GH-deficient youngsters. While purification technologies improved, there was a coincident reduction in the availability of donated human pituitary glands. Consequently, there was still a scarcity of hGH.

The advent of rDNA technologies or genetic engineering has provided an alternative to using cadaveric human pituitary GH. Genetically engineered hGH has now been developed by at least four biotechnology companies. In 1985, a rDNA-derived GH or methionyl hGH (Met-hGH) was approved by the U.S. Food and Drug Administration (FDA) for therapeutic use. The commercialization of Met-hGH was undoubtedly hastened by the fact that the FDA suspended the distribution of cadaveric pituitary hGH, due to the suspicion that some of the cadaveric preparations may have been contaminated with a slow virus that causes Creutzfeldt–Jakob disease. Creutzfeldt–Jakob disease is a rare, fatal disease characterized by subacute spongiform encephalopathy, leading to progressively severe dementia with myoclonus.

In addition to vastly increasing the amount of therapeutically available hGH, the

Michael J. Thomas • Department of Pharmacology and Toxicology, West Virginia University School of Medicine, Morgantown, West Virginia 26506. *John A. Thomas* • Department of Pharmacology, University of Texas Health Science Center, San Antonio, Texas 78284.

rDNA-derived hGH will eliminate the risk of acquiring transmissable viral contaminants present in cadaveric hGH preparations. Further, the therapeutic indications for its use, which were once quite narrow and restricted to a subpopulation of children with hypopituitarism, can now be prudently expanded to include children with so-called normal variant short stature (NVSS). NVSS youngsters may constitute as many as 40% of children in the United States, i.e., those who are below the third percentile in predicted body height.

The potential for overzealous therapeutic use of hGH due to the newly realized abundance of supplies has led to concern about its medical misuse and its outright abuse by athletes attempting to gain weight and height. The increased availability of hGH has also prompted suggestions that this hormone be restricted and be prescribed only by pediatric endocrinologists in order to minimize its abuse. The hormone should not be used by normal individuals possesing normal circulating levels of this hormone. Prolonged elevated levels of hGH are manifested by the characteristic pathological changes of acromegaly, but the potential long-term side effects of supraphysiological injections of hGH are yet to be established.

2. REGULATION OF GROWTH HORMONE SECRETION

GH is secreted by acidophilic cells (somatotrophs) of the anterior pituitary (adenohypophysis) in response to a variety of stimuli. The most important regulators of growth hormone secretion are two hypothalamic hormones, growth-hormone-releasing hormone (GHRH) and somatostatin (SS).[2] GHRH and SS are both peptide hormones (57 amino acids and 14 amino acids in length, respectively) which are released by the hypothalamus into the hypophyseal portal circulation and delivered to the anterior pituitary. GHRH acts at a receptor on somatotrophs and stimulates GH production and release, and SS inhibits GH release. Modulation of GH secretion is regulated by the release of these two hormones. Neuronal secretion of GHRH seems to be inherently episodic and is affected by a variety of diverse stimuli. The secretion of GHRH is enhanced by dopaminergic and serotonergic neuronal pathways. Alpha-adrenergic stimulation facilitates GHRH secretion, whereas beta-adrenergic stimulation suppresses GHRH secretion. Such a scheme for the modulation of GH can be depicted graphically as in Fig. 1.

The release of GH leads to the release of somatomedins, (principally insulin-like growth factor I (ILGF-I), from the liver and other tissues, ILGF-I can modulate some of the growth effects of GH on target tissues. It can inhibit the secretion of GH by stimulating somatostatin release from the hypothalamus, and can also directly antagonize GHRH effects on GH release.

Several physiological stimuli affect GH release, including stress, hypoglycemia, and sleep. Exercise-mediated hypoglycemia and vigorous physical activity can stimulate GH secretion. Severe psychological deprivation, hypothyroidism, hypocaloric malnutrition, chronic renal disease, and chromosomal and metabolic abnormalities are pathological conditions that are capable of interfering with GH secretion. Many of these pathological states cause growth retardation as evidenced by short stature. Thus,

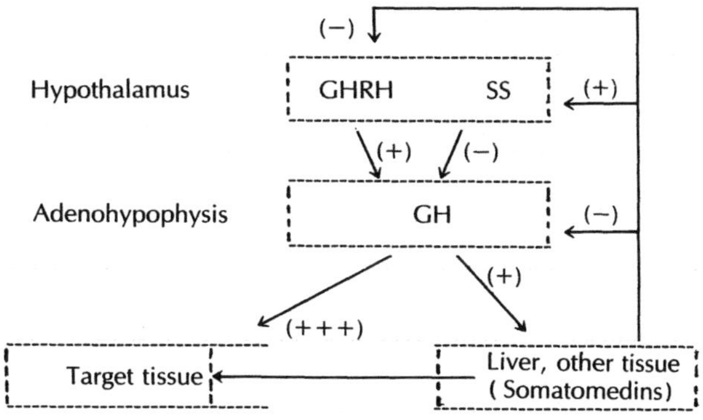

Figure 1. Scheme for the modulation of GH.

modulation of GH secretion is influenced by several physiological and pathological factors.

3. CHEMISTRY

GH from a number of mammalian species has been isolated and characterized. The amino acid sequence of GH varies from species to species (Table 1). The primary structure of hGH was elucidated by Li and his coworkers in the late 1960s. Of all the biologically active adenohypophyseal hormones, GH is probably the most abundant.

Human GH is a single-chain molecule consisting of 191 amino acid residues (Fig. 2). It contains two intrachain disulfide bonds. The molecule is predominantly alpha-helical in secondary structure. Many growth hormones from other species have been well characterized (e.g., rat, bovine, ovine, elephant, and monkey), and while they share some common structural features, the amino acid sequences are significantly

Table 1. Comparison of Selected Mammalian Growth Hormones

Species	Source	Number of amino acids
Rat	Pituitary	190
Bovine	Pituitary	195
Ovine	Pituitary	195
Elephant	Pituitary	191
Monkey	Pituitary	191
Man	Pituitary	191
Man	rDNA (*E. coli*)	192
Man	rDNA	191

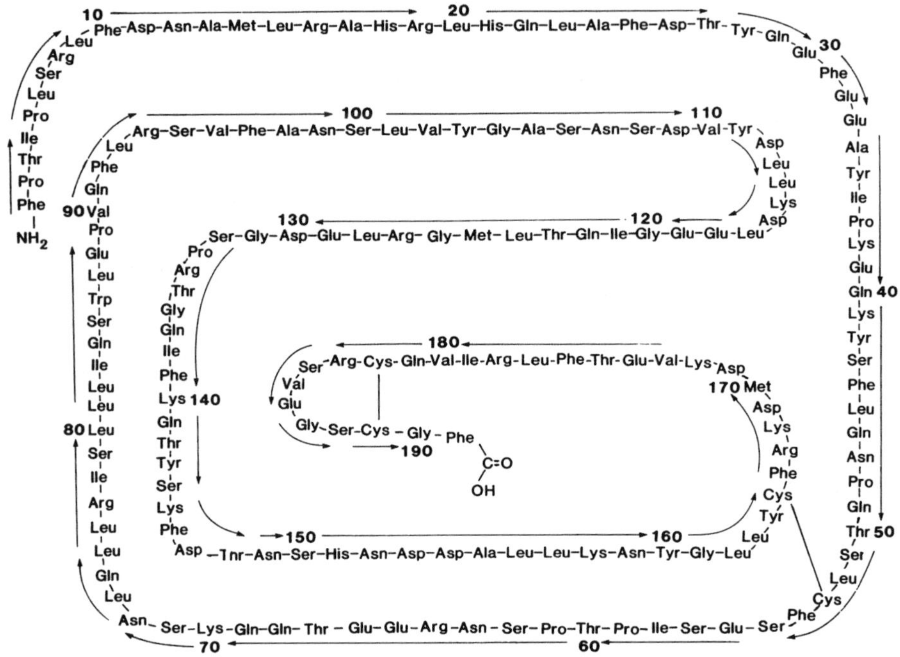

Figure 2. Primary structure of human growth hormone.

different, so that biological activity does not transcend species lines. Hence, these growth hormones are biologically ineffective in humans. Monkey GH most closely resembles human GH; however, four amino acids are different in the primary structure, and biological activity in humans is minimal.[3] Similarly, elephant GH is 191 amino acid residues which impart growth-promoting action.[4] However, it is interesting to note that the initial 20-amino-acid sequence from rat GH has been employed as a "signal peptide" sequence in the recombinant expression of Met-hGH from *E. coli*.

The primary and secondary structure of GH is similar to that of two other hormones, chorionic somatomammotropin and, to a lesser extent, prolactin. These three hormones are immunologically and biologically cross-reactive, suggesting common structural features that bind and recognize antibodies and receptors. These three hormones are part of a multigene cluster which bears a high degree of nucleic acid sequence homology. These genes may have evolved from a common ancestral gene which duplicated millions of years ago. In humans, there are two copies of the GH gene, GH "N" gene (hGH-I) and GH "V" gene (hGH-II). Only hGH-I gene is expressed into growth hormone, since the hGH-II gene cannot substitute in cases of GH "N" gene deficiency.

Several molecular forms of hGH are found in extracts obtained from the human pituitary gland. The predominant circulating form of GH is a 22-kilodalton peptide, but a smaller 20-kilodalton (20K) variant composes 5% to 15% of circulating plasma GH. The smaller 20K variant is detected in the sera of normal and acromegalic individuals.

The 20K variant differs from the 22K GH by 15 amino acids (residues 32 to 46). This may be due to a different mRNA splicing process which deletes these codons in GH mRNA processing. With that exception, the 22K and 20K GH variants are structurally identical, but they exhibit dissimilar metabolic actions. In the plasma, GH can circulate as large aggregates 40 to 100 kilodaltons in size, but the physiological significance is not known. GH is proteolytically cleaved to inaction fragments so that the plasma half-life is only 20 to 30 min.

Biosynthetic Met-hGH (e.g., Somatrem) was developed using rDNA technologies. Met-hGH can be produced in the bacteria *E. coli* (K12) using recombinant plasmids containing the cloned GH gene. Using conventional fermentation techniques, bacteria containing the recombinant GH plasmid can produce Met-hGH in large quantities that can be purified. The Met-hGH can be used as hormonal replacement therapy in children with growth hormone deficiencies. Analysis of the amino acid composition of the rDNA-derived Met-hGH reveals a protein that is comparable to that of the natural, endogenous hGH, with the only difference being the additional methionine at the N-terminal end of the peptide.

Earlier rDNA technologies employed prokaryotic cell systems (e.g., *E. coli*) to produce GH for hormonal replacement therapy. Consequently, the bacterially derived GH was a 192-amino-acid peptide with an N-terminal methionine. More recently, eukaryotic expression vectors have been developed that can produce large quantities of the endogenous 191-amino-acid GH, without the extra methionine. Evidence to date indicates pharmacological equivalency of the 191- and 192-amino-acid forms of GH, although some questions have arisen regarding antigenicity and provocation of antibodies.

4. PHYSIOLOGICAL AND METABOLIC EFFECTS OF GROWTH HORMONE

GH has a multitude of physiological and metabolic effects in the body (Table 2). Its primary function is to promote protein synthesis and cellular growth.[5] The anabolic effects of GH are complex and vary among different tissues. Prior to closure of the epiphyseal end plates, GH can stimulate linear skeletal growth.[6] GH can stimulate the proliferation of chondrocytes in the epiphyseal cartilage, which then allows the osteoblasts to lay down new bone matrix at the ends of long bones.[7] After epiphyseal plate fusion occurs at puberty, linear bone growth is no longer possible, but excessive GH can thicken bone periosteum, leading to a condition known as acromegaly.[8] In addition to bone, GH can stimulate growth in other tissues. GH causes an increase in skeletal muscle mass and, to a lesser extent, in cardiac and smooth muscle. Organ enlargement in response to GH is seen in the liver, thymus, and lymph nodes, and a slight enlargement is seen in the gonads, adrenals, and thyroid.[9]

In most tissues, GH stimulates amino acid uptake and protein synthesis.[5] GH induction of protein synthesis seems to occur at the transcriptional and translational levels, since levels of rRNA and mRNA increase following GH administration.[6] The intracellular signals that mediate the nuclear and ribosomal events of protein synthesis

Table 2. Biological Effects of Human Growth Hormone

Anatomical actions
Accelerates linear bone growth
Diminishes adipose mass
Increases enlargement of lean body mass
Metabolic actions
Enhances amino acid transport
Promotes protein anabolism
Stimulates DNA/RNA synthesis
Increases polyamine synthesis
Stimulates lipolysis
"Diabetogenic"
Physiological actions
Increases basal metabolic rate
Stimulates osteogenesis
Stimulates erythropoiesis
Expands extracellular fluid space
Increases renal blood flow and glomerular filtration rate
Increases tubular resorption of PO_4

induction by GH are not known. The anabolic effect of GH on body tissues results in a decrease in the circulating plasma levels of amino acids and a decrease in blood urea nitrogen (BUN), which leads to nitrogen retention and a positive nitrogen balance.[9] The body also retains many minerals and ions in response to GH. Levels of plasma phosphorus increase. Sodium, potassium, and chloride ions are retained by the kidney, and plasma volume expands as a result of a direct tubular effect of GH that increases renal sodium pump activity *in vitro*. Calcium is also retained by the kidney, in addition to its increased gastrointestinal absorption, due to the effects of GH. Also, a positive balance of magnesium is associated with these responses.[9]

The metabolic effects of GH are very complex, and not all of the metabolic effects may be physiologically significant. Other metabolic regulators may be more important in maintaining metabolic homeostasis, and the metabolic effects of GH may become important only in individuals receiving GH therapy or in disease states (e.g., GH-secreting tumors). The effects of GH on carbohydrate metabolism are opposite that of insulin. Thus, GH has been termed a ''diabetogenic'' or ''anti-insulin'' hormone. GH can produce hyperglycemia, which can exacerbate a diabetic condition in susceptible individuals.[6,10] GH triggers the release of glucose from hepatic glycogen stores, but it blocks glucose uptake and transport into tissues such as muscle. GH can stimulate a slight increase in the basal level of insulin, but this is unable to facilitate glucose uptake into tissues due to the lipolytic effect of GH. In adipose tissue, GH mobilizes triglyceride breakdown into fatty acids and glycerol. Ketogenesis can occur when hepatic oxidation of free fatty acids produces ketone bodies. The increase in free fatty acids can also antagonize carbohydrate metabolism and stimulate gluconeogenesis.[6]

GH has a variety of other miscellaneous actions on different body tissues. In bone marrow stromal cells, GH can stimulate erythropoiesis and lymphopoiesis, but not granulopoiesis.[6] GH can also stimulate the release of somatomedins from several tissues, most notably hepatocytes and fibroblasts.[11] As will be discussed below, the somatomedins are growth factors which may be very important mediators in the molecular mechanisms of action of GH.

5. GROWTH HORMONE RECEPTOR AND INTRACELLULAR CHANGES

Like other hormones, GH interacts with a receptor on a target cell to produce its physiological effects. However, efforts to characterize the nature of the GH receptor have been difficult for several reasons. One of the problems has been the discrepancy between the *in vivo* and *in vitro* effects of GH.[6,12] GH has variable effects upon the growth of cell cultures, depending upon the media and incubation conditions. A consistent change in cellular metabolism has been difficult to demonstrate. This difficulty may be due to multiple forms of the GH peptide (e.g.. the 20K or 22K variants) having different effects in different tissues.[11] Other factors, such as the somatomedins, may be modulating the interaction of GH and its receptor in different tissues.[6] Another possibility could be the existence of multiple forms of the GH receptor in various target tissues.[7] GH receptor heterogeneity could be due to different receptor subunits or different signal transduction mechanisms. Another problem in identifying the GH receptor has been the lack of a receptor ligand other than proteolytic fragments of GH.[7] Currently, no effective GH receptor agonist or antagonist exists that is specific enough for receptor binding studies.[7] Attempts at producing a monoclonal antibody to the GHs have been met with limited success. Clearly, more research is needed to fully characterize the GH receptor and to elucidate the cellular mechanism of action.

The GH receptor is widely distributed throughout the body. The receptor has been identified on the cell surface membranes of of hepatocytes, adipocytes, fibroblasts, lymphocytes, and chondrocytes.[7] Under nondenaturing conditions, the GH receptor of a human lymphocyte cell line appears to have a molecular weight in excess of 200 kilodaltons, but using sodium dodecyl sulfate (SDS) gel electrophoresis, the apparent molecular weight of the receptor is 108 kilodaltons.[7] The GH receptor may be composed of subunits linked by disulfide bonds, but this has not been fully characterized. GH receptors appear to have carbohydrate residues attached to the extracellular surface, but it is not clear whether the carbohydrate moiety is required for biological activity. The binding affinity of GH for the receptor is not altered in the absence of the carbohydrate moiety.[7] There is some evidence that GH may be internalized by the GH receptor.[13] The biological significance of receptor-mediated endocytosis and degradation of GH by the target cell is not understood.

Other mechanisms for signal transduction of GH have been proposed. Like the receptors for many other hormones and growth factors, the GH receptor may possess tyrosine kinase activity on its cytoplasmic surface. Recently, *in vitro* experiments with rat hepatocytes showed that addition of GH to the media resulted in the phosphorylation of certain proteins which were not affected by the addition of other hormones.[14]

Phosphorylation of intracellular proteins has been shown to be an important event in proliferation, differentiation, and growth processes triggered by growth factors.[15] Phosphorylation can alter enzymatic activity and cytoskeletal mobility, and may modulate events in the nucleus, such as gene expression. Phosphoinositide metabolism, a common signal transduction mechanism which regulates protein kinase C activity, is probably not involved in the cellular mechanism of GH action.[16] Many researchers have looked for changes in the intracellular levels of cyclic nucleotides in response to GH. The intracellular messenger role of cyclic nucleotides in GH receptor transduction mechanisms is still unclear. In some tissues, it is possible to show that GH causes a decrease in adenylate cyclase activity and cAMP levels.[6] In other tissues, no effect is observed. A role for cGMP is unclear, but it may mediate the inhibitory effect of GH.[6] Many of the new molecular biology techniques may facilitate elucidation of these problems.

6. THE INTERACTION OF GROWTH HORMONE AND SOMATOMEDINS

Many of the physiological effects of GH may be mediated by a class of polypeptides known as somatomedins, or insulin-like growth factors (ILGFs).[17] The somatomedin hypothesis accounts for the experimental observation that growth and mitotic activity of cartilage are dependent upon GH *in vivo,* but there is no effect of GH upon this tissue *in vitro.*[6] Addition of somatomedins to cartilage tissue *in vitro* will elicit growth and cell division. Somatomedins are thought to mediate the stimulatory effect of GH in certain target tissues.[12] Two somatomedins have been isolated and characterized and their cDNAs cloned. Somatomedin C, more commonly identified as ILGF-I, is a 70-amino-acid single-peptide chain with three disulfide bonds.[11] The levels of ILGF-I are largely GH dependent.[12] In GH-deficient individuals, the levels of ILGF-I are very low, but rise upon administration of GH.[11] In disease states of growth hormone excess, such as acromegaly, the level of ILGF-I is elevated.[18,19] ILGF-II, or "multiplication stimulating activity" (MSA), is a closely related 67-amino-acid single-peptide chain which can also stimulate growth and cell division in target tissues, although it is not as potent as ILGF-I. Unlike ILGF-I, ILGF-II levels do not appear to be dependent upon GH levels.[11,12]

Both ILGF-I and ILGF-II bear approximately 50% structural homology to the proinsulin amino acid sequence.[12] Thus, the ILGFs possess insulin-like effects on insulin target tissues, which include stimulation of glucose transport, glycogen synthesis, and glycolysis. In large doses, ILGFs can produce a hypoglycemic state *in vivo.*[12,20]

The somatomedins are produced primarily in the liver. ILGF-I and ILGF-II are originally synthesized as large precursors (130 and 180 amino acids long, respectively) which are proteolytically processed prior to secretion from the cell. Somatomedins are not stored in secretory granules; rather, they are steadily secreted at low basal levels.[12] There is some evidence that growth hormone modulates the expression of the ILGF-I gene.[21] Once the somatomedins are secreted into the circulation, they are highly bound by at least two plasma protein carrier molecules. The plasma protein carriers are also synthesized by the liver and are referred to as ILGF binding proteins. The ILGF binding proteins have molecular weights of approximately 50 and 150 kilodaltons. and they protect the somatomedins from proteolysis. thus increasing the plasma half-life.[12] When bound to ILGF binding proteins, the somatomedins cannot readily interact with target tissues, so some mechanism must account for delivery of the somatomedins to the site of action. GH can influence the levels of ILGF binding proteins. In GH-deficient individuals, the larger 150-kilodalton protein is lacking. Administration of GH to these individuals will lead to the reappearance of the 150-kilodalton protein.[12] Thus, GH may play a modulatory role in the delivery and bioavailability of somatomedins to target tissues.[20,22]

Both ILGF-I and ILGF-II act at receptors on the cell surface of target tissues. Three membrane-bound receptors are responsible for the cellular effects of ILGFs: the insulin receptor, the ILGF-I receptor, and the ILGF-II receptor.[11] ILGF-I preferentially binds to the ILGF-I receptor, but it can also cross-react with the insulin and ILGF-II receptors. The cross-reactivity of ILGF-I with the insulin receptor may account for the insulin-like effects observed *in vivo.*[12] ILGF-II binds to the ILGF-II receptor, but may cross-react with the ILGF-I receptor to a lesser degree. The structure of the ILGF-I receptor is similar to the structure of the insulin receptor. Both receptors are composed of subunits linked by disulfide bonds and possess tyrosine kinase activity on their cytoplasmic surface. The ILGF-II receptor, on the other hand, has a single polypeptide structure and does not appear to possess kinase activity on the cytoplasmic surface of the membrane.[11] ILGF receptors are widely distributed and appear to be present in all tissues studied thus far. They are especially prominent in placental tissues.[10] In addition. ILGF-II receptors are densely distributed in the liver.[10,12]

The cellular and physiological effects of the somatomedins are complex and not fully understood. One of the earliest noted effects of the somatomedins was sulfation activity (^{35}S incorporation) on cartilage proteoglycans incubated with serum *in vitro.* This activity was absent in the serum of hypophysectomized animals, and addition of GH to the incubation medium could not restore sulfation activity. Only serum of hypophxsectomized animals treated with GH replacement therapy possessed sulfation activity on cartilage proteoglycans *in vitro.*[11,12] In addition, somatomedins were later shown to cause an increase in the synthesis of proteoglycans and other components of the cartilage matrix.

Early experiments with the somatomedins were troubled by impurities, but ILGF-I and ILGF-II were eventually purified to homogeneity. *In vitro* tissue culture experiments reveal that ILGF-I and ILGF-II can stimulate DNA synthesis in a wide variety of cell types.[12] ILGFs can stimulate mitogenesis, but are less potent mitogens than platelet-derived growth factor (PDGF) and other growth factors. The effects of ILGFs and PDGF on DNA synthesis appear to be additive, implying that these effects are mediated through different receptors and different intracellular changes.[12] Similarly, epidermal growth factor (EGF) and ILGF-I can synergistically stimulate the proliferation of certain mesenchymal cells.[12] In addition to their proliferation effects on mesenchymal cells, ILGFs can stimulate differentiation of these cells *in vitro.* The somatomedins can stimulate myoblast differentiation and myotube formation.[12]

ILGF-I is also capable of stimulating colony formation and differentiation of erythroid cells in murine hematopoietic tissue, effects similar to those of erythropoietin.[12] Like thyroid hormone, ILGF-I may play a role in bone growth and development by stimulating the differentiation of an osteoblast-like cell in newborn rats. Yet, not all differentiation effects are solely mediated by ILGF-I. GH, but not ILGF-I, is capable of stimulating the differentiation of pre-adipocytes to adipocytes *in vitro*. In addition, this GH treatment seems to sensitize the mitogenic response of the adipocytes to ILGF-I.[23] GH may interact directly with target tissue to modulate the cellular effects of the somatomedins. To elucidate whether GH or ILGF-I is primarily responsible for the *in vivo* effects observed on growth, Zapf *et al.* implanted osmotic minipumps subcutaneously into hypophysectomized rats.[20] Doses of ILGF-I, ILGF-II, or GH were continuously infused into the animals for 6 days. Both ILGF-I and GH caused increases in body weight, tibial epiphyseal width, and thymidine incorporation into costal cartilage, whereas ILGF-II had little effect on these parameters.[12,20] Thus, ILGF-I seems capable of mediating the effects of GH *in vivo,* but it is not clear if GH may further modulate the physiological response in a normal individual. When ILGF-I is given subcutaneously or intravenously, its metabolic effects appear to be more prominent than its growth effects, which are less substantial.[24] Perhaps GH and ILGFs may interact with their respective receptors and cause different metabolic changes at different phases of the cell cycle. Both GH and the somatomedins appear to have distinct direct effects on tissue growth and develoqment, which interact to produce the overall physiological responses.

7. CLINICAL FEATURES OF ABNORMAL GROWTH HORMONE PRODUCTION

Abnormalities in the secretion or regulation of GH can lead to pathological disease states. In GH-deficient states, children fail to attain normal stature. Typically, these individuals are short (greater than 3 standard deviations below the norm), have varying degrees of bone retardation, have excessive skinfold thickness (about the 90th percentile), and may have a characteristic "pinched" facies.[25] GH-deficient individuals can present with a spectrum of appearances, with those less severely deficient assuming a more normal appearance. GH-deficient individuals will present with growth velocity charts below the normal limits of anthropometric assessment.[25,26] While there are many causes of short stature (genetic, nutritional, psychosocial), GH deficiency is most common. Serum GH levels must be determined (usually done by radioimmunoassay), and further provocative testing may be indicated to ascertain pituitary integrity.[19]

In contrast to the short stature caused by GH deficiency, excessive GH production results in skeletal, soft tissue, and visceral enlargement.[8] This condition is known as acromegaly, and occurs with an annual incidence of approximately 3 per 1 million.[8] If excessive GH production occurs prior to closure of the epiphyseal plates at adolescence, these children rapidly grow to excessively tall stature, a condition known as gigantism.[27] More commonly, the excessive GH production occurs at adulthood, after epiphyseal plate closure. and the features of acromegaly result. Unlike gigantism, the features of acromegaly develop more insidiously, sometimes taking years to present clinically.[10] The most prominent physical features are enlargement of the hands, feet, and face. The "acromegalic facies" is due to the effects of GH on the membranous bones in the skull, and patients with acromegaly will characteristically have a large protruding jaw (prognathism); accentuated, thickened supraorbital and frontal ridges; and an enlarged, flattened nose.[8] Excessive GH levels may also cause changes in the vertebrae, leading to a kyphosis or "hunchback" appearance. In addition to skeletal derangements, patients with acromegaly often have enlarged viscera and soft tissues. Thickened lips and a large tongue often add to the features of acromegalic facies, and the kidneys, liver, heart, spleen, and other internal organs may become enlarged.[10] Acromegaly may produce metabolic changes including glucose intolerance (sometimes mimicking diabetes mellitus), osteoporosis, and hypertension. The patient may have increased amounts of body hair (hirsutism), and sometimes gynecomastia and lactation can occur.[10] A small percentage of patients experience visual field defects (bitemporal hemianopsia).[10]

8. PATHOLOGY OF GROWTH HORMONE PRODUCTION

8.1. Growth Hormone Deficiency

GH deficiencies have several underlying etiologies. They can occur due to defects at the hypothalamic, pituitary, or target tissue level.[25] These disorders can be either congenital or acquired. Most can be treated with GH replacement therapy, but identification of the underlying etiology is imperative for effective treatment and management of the GH-deficient patient.

The most common cause of GH deficiency is a secondary deficiency due to a hypothalamic defect.[25] The hypothalamus regulates GH secretion from the anterior pituitary by releasing two peptide hormones (GHRH and SS) into the hypophyseal portal circulation. GHRH stimulates GH release and SS inhibits GH release.[2,28,29] Hypothalamic control of GH secretion can be disrupted by several mechanisms. In some instances, there is a defective secretion of GHRH which can be transmitted as an autosomal recessive trait, but the genetic defect is not known.[11] Most causes of hypothalamic dysfunction are idiopathic. Congenital causes include developmental brain midline abnormalities, sometimes associated with hydrocephalus. Meningitis, granulomas, infections, and traumatic delivery at birth may damage the hypothalamus. Hypothalamic tumors such as craniopharyngiomas, hamartomas, and neurofibromas can lead to GH deficiency.[25] Hypothalamic defects can often be radiographically detected using computerized tomography (CT) scanning techniques. Pituitary gland integrity can be determined by provocative pharmacological stimuli of GH secretion; an increase in serum GH will indicate hypothalamic dysfunction in GH-deficient individuals.[10,25]

Hypopituitarism is another cause of GH deficiency; however, pituitary insufficiency rarely manifests as an isolated lack of GH.[8] Serum levels of all adenohypophyseal hormones will aid in the differential diagnosis of hypopituitarism. The majority of hypopiuitarism cases are idiopathic; however, developmental brain abnormalities (e.g., anencephaly, holoprosencephaly) may be causes of pituitary aplasia or hypoplasia. There is an increased incidence of hypopituitarism in individuals with cleft lip or palate. In certain rare instances, absence of GH secretion can be due to a 7.5-kilobase deletion of the GH gene, which can be inherited in autosomal recessive pattern.[10] Nonsecretory adenomas account for a large majority of destructive pituitary lesions, followed by craniopharyngiomas and optic nerve gliomas.[8,25] Sheehan's pituitary necrosis (also known as postpartum pituitary necrosis) is due to infarction of the anterior pituitary following obstetric hemmorhage or shock.[8] Empty sella syndrome is an uncommon disorder with several etiologies, but usually is due to a congenitally incomplete diaphragma sella, with subsequent intrasellar cisternal herniation and compression of the pituitary gland.[8] Like the hypothalamus, the pituitary can be adversely affected by infections, meningitis, granulomas, and traumatic delivery at birth. Cranial irradiation, usually received as part of radiation therapy for inoperable brain tumors, can result in pituitary dysfunction. Diagnosis of many pituitary disorders can be made with CT scanning techniques, which can reveal anatomic abnormalities. Radioimmunoassays of adenohypophyseal hormones can reveal changes in normal serum levels. GH deficiency due to pituitary dysfunction usually will not respond to provocative pharmacological stimuli.[11,25]

The last category of growth disorders comprises individuals who do not necessarily have decreased levels of GH; their short stature is usually the result of some unknown defect. Laron dwarfism is an autosomal recessive trait where GH levels are elevated, but serum ILGF-I levels are depressed to levels seen in hypopituitarism and cannot be stimulated by administration of GH.[10] Similarly, African Pygmies have normal serum GH levels, but low serum ILGF-I levels.[12] In rarer instances, individuals of short stature may have a biologically inactive form of GH, but the molecular defect in the hormone, receptor, or intracellular changes in the target tissue has not been identified.[11] GH replacement therapy is not beneficial in treating these individuals.

8.2. Growth Hormone Hypersecretion

Acromegaly or gigantism is nearly always due to a GH-secreting adenoma.[27] These benign tumors rarely become malignant and usually occur in the anterior pituitary. Their presence must be eradicated in these individuals, usually surgically, in order to preserve normal pituitary function.[30] Alternatively, the pituitary may be irradiated, destroying the tumor and surrounding tissue, but these patients must be managed with hormone replacement therapy. Recently, somatostatin analogues and other pharmacological agents have been used successfully to treat patients with mild acromegaly.

There are several types of GH-producing adenomas. GH-producing adenomas account for approximately 30% of all adenomas, which can also secrete prolactin or ACTH.[27] GH-producing adenomas usually coproduce other hormones such as prolactin and glycoprotein hormones, but certain adenoma subtypes exist which exclusively produce GH. Upon histological examination, the adenomas can appear densely or sparsely granulated, giving an eosinophilic or chromophobic appearance, respectively. No correlation between histological appearance of the adenoma and severity of the acromegaly can be noted.[27]

Elevated levels of serum ILGF-I occur in acromegaly. While the pathophysiological significance of this elevation is not understood, the severity of acromegaly correlates well with serum ILGF-I levels.[18,31]

Rarely, GHRH overproduction can produce acromegaly and gigantism. GHRH can be secreted from gangliocytomas, usually in the hypothalamus, and they typically produce sellar enlargement.[27] Ectopic GHRH production is even rarer; however, it is of interest to point out that isolation and purification of GHRH from a pancreatic islet cell tumor that produced GHRH in a patient occurred in 1982.

9. ASSESSMENT OF GROWTH HORMONE PRODUCTION

Accurate measurement of endogenous GH production is of paramount importance to the diagnosis of GH deficiency in children of short stature. The recent availability of rDNA-derived hGH has prompted therapy in many short-statured individuals who may not be GH deficient. Selection of candidates for GH therapy is usually based upon responses to a battery of provocative pharmacological or physiological stimuli designed to transiently increase serum levels of GH. A blunted GH response to two or more stimuli is usually indicative of GH deficiency. While the definition of a "subnormal" response can vary among laboratories, the NIH standard has been arbitrarily defined as a GH serum level less than 7 ng/ml, following pharmacological or physiological stimuli.[11] Subjects may have to be tested multiple times in order to detect blunted GH secretion.

Several pharmacological stimuli have been used to test GH secretion (Table 3).[11,25] Because hypoglycemia can trigger GH release, administration of insulin (i.v.) to induce hypoglycemia can be used. A 50% fall in blood glucose is necessary for stimulation of GH release to occur. Depending upon insulin dosage, serum levels of GH levels will peak 45 to 75 minutes after insulin administration. This method is very reliable; however, precautions must be taken to administer glucose if blood glucose levels drop too rapidly. Clonidine, a centrally acting sympatholytic agent, can also be used to stimulate GH release. This test has the advantage of few side effects. Arginine infusion is also commonly employed to trigger GH release. Other pharmacological agents used to stimulate GH release include L-DOPA, glucagon, prostaglandin E_2, and bombesin. Sometimes propranolol (given 30 minutes prior to the primary stimulus) can be used to potentiate the responses to insulin. arginine, or glucagon. GHRH has recently been purified and may become widely used to stimulate GH secretion. Because most of these pharmacological tests carry a 15% false negative rate, it is necessary to perform more than one kind of test.[25]

Physiological stimuli of GH secretion can also be used to assess GH production in the short-statured individual.[11] GH secretion can be elicited by exercise; in a fasting patient, 15 minutes of moderate exercise, followed by 5 minutes of vigorous exercise will produce a rise in serum GH levels approximately 30 minutes after exercise is

Table 3. Factors/Agents Affecting Serum Growth Hormone Levels[a]

Blood levels increased by:
GHRH
TRH
ADH
Substance P
Endorphins
Enkephalins
Insulin (hypoglycemia)[b]
Norepinephrine
Epinephrine
Serotonin
Prostaglandins
Desoxyglucose
Apomorphine
L-DOPA[b]
Clonidine[b]
Arginine[b]
Beta-adrenergic antagonists[b]
Bromocriptine (normal individual)
Blood levels decreased by:
Somatostatin
ILGF-I
Bromocriptine (acromegaly)

[a]Modified from Thomas and Keenan.[5]
[b]Can be used as a provocative test agent for the diagnosis of growth hormone disorders.

begun. GH secretion is also induced by deep sleep (stage IV), and electroencephalographic (EEG) monitoring can be used to determine when GH secretion should begin.

Provocative testing of GH secretion may not always be a reliable indication of endogenous GH secretion. In some cases, determination of a mean 24-h GH concentration, coupled with serum ILGF-I levels, may be a better screening test for detection of false negatives.[32]

Measurement of GH is routinely performed using radioimmunoassay.[19] It is the method of choice for detection of hypopituitarism and acromegaly. Diagnosis of pituitary dwarfism on the basis of serum GH levels may be difficult, because these individuals have serum levels less than 1.0 ng/ml, whereas the normal range is between 1.0 and 5.0 ng/ml range, but there is variability above and below this range. [19] Therefore, provocative testing of GH secretion is indicated. Typically, acromegaly patients have serum GH levels in the 25- to 50-ng/ml.[19] Therefore, provocative testing of GH secretion is indicated. Typically, acromegaly patients have serum GH levels in the 25- to 50-ng/ml range, but there is variability above and below this range.[19]

Sometimes, serum ILGF-I levels are useful in diagnosing dwarfism (especially

Laron Dwarfism) and acromegaly. Radioimmunoassay techniques exist for both ILGF-I and ILGF-II, though serum levels of ILGF-II are rarely helpful. Serum ILGF-I binding proteins can be a problem in obtaining accurate serum ILGF-I levels using radioimmunoassay.[18]

10. GROWTH HORMONE THERAPY

GH replacement therapy is indicated for several disorders resulting in short stature (Table 4). Nearly all children of short stature due to GH deficiency will benefit from growth hormone.[10,11,33] Recently, GH was successfully used to treat short stature of patients with Turner's syndrome.[34] FDA approval of biosynthetic Met-hGH will provide clinicians with an unlimited supply to treat individuals with short stature. Met-hGH is equipotent to the endogenous form in both *in vitro*[35] and clinical trials.[36–41] The risk of acquiring Creutzfeldt–Jakob disease, which has been associated with use of GH derived from cadaveric pituitaries, is not evident with use of Met-hGH.[42] Concern about GH abuse has already been expressed.[43]

GH is effective in treating individuals of short stature only before the closure of epiphyseal plates at puberty. Little beneficial effect is observed in short-statured individuals post-adolescence. Several commercial hGH preparations are available (Table 5). GH is administered intramuscularly (or subcutaneously) three times a week. Maximum dosage is 0.1 mg/kg, but the dosage will vary with the individual.[1,11] Typically, young children respond better than older children, and children with severe GH deficiency seem to benefit the most.[11] The growth velocity rate in children given GH usually doubles during their first year of treatment.[10] Sometimes, additional hormonal

Table 4. Possible Clinical Indications for Human Growth Hormone[a]

Hormonally deficient or endocrine related
Short stature
Infantile hypoglycemia
Turner's syndrome
Non-endocrine related
Wound healing
Burn trauma
Stress ulcers
Cartilage healing
Fracture healing
Osteoporosis[b]
Juvenile rheumatoid arthritis
Hypercholesterolemia (?)
Obesity (?)

[a]Modified from Thomas and Keenan.[5,46]
[b]Also hormone related.

Table 5. Human Growth Hormone Preparations[a]

Common name	Trade name(s)	Source
hGH (somatropin)	Crescorman, Asellacrin	Human pituitary
hGH	Humatrope	rDNA
Met-hGH (somatrem)	Somatonorm, Protropin	rDNA

[a]Additional readings in ref. 47.

replacement therapy is necessary for hypopituitarism. Treatment with androgens (for males) or estrogens (for females) may be necessary at puberty to stimulate sexual maturity.[11]

Adverse side effects to GH are uncommon. While allergic reactions to GH are rare, long-term GH therapy can elicit antibodies to GH, rendering these individuals less responsive to the beneficial effects of GH replacement.[11,44] Usually the antibody titers diminish upon discontinuation of GH therapy, but antibody levels must be monitored when therapy is resumed, usually after 4 to 6 months.[11,44] Contamination of rDNA Met-hGH with *E. coli* polypeptide can increase antigenicity of the GH.[36–41] The frequency of antibody production thus depends upon the preparation, but can range from 5–10% to as high as 60% of patients receiving GH therapy.[11] There appears to be a slightly higher incidence of antibody formation to Met-hGH than to hGH.[45] A small percentage (<5%) of patients can develop hypothyroidism during treatment.[11]

11. SUMMARY

The concept of hormone replacement therapy can no longer be considered revolutionary. Indeed, insulin therapy in the medical management of diabetes mellitus was introduced over 50 years ago. Likewise, natural and synthetic estrogens have been used in the treatment of a variety of gynecologic disorders as has thyroxine replacement in the treatment of myxedema.

Unlike the therapeutic successes enjoyed by the patient with diabetes receiving animal insulins, hypopituitarism in children cannot be successfully treated with GH obtained either from subhuman primates or domestic animals. Assuredly, rDNA technologies now offer the medical community unlimited supplies of either hGH or met-hGH.

The central regulation of GH is complex and still is not fully understood. Many physiological stimuli. including exercise, affect GH secretion. Recently, considerable interest has been focused on the role of various growth factors and related polypeptides that seem to act in regulating cellular metabolism. Finally, continued research will undoubtedly lead to a better understanding of the nature of the growth hormone receptor and to what extent various biochemical and pathological changes can affect its function.

REFERENCES

1. Raiti S, Tolman RA (eds): *Human Growth Hormone*. New York, Plenum Medical Book Co., 1986.
2. Thorner MO, Vance ML, Evans WS, et al: Physiological and clinical studies of GRF and GH. *Recent Prog Horm Res* 42:589–640, 1986.
3. Li CH, Chung C, Hans-Werner L, Stein S: The primary structure of monkey pituitary growth hormone. *Arch Biochem Biophys* 245:287–291, 1986.
4. Li CH, Bewley TA, Chung D, Oosthuizen MMJ: Elephant growth hormone. *Int J Peptide Prot Res* 29:62–67, 1987.
5. Thomas JA, Keenan EJ: *Principles of Endocrine Pharmacology*. New York, Plenum Publishing Co., 1986.
6. Isaksson OGP, Eden S, Jansson J-O: Mode of action of pituitary growth hormone on target cells. *Annu Rev Physiol* 47:483–499, 1985.
7. Hughes JP, Friesen HG: The nature and regulation of the receptors for pituitary growth hormone. *Annu Rev Physiol* 47:469–482, 1985.
8. Robbins SL, Cotran RS, Kumar V: *Pathologic Basis of Disease,* ed 3. Philadelphia, W.B. Saunders Co., 1984, pp 1192–1200.
9. Murad F, Haynes RC Jr: Adenohypophyseal hormones and related substances, in Gilman AG, Goodman LS, Rall TW, Murad F (eds): *The Pharmacological Basis of Therapeutics,* ed 7. New York, Macmillan Publishing Co., 1985, pp 1362–1388.
10. Daughaday WH: The anterior pituitary, in Wilson JD, Foster DW (eds): *Williams Textbook of Endocrinology,* ed 7. Philadelphia, W. B. Saunders Co., 1985, pp 568–613.
11. Underwood LE, Van Wyk JJ: Normal and aberrant growth, in Wilson JD, Foster DW (eds): *Williams Textbook of Endocrinology,* ed 7. Philadelphia, W.B. Saunders Co., 1985, pp 155–205.
12. Froesch ER, Schmid C, Schwander J, Zapf J: Actions of insulin-like growth factors. *Annu Rev Physiol* 47:443–467, 1985.
13. Weyer B, Sonne O: Receptor-mediated degradation of human growth hormone in rat adipocytes and cultured human lymphocytes (IM-9). *Mol Cell Endocrinol* 41:85–92, 1985.
14. Yamada K, Lipson K, Marino MW, Donner DB: Effect of growth hormone on protein phosphorylation in isolated rat hepatocytes. *Biochemistry* 26:715–721, 1987.
15. Hunter T, Alexander CB, Cooper JA: Protein phosphorylation and growth control, in *Growth Factors in Biology and Medicine* (Ciba Foundation Symposium 116). London, Pitman, 1985, pp 188–204.
16. Gertler A, Friesen HG: Human growth hormone-stimulated mitogenesis of Nb2 node lymphoma cells is not mediated by an immediate acceleration of phosphoinositide metabolism. *Mol Cell Endocrinol* 48:221–228, 1986.
17. Mittra I: Somatomedins and proteolytic bioactiviation of prolactin and growth hormone. *Cell* 38:347–348, 1984.
18. Clemmons DR, Underwood LE: Somatomedin-C/insulin-like growth factor I in acromegaly. *Clin Endocrinol Metab* 15(3):629–653, 1986.
19. Christy NP: The anterior pituitary: assessment of anterior pituitary function, in Wyngaarden JB, Smith LH Jr (eds): *Cecil's Textbook of Medicine, ed 16. Philadelphia, W. B. Saunders Co., 1982, pp 1172–1174.*
20. *Zapf J, Schoenle E, Froesch ER: In vivo effects of the insulin-like growth factors (IGFs) in the hypophysectomized rat: comparison with human growth hormone and the possible role of the specific IGF carrier proteins, in Growth Factors in Biology and Medicine* (CIBA Foundation Symposium 116). London, Pitman, 1985, pp 169–187.
21. Mathews LS, Norstedt G, Palmiter RS: Regulation of insulin-like growth factor-I gene expression by growth hormone. *Proc Natl Acad Sci USA* 83(24):9343–9347, 1987.
22. Grant MB, Schmetz I, Russell B, et al: Changes in insulin-like growth factors I and II and their binding protein after a single intramuscular injection of growth hormone. *J Clin Endocrinol Metab* 63(4):981–984, 1986.
23. Zezulak KM, Green H: The generation of insulin-like growth factor-I-sensitive cells by growth hormone action. *Science* 233:551–553, 1986.

24. Skottner A, Fryklund L, Hansson HA: Experimental research on IGF-1. *Acta Paediatr Scand* 325(suppl):107–114, 1986.
25. Brook CGD, Hindmarsh PC, Smith PJ, Stanhope R: Clinical features and investigation of growth hormone deficiency. *Clin Endocrinol Metab* 15(3):479–493, 1986.
26. Schaff-Blass E, Burstein S, Rosenfield RL: Advances in diagnosis and treatment of short stature, with special reference to the role of growth hormone. *J Pediatr* 104:801–813, 1984.
27. Scheithauer BW, Kovacs K, Randall RV, et al: Pathology of excessive production of growth hormone. *Clin Endocrinol Metab* 15(3):655–681, 1986.
28. Bercu BB, Diamond FB: Growth hormone neurosecretory dysfunction. *Clin Endocrinol Metab* 15(3):537–590, 1986.
29. Grossman A, Savage MO, Besser GM: Growth hormone releasing hormone. *Clin Endocrinol Metab* 15(3):607–627, 1986.
30. Wass JAH, Laws ER Jr, Randall RV, Sheline GE: The treatment of acromegaly. *Clin Endocrinol Metab* 15(3):683–707, 1986.
31. Oppizzi G, Petroncini MM, Dallabonzana D, et al: Relationship between somatomedin-C and growth hormone levels in acromegaly: basal and dynamic evaluation. *J Clin Endocrinol Metab* 63(6):1348–1353, 1986.
32. Bercu BB, Shulman D, Root AW, Spiliotis BE: Growth hormone (GH) provocative testing frequently does not reflect endogenous GH secretion. *J Clin Endocrinol Metab* 63(3):709–716, 1986.
33. Albertsson-Wikland K: Growth hormone treatment in short children. *Acta Paediatr Scand* 325(suppl):64–70, 1986.
34. Takano K, Hizuka N, Shizume K: Treatment of Turner's syndrome with methionyl human growth hormone for six months. *Acta Endocrinol* 112:130–137, 1986.
35. Schwartz J, Foster CM: Pituitary and recombinant deoxyribonucleic derived human growth hormones alter glucose metabolism in 3T3 adipocytes. *J Clin Endocrinol Metab* 62(4):791–794, 1986.
36. Bierich JR: Treatment of pituitary dwarfism with biosynthetic growth hormone. *Acta Paediatr Scand* 325(suppl):13–18, 1986.
37. Girard F, Gourmelen M: Clinical experience with somatonorm. *Acta Paediatr Scand* 325(suppl):29–32, 1986.
38. Milner RDG: Clinical experience with somatren: UK preliminary report. *Acta Paediatr Scand* 325(suppl):25–28, 1986.
39. Takano K, Shizume K: Clinical experience with somatrem in Japan. *Acta Paediatr Scand* 325(suppl):19–24, 1986.
40. Vicens-Calvet E, Potau N, Carracosa A, et al: Clinical experience with somatrem in growth hormone deficiency. *Acta Paediatr Scand* 325(suppl):33–40, 1986.
41. Westphal O: Experiences of somatonorm in Sweden. *Acta Paediatr Scand* 325(suppl):41–44, 1986.
42. Brown P, Gajdusek DC, Gibbs CJ, Asher DM: Potential epidemic of Creutzfeldt–Jakob disease from human growth hormone therapy. *N Engl J Med* 313:728–731, 1985.
43. Underwood LE: Report on the conference on uses and possible abuses of biosynthetic human growth hormone. *N Engl J Med* 311:606–608, 1984.
44. Andersson R: Immunological aspects of growth hormone. *Acta Paediatr Scand* 325(suppl):48–54, 1986.
45. Kaplan SL: Current status of the treatment of growth hormone deficiencies. 68th Annual Meeting Endocrine Society Proceedings, June, 1986.
46. Ranke MB, Bierich JR: Treatment of growth hormone deficiency. *Clin Endocrinol Metab* 15(3):495–510, 1986.
47. Fryklund LM, Bierich JR, Ranke MB: Recombinant human growth hormone. *Clin Endocrinol Metab* 15(3):511–535, 1986.

14

CNS Stimulants and Athletic Performance

Galen R. Wenger

1. INTRODUCTION

In an effort to find a short cut that will reduce the time and effort required to become competitive or to meet the challenge of the moment, it has been all too common an occurrence in the history of man to try chemicals of various types to improve both mental and physical performance. Examples of this range from students trying to obtain a better grade, to athletes trying to shave seconds off the time required to perform an athletic feat, to the military's use of chemicals to help soldiers perform heroic feats of endurance in an effort to defeat the enemy. The first reported use of drugs to increase or improve athletic performance predates the birth of Christ. It is reported in the writings of Homer that Greek athletes consumed mushrooms prior to athletic events to improve their performance. More recently, during the nineteenth century, there were widespread reports of athletes using caffeine, alcohol, nitroglycerine, ethyl ether, and opium.[1] However, it was not until the unfortunate death of a Danish cyclist during the 1960 Olympic Games in Rome that the attention of the world was drawn to this serious problem. Today, drug use by athletes involves several classes of drugs; however, this chapter will restrict itself to a discussion of the use of three drugs or drug classes: amphetamines, cocaine, and caffeine.

1.1. General Pharmacology

For a full discussion of the general pharmacology of the three classes of drugs to be discussed in this chapter, the reader is encouraged to go to a standard pharmacology textbook such as *Goodman and Gilman's The Pharmacological Basis of Therapeutics*.[2] The pharmacology presented here will be a brief synopsis of the pharmacology of each drug class relevant to its effects on endurance and physical performance.

Galen R. Wenger • Department of Pharmacology, University of Arkansas for Medical Sciences, Little Rock, Arkansas 72205.

1.1.1. Amphetamines

Amphetamine was first synthesized in 1887 and is the prototype drug of the class generally referred to as psychomotor stimulants. Amphetamine exists in both the *d*-form and the *l*-form. With respect to central nervous system (CNS) excitatory effects, the *d*-form is 3 to 4 times more potent than the *l*-form. Several methylated derivatives exist, with the most widely studied being methamphetamine. The activity of methamphetamine at low doses is almost exclusively limited to the CNS. At higher doses, some peripheral activity is observed.[2]

The effect of amphetamine on the cardiovascular system is an increase in both systolic and diastolic blood pressure and an increase in heart rate. As the dose of amphetamine is increased, the positive ionotropic effect is reduced, presumably through a reflex action.[2,3] The *l*-isomer of amphetamine is more potent than the *d*-isomer with respect to its cardiovascular effects.

The CNS effect of amphetamine is a general stimulation. Activity in the medullary respiratory center, spinal cord, and reticular formation is increased. The EEG is accelerated and desynchronized. The psychic effects of amphetamine in man following doses of 10 to 30 mg are characterized by wakefulness, alertness, a decreased sense of fatigue, elevation of mood, self-confidence, elation, euphoria, and increases in motor and speech activity.[2]

The mechanism of action for the peripheral and CNS activity of the amphetamines is primarily an indirect effect mediated by a release of norepinephrine, dopamine, and possibly even serotonin from nerve endings. In addition, there is some support in the literature for a direct effect of amphetamine on central serotonergic receptors.[4]

Although amphetamine is well known for its ability to suppress appetite, amphetamine has only minimal effects on total body metabolism.

Amphetamine is well absorbed following oral and intramuscular administration. It has a moderately long duration of action with an estimated total elimination half-life in man of about 20 h.[5]

1.1.2. Cocaine

Cocaine is a naturally occurring chemical isolated from the leaves of the coca plant (*Erythroxylon coca*), which grows in the Andes Mountains of Peru. For several centuries, the local inhabitants of these mountains have chewed on the leaves of the plant. In fact, it is estimated that almost nine million kilograms of leaves are consumed annually by the two million inhabitants of the region.[2] The popularity of cocaine has waxed and waned through the centuries. It has been, at times, hailed as a ''magical drug'' capable of curing a variety of mood disorders as well as alcohol and morphine addiction. At other times, it has been placed under such tight legal restrictions as to make its use by humans legally impossible. Clearly, the reason for the high degree of consumption of the coca leaves by the inhabitants of the Andes, its wide acceptance as a ''magical drug,'' and the legal restrictions on its use are probably more closely related to its mood-altering and reinforcing properties than to any therapeutic benefit of the drug.

The most important therapeutic activity of cocaine is its activity as a local anesthetic. Aside from this local anesthetic activity, its most prominent effects are on the

CNS. In man, the effect of cocaine on the CNS is a generalized stimulation. The initial effect upon administration is euphoria and a feeling of well-being, although dysphoria is sometimes reported. Cocaine abusers describe the euphoria produced by cocaine in terms which are almost identical to the description of the euphoria produced by amphetamine given by amphetamine abusers. Experienced cocaine abusers given cocaine or *d*-amphetamine intravenously frequently cannot distinguish the two drugs.[6] No effect on motor function is observed at low doses. However, as the dose is increased, tremors and potentially lethal convulsions may be seen. The stimulation is followed by a depression, and eventually the respiratory centers become depressed. At high doses, the cause of death is respiratory depression.

The effects of low to moderate doses of cocaine on the cardiovascular system of man are similar to those of amphetamine. At low doses, a bradycardia is sometimes seen due to a central vagal stimulation. However, as the dose is increased, the heart rate and mean blood pressure increase.[7,8] At high doses, acute myocardial infarctions, often associated with potentially lethal arrhythmias, have been reported.[9,10]

The mechanism of action for the CNS effects and probably some of the cardiovascular effects of cocaine appears to be related to its ability to block the neuronal reuptake of catecholamines at nerve endings. Thus, cocaine causes a potentiation or at least an increase in the duration of action of catecholamines in the synaptic cleft.

Cocaine is well absorbed from all sites following application, including nasal and gastrointestinal mucosa and the lungs.[2] However, due to its vasoconstrictor properties, its absorption is somewhat self-limiting. Once absorbed into the bloodstream, cocaine is rapidly metabolized by plasma esterases and in some species by hepatic enzymes. The plasma half-life in man is approximately 1 h.[11]

1.1.3. Caffeine

Caffeine, like cocaine, is a naturally occurring compound found in the fruit of *Coffea arabica* and related species. Caffeine is also found in other plants including the leaves of *Thea sinensis* (tea). It is commonly used in the form of an ingredient in various beverages by people of all ages.

Caffeine has a significant stimulatory effect on the CNS. It is reported to decrease drowsiness and promote a more rapid and clearer thought process. Goldstein *et al.*[12] reported that humans consuming 85 to 250 mg of caffeine demonstrated an increased capacity for sustained intellectual effort and a decreased reaction time. However, fine motor coordination and the ability to judge the length of time was severely affected. Caffeine also stimulates the medullary respiratory centers, as well as producing a centrally mediated emesis.[2]

Caffeine produces a tachycardia at high doses and a transient increase in cardiac output. It causes a dilatation of most peripheral blood vessels, which, along with the increase in cardiac output, results in an increase in peripheral blood flow. In contrast, caffeine produces a constriction in cerebral blood vessels.

Caffeine has significant effects on body metabolism. It induces a significant mobilization of free fatty acids and the utilization of fat as the primary energy substrate. This results in a sparing of muscle glycogen.[13]

The mechanism of action for caffeine is not fully understood. Caffeine can be shown to have at least three different effects that could account for its activity. It has been shown *in vitro* that caffeine is capable of (1) producing a translocation of intracellular calcium, (2) inhibiting phosphodiesterase, thus leading to an accumulatin of cyclic nucleotides, and (3) blocking the actions of adenosine at the adenosine receptor.[2] At the present time, it is thought that the first two activities are unlikely to explain the activity of caffeine *in vivo*. These effects are only seen at concentrations higher than those which are thought to be achieved following therapeutic doses.[14] Thus, the activity of caffeine at the adenosine receptor is thought to be the most likely candidate for the mechanism of action of caffeine. However, it is not known if this mechanism is responsible for all of caffeine's effects.

Caffeine is well absorbed orally, rectally, or parenterally. Following oral administration, peak blood levels are achieved in about 1 h, and caffeine has a plasma half-life in man of about 3.5 h.

1.2. Abuse, Tolerance, and Physical Dependence

An important aspect of the drugs in question is their direct reinforcing properties or abuse potential. One must always remember that drugs might be used by athletes because of their reinforcing properties, independent of their effects on athletic performance. For all three classes of drugs, abuse, tolerance, and physical dependence are well known. Amphetamine and cocaine have many similarities in this respect and will be discussed together.

1.2.1. Amphetamine and Cocaine

Both cocaine and amphetamine are self-administered by humans for nontherapeutic reasons. Both are reported by users to produce a feeling of decreased fatigue, euphoria, and a feeling of well-being. Unlike the opioids, cocaine and amphetamine are frequently self-administered in bouts of use (''runs'') with significant drug-free periods between bouts. During these bouts, toxic reactions are not uncommon, frequently taking the form of hyperactivity accompanied by paranoid thought processes. However, upon discontinuation of drug intake, there frequently are no consequences. This difference in abuse pattern compared to opioids has made it difficult to characterize the development of tolerance and physical dependence in humans.

There is a development of tolerance to some of the effects of amphetamine and cocaine, but the tolerance does not develop equally to all of the effects of these drugs. Tolerance frequently develops to the euphoric effects of amphetamine, and because of this, abusers frequently increase the dose. However, the incidence of toxic psychotic-like reactions increases at higher doses. There are some reports in the literature that a reverse tolerance or sensitization to some of the effects develops with repeated exposure to amphetamine and cocaine. For recent reviews on the subject of tolerance and sensitization to psychomotor stimulants, see Post,[15] Post and Contel,[16] and Demellweek and Goudie.[17]

Physical dependence is frequently, by definition, said to be present if one observes a characteristic withdrawal syndrome upon the abrupt discontinuation of drug intake. This definition largely comes from the well-documented events surrounding the discontinuation of opioid intake, and some controversy exists as to how this definition applies to the psychomotor stimulants such as amphetamine and cocaine. Most workers are in agreement that upon abrupt discontinuation of amphetamine or cocaine intake, an opioid-like withdrawal syndrome is not observed. However, there is less agreement about what to call the syndrome that is observed. Subjects who abruptly stop intake of amphetamine or cocaine frequently report an increased craving for the drug, prolonged periods of sleep, general fatigue, hyperphagia, and depression.

1.2.2. Caffeine

It is difficult to apply the term abuse potential to caffeine because it is legally available and widely used in most societies in the form of an ingredient in various beverages. It is not always clear why the beverage is consumed or even if the caffeine in the beverage has anything to do with its consumption. Barone and Roberts[18] have estimated a mean daily intake of 3 mg/kg per day for all adults in the United States and Canada. The abuse of caffeine becomes clearer when caffeine is taken apart from a beverage without a valid medical reason. However, such fine distinctions concerning recreational drug intake are ambiguous, at best. Suffice it to say that such widespread use across societies either as an in a beverage or otherwise is evidence of an abuse potential.

Tolerance to the effects of caffeine does occur. It has been shown to develop to the cardiovascular[19] as well as the behavioral effects.[12] In heavy users, there also is a characteristic withdrawal syndrome,[12] indicating physical dependence.

2. THE MAGNITUDE OF DRUG EFFECTS ON ATHLETIC PERFORMANCE

The competitive nature of athletic events forces the participants to strive to do their best. Athletes will train for long periods of time to better their previous time in an athletic event by less than a second. In a similar manner, governments force their military troops to train to a high degree of physical fitness in an effort to gain an advantage over the enemy. While perhaps of greater importance in years gone by, an army that could move its foot soldiers faster and over greater distances gained a considerable advantage over the enemy. In these and other situations, the motivation to win or improve on one's past performance is exceedingly strong, and frequently man has resorted to the use of drugs or chemical agents to improve performance.

As pointed out by Coyle,[20] by far the most effective means of improving physical performance is a good training program. Coyle estimates that in previously sedentary individuals, improvements in muscle strength or speed in long-distance running events can be improved by 50% following the appropriate training program. As will be seen later in this chapter, there are very few reports of drugs improving performance by more than 10%, and in fact, the improvement in well-trained individuals shown by most studies is not even close to 10%. However, while it is true for most biological studies that a change of less than 10% is considered trivial, in many athletic events an improvement in performance of far less than 10% represents the difference between a winner and an also-ran. To put this argument another way, Laties and Weiss[21] pointed out that the improvement in the time required to complete the mile run was less than 15% during the 100-year period from the 1860s to the 1960s. To take an example over a shorter and more recent period of time, Roger Banister broke the 4-min mile barrier in 1954 (3:59.4). Between Banister's performance and the 1981 performance of Sebastian Coe (3:47.33), 15 different athletes held the new best time. In many of these 15 different world-record-breaking performances, the improvement in time was less than 1 s. The current record time set by Steve Cram (3:46.32) in July of 1985 represents a 5.46% improvement over Banister's 1954 performance, and a 0.4% improvement over Coe's 1981 performance, or an average improvement of less than 0.2% per year. The point of all of this is that a drug or chemical capable of improving a well-trained athlete's performance by less than 1% accomplishes what years of training could not. Thus, even if these effects are so small as to be of no significance by most biological standards, and may not even reach the magnitude required for statistical significance, such a small improvement in performance could give an athlete a tremendous advantage.

2.1. The Problem of the Researcher

The magnitude of the effect of drugs on performance presents some real problems for those studying performance enhancers. It is of extreme importance that baseline variability be reduced as much as possible. Subjects living a mostly sedentary lifestyle and even weekend athletes would be expected to show considerable day-to-day variation in performance on events requiring maximal endurance and/or speed. Furthermore, with repeated testing of an individual subject, there will be an improvement in performance due to the effect of training. From a practical point of view, therefore, this means that subjects studied must be well-trained athletes at the start of the experiment in order to ensure that their performance will not change significantly over the course of the experiment. There also is the question of whether drugs are capable of improving performance over and above what can be achieved through years of training. Drug results may differ between studies conducted in weekend athletes and in world-class athletes. For these reasons, the investigator frequently would like to conduct experiments with as close as possible to world-class athletes. However, athletes of this caliber, and coaches of such athletes, are reluctant to jeopardize their standing in the athletic community by using drugs which are banned by various athletic committees. The truth of the matter is that, as in horse racing, many of these experiments may have already been done in a pseudoscientific fashion. However, it is unlikely that the participants will divulge the information.

Finally, a note on terminology. Although the title of this work focuses on athletic performance, not all the studies to be discussed were true measures of performance in athletic competition. However. the studies all involve measures of endurance and physical performance, features common to all athletic events. Consequently, "endurance and physical performance" will be used interchangeably with "athletic performance" in the remainder of this chapter.

3. EFFECTS OF CAFFEINE ON ENDURANCE AND PHYSICAL PERFORMANCE

Caffeine has long been considered to have the potential for enhancing endurance and physical performance. However, literature on the effects of caffeine has not been in total agreement. This lack of agreement on the subject is reflected in the conflicting rulings issued by various national and international athletic committees concerning the legality of caffeine use prior to athletic events. In 1939, Boje[22] stated that the use of pure caffeine, or preparations with high caffeine content, in conjunction with athletic competition should be prohibited. In 1962, a study conducted among Italian athletes reported that caffeine was one of the most common doping agents used by athletes.[23] Subsequently, its use was banned in athletic competition. In the 1970 British Commonwealth Games, caffeine in the amounts present in a cup of coffee was not regarded as a doping agent.[24] Finally, Fischbach[25] was successful in convincing the International Olympic Committee that caffeine was not a doping agent, and caffeine was removed from the banned list prior to the 1972 Olympic Games. Since that time, the International Olympic Committee has changed its mind and once again placed caffeine back on the list, but blood caffeine levels below 15 μ/ml are considered legal.

A review of the literature on the effects of caffeine on endurance and physical performance is complicated by several problems. First of all, there are only a few studies in which more than one dose has been used. Consequently, it is difficult to obtain a good dose–response relationship. Secondly, many studies do not indicate whether or not their subjects were regular users of caffeine-containing beverages. Such regular use frequently is associated with tolerance to the effects of caffeine. Some studies state that subjects were not allowed to consume caffeine-containing beverages for 24 hours prior to the test session. This probably is not a sufficient time to control for any tolerance effects. Unfortunately, the frequent failure to run more than one dose makes the assessment of tolerance impossible.

3.1. Studies Showing Positive Effects with Caffeine

Rivers and Webber[26] were among the earliest investigators to study the effects of caffeine using a placebo control. Participating as their own subjects, each pulled on a weight with a finger (using a Mosso ergograph) after administration of either 500 mg of caffeine citrate or placebo. Even though they did not know whether they had been given the placebo or caffeine, a consistent increase in work output was observed in those sessions in which caffeine had been administered prior to testing. It must be emphasized that only two subjects were included in this study.

A considerable amount of work was conducted on the effects of drugs on the endurance and physical performance of the armed forces during World War II. This work was largely stimulated by reports that the Germans were using methamphetamine to prolong the endurance of their troops. One of the most extensive studies involving caffeine was performed by Seashore and Ivy.[27] In all but two of these studies, the subjects were military personnel studied under, as nearly as possible, military field conditions. In all, four drug conditions were studied: 450 mg caffeine sodium benzoate, 10 mg amphetamine, 5 mg methamphetamine, and placebo. These studies involved long forced marches followed by all-night guard duty, driving a truck for 18 to 20 hours/day, operating a tank for 5 hours/day in the desert, or other equally demanding work assignments. The drugs were generally superior to placebo in their effects on subjective ratings of fatigue and objective measures of motor performance. However, the drug effects on subjective symptoms of fatigue were more pronounced than the effects on motor function.

Foltz *et al.*[28] studied the effects of caffeine on the work output of exhausted subjects. Four subjects rode a bicycle ergometer to the point of exhaustion at a work load of 1235 kg/min. After resting for 10 minutes, either 500 mg of caffeine or placebo were administered intravenously, and the subjects again rode to exhaustion. In two of the four subjects, caffeine increased the work output compared to placebo. When the two subjects who failed to show a response to 500 mg of caffeine were tested again at a dose of 1 g of caffeine, they showed the same increase in work output as seen at the lower dose in the other subjects. The same investigators[29] reported a similar experiment comparing 500 mg of caffeine sodium benzoate with 5 mg of methamphetamine and 10 mg of amphetamine. As in the previous study, caffeine increased work output, but it did not increase work output as much as methamphetamine. Only two subjects received amphetamine and the results were questionable.

Asmussen and Boje[30] studied the effects of 300 mg of caffeine on the work output of healthy athletes performing two maximal work tasks on a bicycle ergometer. The effect of caffeine was to increase the work output, which the authors concluded was due to caffeine's ability to mask fatigue. Another study by Berglund and Hemmingsson[31] studied the effects of caffeine on the performance of 14 well-trained cross-country skiers racing at altitudes of 300 and 2900 m. In a double-blind study, each skier raced twice at both altitudes: once after placebo and once after caffeine was administered. Caffeine (6 mg/kg) was found to increase the skiers' speed by 1.7% ($P < 0.05$) compared to placebo performance at the 300-m altitude, and at 2900 m, the effect of caffeine was a 3.2% increase over placebo.

In a study on the effects of caffeine on treadmill performance, McNaughton[32] ran 12 subjects on a treadmill at a level which initially produced an oxygen uptake equivalent to 75% of maximum, and this level was maintained while the subjects ran to exhaustion. Caffeine at a dose of 10 mg/kg was without significant effect, but at a dose of 15 mg/kg, the subjects showed a 4.8% increase in the length of time required to run to exhaustion compared to placebo ($P < 0.05$). In two related studies,[33,34] 9 competitive cyclists were exercised to exhaustion on a bicycle ergometer. In one study,[33] the subjects were exercised at 80% of maximum oxygen uptake. After a dose of 330 mg of caffeine, the cyclists were able to ride for 90.2s (SE ± 7.2) compared to 75.5s (SE ± 5.1) after placebo. This represents a 19% improvement over a placebo. In the second study,[34] the cyclists rode an adjusting ergometer at a constant rate of 80 rpm for 2 hr. The resistance of the ergometer was constantly adjusted based on the muscular effort throughout the 360-degree cycle and an estimate of work determined. Each cyclist was given 250 mg of caffeine or a placebo 60 min prior to the start of the exercise period. An additional 250 mg of caffeine or placebo was administered at 15-min intervals over the course of the first 90 min of the experiment. The caffeine treatment resulted in a 7.4% increase in work production and a 7.3% increase in the maximum uptake of oxygen.

There has been one study that has specifically looked at the issue of caffeine tolerance in the context of the effects of caffeine on athletic performance.[35] Six women who were habitual caffeine users (>600 mg/day) were exercised at 75% of maximum oxygen uptake for 1 h. Each woman was tested once following administration of a placebo and once after a caffeine dose of 5 mg/kg body weight. During these initial tests, the subjects were allowed to maintain their normal caffeine intake. After these initial tests, all subjects were withdrawn from caffeine for 4 days. Each subject was then tested under the same conditions following either placebo or 5 mg/kg of caffeine. The 5 mg/kg-dose of caffeine following the withdrawal period resulted in a 0.17-liter/min increase in oxygen uptake compared to placebo or compared to the caffeine test session prior to withdrawal.

3.2. Studies Showing No Effect of Caffeine

There are also a number of studies reporting that caffeine has no significant effects on endurance and physical performance. Foltz *et al.*[36] failed to demonstrate any significant effects of caffeine in an experiment with 23 physically untrained subjects. Each subject was loaded with a knapsack containing a weight equal to one-third of his body weight. The subject stepped up and down a 16-in step every 3 seconds until he could no longer maintain this rate. After the subject rested, he again worked to exhaustion. On each experimental work day, the subjects worked 3 periods. One hour before the first work period, the subjects were given either 10 mg of amphetamine, 500 mg of caffeine sodium benzoate, or placebo. However, due to the fact that with practice, the subjects' performance improved significantly over the course of the experiment, no significant drug effects were observed. While this report neither confirms nor refutes the significant drug effects reported earlier, it shows clearly the importance of the stability of the baseline performance.

In a study on the effect of caffeine and amphetamine on the performance of subjects pulling a weight with their finger (Mosso ergograph), Alles and Feigen[37] were unable to show any significant effects of 100, 200, or 400 mg of caffeine. A similar result was obtained in a study by Haldi and Wynn.[38] These investigators studied the influence of 250 mg of caffeine alkaloid on the 100-yard swimming performance of 12 men. No beneficial or detrimental effects of caffeine were observed.

In more recent work, Ganslen *et al.*[39] studied the performance of 5 subjects on a treadmill test. A dose of 200 mg of caffeine had no effect on aerobic capacity or work. In a similar study by Margaria *et al.*,[40] 100 or 250 mg of caffeine were administered in 5 separate trials to 3 trained subjects. On a treadmill test to exhaustion, no effects of caffeine on oxygen uptake or performance time were observed. Perkins and Williams[41] studied the effects of caffeine on the performance of 14 female undergraduate students riding an electric bicycle ergometer. Caffeine at doses of 4, 7, and 10 mg/kg had no effect on resting heart rate, submaximal exercise heart rate, maximal heart rate, and ratings of perceived exertion. However, as the authors note, this study did not control for possible caffeine tolerance since the subjects were only instructed not to consume caffeine-containing beverages for 24 h prior to the test. Another study using a bicycle ergometer[42] evaluated the effects of 5 mg/kg (mean dose of 372 mg) of caffeine or placebo. Subjects were given drug or placebo 1 h before the start of the test. The subject began pedaling at a work load of 30 W; every 3 min, the work load was increased by 30 W until the subject could not maintain the desired work load. No effect was observed on the time to exhaution (caffeine = 22.3 ± 0.8 min vs. placebo = 21.9 ± 0.7 min).

In a study of the effects of caffeine on the maximum voluntary contraction of the dominant knee extension and flexion muscle in 12 college track sprinters, Bond *et al.*[43] administered either placebo or 5 mg/kg of caffeine 60 min prior to the test. No significant effects of caffeine were noted on peak torque or power of the leg movement. Finally, Casal and Leon[44] studied the effects of 400 mg of caffeine (mean dose of 5.9 mg/kg) or placebo in 9 sub-3-h marathon runners. One hour before a 45-min run on a treadmill at 75% of maximum oxygen uptake, each subject was given either drug or placebo. Two placebos were used: a 350-ml cup of warm water or a 350-ml cup of decaffeinated coffee. No differences in ratings of perceived exertion were observed between the dose of caffeine and the decaffeinated coffee placebo, but following both the caffeinated and decaffeinated coffee, the ratings of perceived exertion were lower than following the cup of warm water placebo. These results indicate either that decaffeinated coffee may have some other active ingredients which reduce levels of perceived exertion or that subjective ratings of perceived exertion may be influenced by a significant placebo effect.

3.3. Conclusions and Possible Mechanisms for the Effects of Caffeine on Endurance and Physical Performance

If one examines the reports described above on the effects of caffeine on endurance and physical performance, there are several conclusions which can be drawn. The first is that there is some confusion due to the lack of good dose–response data. There are 10 studies showing caffeine to have a positive effect and 9 studies showing caffeine to have no effect. However, most of these studies used only one dose of caffeine. In the 10 studies showing a positive effect, the doses ranged from 300 to 1000 mg (4.2 to 14.3 mg/kg in a 70-kg man). However, only 3 of the 10 studies used doses lower than 400 mg (5.7 mg/kg in a 70-kg man).[30,33,35] In the 9 studies showing no effect, the doses ranged from 100 to 700 mg (1.4 to 10 mg/kg in a 70-kg man), and only 2 of these[36,41] were above 400 mg. The study by Foltz *et al.*[36] used a dose of 500 mg, but no significant effects of caffeine were seen because of a training effect seen in the subjects over the course of the experiment. In the other study[41] which failed to show an effect, doses of 4, 7, and 10 mg/kg were used. However, the authors questioned their own results on the basis of caffeine tolerance in the subjects. Thus, one is left with the conclusion that caffeine probably is capable of increasing endurance and physical performance at high doses (>400 mg).

There are at least two possible mechanisms for this effect of caffeine at high doses. First of all, at these high doses there are significant CNS effects. Central stimulation could be a significant factor in reducing levels of perceived exertion and fatigue. In addition, there may be a significant peripheral effect. O'Neil *et al.*[45] point out that during exercise, glucose and fatty acids are the two primary sources of energy. During exercise, energy can be made available through either aerobic metabolism or anaerobic metabolism. Glucose can be metabolized to yield ATP either by aerobic or anaerobic metabolism whereas fatty acids can only be metabolized by aerobic pathways. When fatty acids are made available to tissues as the energy source, glucose is spared, providing there is sufficient oxygen for aerobic metabolism. Glucose can then be made available and metabolized by anaerobic metabolic pathways at a time when oxygen supply to the tissues is not sufficient to allow aerobic metabolism to occur. Caffeine could thus increase endurance by increasing lipolysis and mobilization of fatty acids. Indeed, there is evidence that such a mechanism is occurring during significant work loads in the presence of caffeine. Costill *et al.*[33] and Ivy *et al.*[34] have both demonstrated that following caffeine administration, lipolysis is increased during the period of physical exercise compared to placebo treatment.

4. EFFECTS OF AMPHETAMINES ON ENDURANCE AND PHYSICAL PERFORMANCE

The history of the investigation of the effects of amphetamines on endurance and physical performance is largely one of science responding to, and reacting to, actions by governments. As mentioned previously, the real impetus for studying performance-enhancing drugs came from work done in the early days of World War II. The German military realized that a drug which could keep soldiers performing at a high level of efficiency would result in a tremendous military advantage. For the most part, research on the effects of amphetamines on performance largely started at that time and ended in the USA with the placing of amphetamines under Schedule II of the Controlled Substance Act in 1972.

4.1. Studies Showing Positive Effects with Amphetamines

In one of the early German studies, Lehman *et al.*[46] performed repeated studies on 3 subjects who rode a bicycle ergometer to exhaustion. Compared to placebo controls, doses of either 5, 10, or 15 mg of methamphetamine were able to increase the time to exhaustion in the 3 subjects. A similar study by Heyrodt and Weissenstein[47] demonstrated that 15 mg of methamphetamine increased the length of time that a female subject could run before collapsing of exhaustion. These initial studies were followed by other reports by British and American scientists. Knoefel[48] had subjects ride a bicycle ergometer under the influence of either amphetamine, *d*-amphetamine, methamphetamine, or *d*-methamphetamine. He reported an increase in work output following 10 mg of methamphetamine. He also reported that the *d*-isomer was more efficacious than the racemic form. In a study mentioned earlier in reference to the effects of caffeine, Foltz *et al.*[29] studied the effects of 10 to 15 mg of amphetamine and 5 mg of methamphetamine in subjects riding a bicycle ergometer to exhaustion. Subjects rode to exhaustion and then rested for 10 minutes. After the 10-minute rest period, the subject rode to exhaustion again. At times ranging from 30 seconds to 30 minutes before the first exercise period, either placebo or drug was administered intravenously. The doses of amphetamine used had no effect, but 5 mg of methamphetamine produced a substantial increase in work output.

Somerville[49] studied the effects of amphetamine under a variety of different conditions. This study may have been the first to show that the effect of amphetamine on performance is somewhat task specific. Somerville reported the results of three experiments. In the first experiment, two groups of soldiers (50 soldiers/group) marched for 17 hours. One hour before the end of the march, one group received 15 mg of amphetamine while the other group received placebo. At the end of the march, the performance of the soldiers was evaluated on an obstacle course and on a rifle range. Amphetamine did not improve the performance in either task. In the second study, subjects participated in a 56-hour military exercise which included both day and night marches. During the last 22 hours of the exercise, one-third of the subjects received a total of 30 mg of amphetamine, one-third received 35 mg of amphetamine, and one-third received placebo. No significant differences were observed in rifle marksmanship, but a small difference was observed between the amphetamine groups and placebo controls in the time required to cover an obstacle course. The third study examined the effects of 20 mg of amphetamine in a group of officers participating in a War Staff Course. Over a period of 72 hours, the subjects had to complete nine exercises in staff duties. During the first 42 hours of the exercise, the subjects did not sleep. Compared to placebo controls, 20 mg of amphetamine given on two occasions during the experiment did not improve performance nor prevent sleep.

Cuthbertson and Knox[50] also performed their studies on military field personnel. In the first experiment, subjects were marched for 18 miles after a 24-hour period without sleep. No difference in the time required to cover the course was found between those soldiers receiving 15 mg of methamphetamine and placebo controls. In the second study, two companies of infantry marched 23 miles. At the end of the march, the men either received placebo, 10 mg of amphetamine, or 15 mg of amphetamine before going to sleep. On the second day of the study, the men marched 20 miles before a skirmish with the "enemy." Following the skirmish, drug or placebo was given before an attack was made on the "enemy." The amphetamine groups reported that they slept less well but were less fatigued in the morning.

In one final study under military conditions, Seashore and Ivy[27] studied the effects of 10 mg of amphetamine, 5 mg of methamphetamine, or placebo. Subjects participated in either of two studies. In the first study, subjects marched 18 to 20 miles followed by guard duty from 6:00 P.M. to approximately 4:00 A.M. In the second study, subjects either trained with a full pack, drove a truck for 18 to 20 hours/day, or operated a tank for 5 hours/day. In general, the subjects administered amphetamines had less fatigue as well as slightly better motor performance, but the effect on fatigue was more pronounced.

Bujas and Petz[51] studied the performance of subjects trying to hold a 8.5-kg load as a measure of static work. When given 15 mg of amphetamine 90 minutes before the start of the experiment, a significant increase, compared to placebo controls, was observed in the duration of time the subjects could hold the load.

In probably the most extensive study done to date on the effects of amphetamines on performance in athletic events, Smith and Beecher[52] concluded that these effects were dependent on the task. In experiment 1, the subjects were 15 college swimmers.

Each subject performed his preferred swimming event twice each day for 12 days. On 4 of the days, each swimmer was given an amphetamine dose of 14 mg/70 kg body weight 2 to 3 hours prior to swimming. On 4 other days, each swimmer was given placebo, and on the remaining 4 days, each swimmer was given a secobarital dose of 100 mg/70 kg body weight. The 12 days were divided into 6 competitive days and 6 individual days. The events performed by the 15 swimmers including the 100-yd butterfly, the 100-yd freestyle, the 200-yd freestyle, the 200-yd butterfly, and the 200-yd backstroke. Following amphetamine, 14 of the 15 swimmers swam faster on the first swim of the day than they did when placebo had been given. The difference, although statistically significant according to the authors, was small (1.6%). On the second swim of each day, only performance in the 100-yd events was improved by amphetamine. When the swimmers performed in competition, the drug effects were smaller.

In the second experiment, the subjects were 9 track men. Three ran 600 yards, three ran 1000 yards, and three ran 1 mile. Experiments 3 and 4 also involved track men, but included other track events and the marathon run. When the authors combined the drug effects across all events, the effects of amphetamine were significant compared to placebo controls.

In experiment 5, collegiate shot-putters and weight throwers were studied. Amphetamine increased both the maximum and mean distances thrown by about 4.4% In the final experiment, experiment 6, 16 swimmers each swam 3 times under the influence of amphetamine and 3 times following placebo. This experiment differed from experiment 1 in that each swimmer was promised a steak dinner if he equaled or bettered his median competition time. Despite the fact that this promise decreased overall times (increased performance), amphetamine still decreased the times of 11 of 16 swimmers compared to placebo.

It is interesting that Smith and Beecher[52] were able to demonstrate significant effects in athletes performing the shot put and weight throw. These are athletic events that do not require a tremendous amount of endurance, and the subjects are usually well rested. Performance in this event represents a brief, sudden expenditure of energy. However, this report is not the only report showing that amphetamine is capable of increasing performance of this type. Hurst *et al.*[53] studied the effect of amphetamine on grip strength. Subjects were required to squeeze a simple dynamometer following either placebo or *d*-amphetamine. Following amphetamine, the subjects were able to squeeze with a force equal to 4.2% more than that observed after placebo.

In more recent studies, Wyndham *et al.*[54] studied the effects of 10 mg of methamphetamine or placebo on the performance of two champion cyclists working on a bicycle ergometer. Each cyclist worked at a work load of 45, 136, 181, 203, and 226 W for 3 minutes. After working for 3 minutes at each work load, the cyclists were allowed to rest for 10 to 20 minutes before resuming at loads approximating maximum work. The maximum work load consisted of 3 minutes of work at 294, 316, 339, and, if possible, 362 W. During this period of maximum work, the cyclists were allowed to rest for 10 to 20 minutes between each of the 3-minute work periods. Following amphetamine, no difference, compared to placebo, could be detected in submaximum or maximum oxygen consumption, heart rate, minute ventilation, or blood lactic acid.

However, after amphetamine, the cyclists were able to cycle at maximum effort for a longer period of time, and in a run to exhaustion, one cyclist was able to increase his time by 61% compared to placebo while the other increased his time by 29%. Both cyclists had marked increases in blood lactic acid following this maximal effort under methamphetamine. Chandler and Blair[55] studied the effects of 15 mg of amphetamine/70 kg body weight in 6 college students. For each subject the following measurements were made: strength. muscular power, running speed, acceleration, aerobic power, and anaerobic capacity. When the data were analyzed, it was shown that amphetamine produced a significant increase in knee extension strength (22%), an increase in acceleration (3.8%), an increase in aerobic capacity (8.5%), an increase in the time to exhaustion (4.6%), an increase in the pre-exercise heart rate (12%), and an increase in the maximum heart rate (2.4%). It is interesting that the largest increase was observed in the test of knee extension strength, and no increases were observed in sprinting speed. These results are consistent with those of Smith and Beecher.[52]

4.2. Studies Showing No Effect of Amphetamines

There have been a few studies that have failed to show any positive effects of the amphetamines on performance. In contrast to the Smith and Beecher study,[52] Haldi and Wynn[38] failed to show any effect of amphetamine in nontrained swimmers in a 100-yd swim. Ninety minutes before swimming, subjects were given either placebo or 5 mg of amphetamine. No significant effects in performance were detected as a function of drug administration. Karpovich[56] failed to demonstrate any significant effects of amphetamine on athletic performance. In subjects performing on a treadmill, swimming, or performing various athletic events, neither 10 mg of amphetamine given 1 hour before testing nor 20 mg of amphetamine given 30 minutes before testing produced any improvement. Williams and Thompson[57] gave either a placebo, 5 mg of amphetamine, 10 mg of amphetamine, or 15 mg of amphetamine to 12 male college students working on a bicycle ergometer. The subjects were given the drug or placebo 2 hours before the start of the experiment. The subjects were instructed to ride the bicycle to exhastion. No difference in the time to exhaustion was observed between placebo and amphetamine treatment. However, there was a significant increase in the maximum heart rate following amphetamine treatment.

4.3. Conclusions and Possible Mechanisms for the Effects of Amphetamines on Endurance and Physical Performance

Based on the reported work on amphetamines, it is quite clear that there is a positive effect of the amphetamines on physical performance and endurance. There are only a few reports failing to see any positive effects on performance or sense of fatigue. In the Haldi and Wynn study,[38] possible reasons for failing to see a beneficial effect include failure to use well-trained athletes and a low dose of amphetamine. In the Karpovich study,[56] positive effects might have been seen if a longer time had elapsed between the time of oral dosing and testing. No obvious reasons are apparent for the failure to see positive effects in the Williams and Thompson study.[57]

The exact mechanisms for the positive effects of amphetamine are not known at this time. Clearly, part of the effect can be attributed to a "behavioral" effect. Smith and Beecher[58] reported that the athletes in their studies reported a feeling of being "revved-up" after amphetamine. In a somewhat less scientific study, Mandel[59] and Mandel *et al.*[60] reported similar types of behavioral changes in professional athletes taking amphetamines. However, there are suggestions that this positive effect is not without its price and possible dangers to health. In both the Chandler and Blair study[55] and the Wyndham *et al.* study,[54] the authors noted that athletes continued to work under the influence of amphetamine even after a significant accumulation of lactic acid in the blood. Tyler[61] and Cuthbertson and Knox[50] reported in their respective studies that soldiers marching under the influence of amphetamine ignored severe foot blisters and were willing to continue marching despite the blisters. Amphetamine's ability to mask this normal reaction to fatigue and excessive work may be of little consequence in short-distance events. However, in events lasting for several hours, failure to be aware of these natural warning signals may be a threat to life and well-being.

5. EFFECTS OF COCAINE ON ENDURANCE AND PHYSICAL PERFORMANCE

Despite the recent attention drawn to the use of cocaine by athletes, there are no studies in the literature, to this author's knowledge, on the effects of cocaine on athletic performance. There are anecdotal reports of tremendous physical endurance displayed by some Indians in the Andes Mountains of Peru who chewed the leaves of the coca plant, but there are no scientific studies. A fact which may argue against a significant effect of cocaine on endurance is its short half-life in man. Unfortunately, the current abuse problems with cocaine will make it very difficult to do the types of experiments required to adequately determine in man the effects of cocaine on endurance and physical performance.

6. SUMMARY

Based upon the available evidence in the literature, it is clear that stimulants such as caffeine and amphetamine can increase endurance and physical performance in man. These effects are usually less than 10%. However, as noted earlier, a 10% improvement may be the difference between national fame and recognition, and oblivion. It also should be noted that there are potential dangers to life and well-being with the use of these agents. There is clear evidence that at least part of the effect of these stimulants is mediated by a failure of the athlete to be aware of his/her physical condition. Failure to heed the normal physiological warning signals may lead to permanent damage. It must also be pointed out that all of the cited literature studied the effects of acute administration of these substances. No data are available on the possible consequences of more chronic use of these substances during athletic performance.

REFERENCES

1. Puffer JC: The use of drugs in swimming. *Clin Sports Med* 5:77–89, 1966.
2. Gilman AG, Goodman LS, Rall TW, et al (eds): *Goodman and Gilman's The Pharmacological Basis of Therapeutics*, ed 7. New York, MacMillan Publishing Co., 1985.
3. Tewes PA, Fischman MW: Effects of *d*-amphetamine and diazepam on fixed-interval, fixed-ratio responding in humans. *J Pharmacol Exp Ther* 221:373–383, 1982.
4. Weiner N: Pharmacology of central nervous system stimulants, in Zarafonetis, CJD (ed): *Drug Abuse: Proceedings of the International Conference*. Philadelphia, Lea & Febiger, 1972, pp 243–251.
5. Bowman WC, Rand MJ: *Textbook of Pharmacology*, ed 2. Oxford, Blackwell Scientific, 1980.
6. Fischman MW, Schuster CR: Cocaine self-administration in humans. *Fed Proc* 41:241–246, 1982.
7. Resnick RB, Kestenbaum RS, Schwartz LD: Acute systemic effects of cocaine in man: a controlled study by intranasal and intravenous routes. *Science* 195:696–699, 1977.
8. Fischman MW, Schuster CR, Resnekov L, et al: Cardiovascular and subjective effects of intravenous cocaine administration in humans. *Arch Gen Psychiat* 33:938–989, 1976.
9. Kossowsky WA, Lyon AF: Cocaine and acute myocardial infarction, a probable connection. *Chest* 86:729–731, 1984.
10. Posternack PF, Calvin SB, Bauman FG: Cocaine-induced angina pectoris and acute myocardial infarction in patients younger than 40 years. *Am J Cardiol* 55:847, 1985.
11. Van Dyke C, Jatlow P, Ungerer J, et al: Oral cocaine: plasma concentrations and central effects. *Science* 200:211–213, 1978.
12. Goldstein A, Warren R, Kaizer S: Psychotropic effects of caffeine in man. I. Individual differences in sensitivity to caffeine-induced wakefulness. *J Pharmacol Exp Ther* 149:156–159, 1965.
13. Rosenblum D, Sutton JR: Drugs and exercise. *Med Clin North Am* 69:177–187, 1985.
14. Rall TW: Evolution of the mechanism of action of methylxanthines: from calcium mobilizers to antagonists of adenosine receptors. *Pharmacologist* 24:277–287, 1982.
15. Post RM: Central stimulants. Clinical and experimental evidence on tolerance and sensitization, in Israel Y, Glaser FB, Kalant H, et al (eds): *Research Advances in Alcohol and Drug Problems*. New York, Plenum Press, 1981, pp 1–65.
16. Post RM, Contel NR: Human and animal studies of cocaine: Implications for development of behavioral pathology, in Creese I (ed): *Stimulants: Neurochemical, Behavioral, and Clinical Perspectives*. New York, Raven Press, 1983, pp 169–203.
17. Demellweek C, Goudie AJ: Behavioral tolerance to amphetamine and other psychostimulants: the case for considering behavioral mechansims. *Psychopharmacologia* 80:287–307, 1983.
18. Barone JJ, Roberts H: Human consumption of caffeine, in Dews PB (ed): *Caffeine*. Berlin, Springer-Verlag, 1984, pp 59–73.
19. Robertson D, Wade D, Workman R, et al: Tolerance to the humoral and hemodynamic effects of caffeine in man. *J Clin Invest* 67:1111–1117, 1981.
20. Coyle EF: Ergogenic aids. *Clin Sports Med* 3:731–742, 1984.
21. Laties VG, Weiss B: The amphetamine margin in sports. *Fed Proc* 40:2689–2692, 1981.
22. Boje O: Doping *Bull Health Org League of Nations* 8:439–369, 1939.
23. Venerando A: Doping pathology and ways to control it. *Medicina dello Sport* 3:972–983, 1963.
24. Medical Commission of the British Commonwealth Games: Prevention and detection of drug taking (doping) at the IX British Commonwealth Games. *Scot Med J* 16:364–368, 1971.
25. Fischbach E: The problem of doping. *Med Monatsschr* 26:377–381, 1972.
26. Rivers W, Webber H: The action of caffeine on the capacity for muscular work. *J Physiol* 36:33–47, 1907.
27. Seashore RH, Ivy AC: Effects of analeptic drugs in relieving fatigue. *Psychol Monogr* 67(15):1–16, 1953.

28. Foltz E, Ivy A. Barborka C: The use of double work periods in the study of fatigue and the influence of caffeine. *Am J Physiol* 136:79–86, 1942.
29. Foltz EE, Ivy AC, Barborka CJ: The influence of amphetamine (benzedrine) sulfate, *d*-desoxyephedrine hydrochloride (pervitin) and caffeine upon work output recovery when rapidly exhausting work is done by trained subjects. *J Lab Clin Med* 28:603–605, 1943.
30. Asmussen E, Boje O: The effect of alcohol and some drugs on the capacity for work. *Acta Physiol Scand* 15:109–113, 1948.
31. Berglund B, Hemmingsson P: Effects of caffeine ingestion on exercise performance at low and high altitudes in cross-country skiers. *Int J Sports Med* 3:234–236, 1982.
32. McNaughton LR: The influence of caffeine ingestion on incremental treadmill running. *Br J Sports Med* 20:109–112, 1986.
33. Costill DK, Dalsky GP, Fink WJ: Effects of caffeine ingestion on metabolism and exercise performance. *Med Sci Sports* 10:155–158, 1978.
34. Ivy JL, Costill DL, Fink WJ, et al: Influence of caffeine and carbohydrate feedings on endurance performance. *Med Sci Sports* 11:6–11, 1979.
35. Fisher SM, McMurray RG, Berry M, et al: Influence of caffeine on exercise performance in habitual caffeine users. *Int J Sports Med* 7:276–280, 1986.
36. Foltz EE, Schiffrin MJ, Ivy AC: The influence of amphetamine (benzedrine) sulfate and caffeine on the performance of rapidly exhausting work by untrained subjects. *J Lab Clin Med* 28:601–603, 1943.
37. Alles GA, Feigen GA: The influence of benzedrine on work decrement and patellar reflex. *Am J Physiol* 136:392–400, 1942.
38. Haldi J, Wynn W: Action of drugs on the efficiency of swimmers. *Research Quart* 17:96–101, 1946.
39. Ganslen RV, Balke B, Nagle F, et al: Effects of some tranquilizing, analeptic and vasodilating drugs on physical work capacity and orthostatic tolerance. *Aerospace Med* 35:630–633, 1964.
40. Margaria R, Nghemo P, Rovelli E: The effect of some drugs on the maximal capacity of athletic performance in man. *Int Z Angew Physiol* 20:281–287, 1964.
41. Perkins R, Williams MH: Effect of caffeine upon maximal muscular endurance of females. *Med Sci Sports* 7:221–224, 1975.
42. Powers SK, Byrd RJ, Tulley R, et al: Effects of caffeine ingestion on metabolism and performance during graded exercise. *Eur J Physiol* 50:301–307, 1983.
43. Bond V, Gresham K, McRae J, et al: Caffeine ingestion and isokinetic strength. *Br J Sports Med* 20:135–137, 1986.
44. Casal DC, Leon AS: Failure of caffeine to affect substrate utilization during prolonged running. *Med Sci Sports Exerc* 17:174–179, 1985.
45. O'Neil FT, Hynak-Hankinson MT, Gorman T: Research and application of current topics in sports nuitrition. *J Am Diet Assoc* 86:1007–1015, 1986.
46. Lehman G, Straub H, Szakall A: Pervitin als leistungssteigerndes Mittel. *Arbeitsphysiologie* 10:680–691, 1939.
47. Heyrodt H, Weissenstein H: Uber Steigerung korperlicher Leistungfahigkeit durch Pervitin. *Arch Exp Pathol Pharmakol* 195:273–275, 1940.
48. Knoefel PK: The influence of phenisopropyl amine and phenisopropyl methyl amine on work output. *Fed Proc* 2:83, 1943.
49. Somerville W: The effect of benzedrine on mental or physical fatigue in soldiers. *Can Med Assoc J* 55:470–476, 1946.
50. Cuthbertson DP, Knox JAC: The effects of analeptics on the fatigued subject. *J Physiol* 106:42–58, 1947.
51. Bujas Z, Petz B: Utjecaj fenamina na economicnast staticnog rada. *Arh Hig Rada* 6:205–208, 1955.
52. Smith GM, Beecher HK: Amphetamine sulfate and athletic performance. I. Objective effects. *JAMA* 170:542–557, 1959.
53. Hurst PN, Radlow R, Bagley SK: The effects of D-amphetamine and chlordiazepoxide upon strength and estimated strength. *Ergonomics* 11:47–52, 1968.
54. Wyndham CH, Rogers GG, Benade AJS, et al: Physiological effects of the amphetamines during exercise. *S Afr Med J* 45:247–252, 1971.
55. Chandler JV, Blair SN: The effect of amphetamines on selected components related to athletic success. *Med Sci Sports Exerc* 12:65–69, 1980.

56. Karpovich PV: Effect of amphetamine sulfate on athletic performance. *JAMA* 170:558–561, 1959.
57. Williams MH, Thompson J: Effect of variant dosages of amphetamine upon endurance. *Research Quart* 44:417–422, 1973.
58. Smith GM, Beecher HK: Amphetamine, secobarbital, and athletic performance. II. Subjective evaluations of performances, mood states, and physical states. *JAMA* 172:1502–1514, 1960.
59. Mandel AJ: *The Nightmare Season*. New York, Random House, 1976.
60. Mandel AJ, Stewart KD, Russo PV: The Sunday syndrome: From kinetics to altered consciousness. *Fed Proc* 40:2693–2698, 1981.
61. Tyler DB: The effect of amphetamine sulfate and some barbiturates on the fatigue produced by prolonged wakefulness. *Am J Physiol* 150:253–262, 1947.

Index

SPRINGER NATURE

GPSR Compliance

The European Union's (EU) General Product Safety Regulation (GPSR) is a set of rules that requires consumer products to be safe and our obligations to ensure this.

If you have any concerns about our products, you can contact us on ProductSafety@springernature.com

In case Publisher is established outside the EU, the EU authorized representative is:

Springer Nature Customer Service Center GmbH
Europaplatz 3
69115 Heidelberg, Germany

MIX
Papier | Fördert
gute Waldnutzung
FSC® C083411

Kolibri 360 GmbH
Ferdinand-Jühlke-Straße 7
99095 Erfurt, Deutschland
produktsicherheit@kolibri360.de